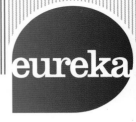
eureka

Physiology

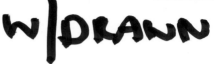
W/DRAWN

Jake P Mann BMedSc MBChB (Hons)
MRCP (UK) MAoMEd
Academic Clinical Fellow in
Paediatrics
Department of Paediatrics
University of Cambridge
Cambridge, UK

David Marples BA BM BCh MA
DPhil PhD
Senior Lecturer in Physiology and
Anatomy
School of Biomedical Sciences
Faculty of Biological Sciences
University of Leeds
Leeds, UK

Series Editors

Janine Henderson MRCPsych
MClinEd
MB BS Programme Director
Hull York Medical School
York, UK

David Oliveira PhD FRCP
Professor of Renal Medicine
St George's, University of London
London, UK

Stephen Parker BSc MS DipMedEd
FRCS
Consultant Breast and General
Paediatric Surgeon
St Mary's Hospital
Newport, UK

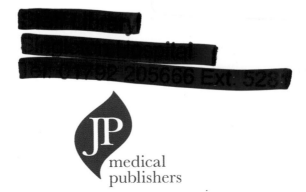
JP
medical
publishers

London • Philadelphia • New Delhi • Panama City

© 2015 JP Medical Ltd.

Published by JP Medical Ltd, 83 Victoria Street, London, SW1H 0HW, UK

Tel: +44 (0)20 3170 8910   Fax: +44 (0)20 3008 6180

Email: info@jpmedpub.com   www.jpmedpub.com

ISBN: 978-1-909836-07-5

British Library Cataloguing in Publication Data
A catalogue record for this book is available from the British Library

Library of Congress Cataloging in Publication Data
A catalog record for this book is available from the Library of Congress

Publisher:	Richard Furn
Development Editors:	Thomas Fletcher, Paul Mayhew, Alison Whitehouse
Editorial Assistants:	Sophie Woolven, Katie Pattullo
Copy Editors:	Kim Howell, Carrie Walker
Graphic narratives:	James Pollitt
Cover design:	Forbes Design
Page design:	Designers Collective

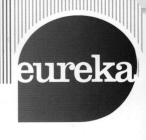

Series Editors' Foreword

Today's medical students need to know a great deal to be effective as tomorrow's doctors. This knowledge includes core science and clinical skills, from understanding biochemical pathways to communicating with patients. Modern medical school curricula integrate this teaching, thereby emphasising how learning in one area can support and reinforce another. At the same time students must acquire sound clinical reasoning skills, working with complex information to understand each individual's unique medical problems.

The *Eureka* series is designed to cover all aspects of today's medical curricula and reinforce this integrated approach. Each book can be used from first year through to qualification. Core biomedical principles are introduced but given relevant clinical context: the authors have always asked themselves, 'why does the aspiring clinician need to know this'?

Each clinical title in the series is grounded in the relevant core science, which is introduced at the start of each book. Each core science title integrates and emphasises clinical relevance throughout. Medical and surgical approaches are included to provide a complete and integrated view of the patient management options available to the clinician. Clinical insights highlight key facts and principles drawn from medical practice. Cases featuring unique graphic narratives are presented with clear explanations that show how experienced clinicians think, enabling students to develop their own clinical reasoning and decision making. Clinical SBAs help with exam revision while starter questions are a unique learning tool designed to stimulate interest in the subject.

Having biomedical principles and clinical applications together in one book will make their connections more explicit and easier to remember. Alongside repeated exposure to patients and practice of clinical and communication skills, we hope *Eureka* will equip medical students for a lifetime of successful clinical practice.

Janine Henderson, David Oliveira, Stephen Parker

About the Series Editors

Janine Henderson is the MB BS undergraduate Programme Director at Hull York Medical School (HYMS). After medical school at the University of Oxford and clinical training in psychiatry, she combined her work as a consultant with postgraduate teaching roles, moving to the new Hull York Medical School in 2004. She has a particular interest in modern educational methods, curriculum design and clinical reasoning.

David Oliveira is Professor of Renal Medicine at St George's, University of London (SGUL), where he served as the MBBS Course Director between 2007 and 2013. Having trained at Cambridge University and the Westminster Hospital he obtained a PhD in cellular immunology and worked as a renal physician before being appointed as Foundation Chair of Renal Medicine at SGUL.

Stephen Parker is a Consultant Breast and General Paediatric Surgeon at St Mary's Hospital, Isle of Wight. He trained at St George's, University of London, and after service in the Royal Navy was appointed as Consultant Surgeon at University Hospital Coventry. He has a particular interest in e-learning and the use of multimedia platforms in medical education.

Preface

Physiology underlies all clinical medical practice. A good understanding is crucial to making a diagnosis, predicting how pathological changes will influence the body and anticipating the effects of treatment.

Eureka Physiology integrates clinical concepts alongside core physiology. It links physiological processes with common pathologies, illustrating the role of cellular and molecular science in medicine. Chapter 1 describes the principles of physiology: cell structure and function. Subsequent chapters cover the physiology of each body system, using clinical cases to provide an insight into how patients present and how they are managed in real life. Throughout the book artworks are used to illustrate key concepts and anatomy, and clinical images show how these translate to clinical practice. Chapter 10 contains exam-style questions to consolidate learning and to use as a revision aid in the run-up to exams.

We hope that this book will give you a grasp of physiology that you can utilise beyond your exams and incorporate into your clinical practice.

Jake Mann, David Marples
April 2015

About the Authors

Jake Mann is an Academic Clinical Fellow in Paediatrics at the University of Cambridge. He teaches a national preclinical science revision course and has authored several educational smartphone apps. He is passionate about integrating core science into clinical practice and engaging students with current scientific research.

David Marples is a Senior Lecturer in anatomy and physiology at the University of Leeds. His major research interests are in renal physiology; specifically the role of aquaporin water channels in fluid-balance disorders. His teaching covers a wide range of physiology and anatomy topics, and his goal is to encourage students to think about how their bodies work in an integrated way.

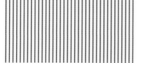

Contents

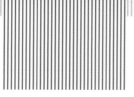

Glossary

5'NT	5' nucleotidase
5-DHT	5-dihydrotestosterone
5-HT	serotonin
5-LO	5-lipoxygenase
A	adenine
AC	adenylate cyclase
ACE	angiotensin-converting enzyme
ACEi	angiotensin-converting enzyme inhibitor
ACh	acetylcholine
AChE	acetylcholine esterase
ACTH	adrenocorticotropic hormone
ADH	antidiuretic hormone (vasopressin)
ADP	adenosine diphosphate
AKI	acute kidney injury (acute renal failure)
α-AdR	α-adrenoceptor
AMP	adenosine monophosphate
AMPA	α-amino 3-hydroxy 5-methyl 4-isoxazolepropionic acid
Ang-II	angiotensin II
ANP	atrial natriuretic peptide
ANS	autonomic nervous system
AP	action potential
APUD	amine precursor uptake and decarboxylation
AQP	aquaporin
AT	anaerobic threshold
ATN	acute tubular necrosis
ATP	adenosine triphosphate
AVN	atrioventricular node
BA	bile acid
β-AdR	β-adrenoceptor
BNP	b-type natriuretic peptide
bpm	beats per minute
Br	bilirubin
BUN	blood urea nitrogen
C	cytosine
CA	carbonic anhydrase
cAMP	cyclic adenosine monophosphate
CCK	cholecystokinin

CDK	cyclin-dependent kinase
CFTR	cystic fibrosis transmembrane conductance regulator
cGMP	cyclic guanosine monophosphate
CICR	calcium-induced calcium release
CK	creatine kinase
CLC	chloride channel
CN	cranial nerve
CNS	central nervous system
CO	cardiac output
CoA	coenzyme A
COPD	chronic obstructive pulmonary disease
COX	cyclo-oxygenase
CR	complement receptor
CRH	corticotrophin-releasing hormone
CT	computerised tomography
CTZ	chemoreceptor trigger zone
CVP	central venous pressure
DAG	diacyl glycerol
DBP	diastolic blood pressure
DCT	distal convoluted tubule
DHEA	dehydroepiandrosterone
DHP	dihydropyridine
DIT	di-iodothyronine
DKA	diabetic ketoacidosis
DMT	divalent metal transporter
DNA	deoxyribonucleic acid
DPP	dipeptidyl peptidase
dTL	descending thick limb (of Loop of Henle)
ECF	extracellular fluid
ECG	electrocardiogram
ECL	enterochromaffin-like
ECM	extracellular matrix
ECV	effective circulating volume
EDV	end-diastolic volume
eGFR	estimated glomerular filtration rate
E_m	resting membrane potential
ENaC	epithelial sodium channel
ENS	enteric nervous system
EPI	extrinsic pathway inhibitor
EPO	erythropoietin

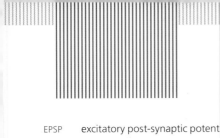

EPSP	excitatory post-synaptic potential	GTN	glyceryl trinitrate
ERV	expiratory reserve volume	GTP	guanosine triphosphate
ESV	end-systolic volume		
ETC	electron transport chain	haemoglobin A	adult haemoglobin
		haemoglobin A2	adult haemoglobin variant
FAD	flavin adenine dinucleotide	haemoglobin F	fetal haemoglobin
$FADH_2$	reduced form of flavin adenine dinucleotide	Hb	haemoglobin
		HDL	high-density lipoprotein
FFA	free fatty acid	HLA	human leucocyte antigen
FII	factor II	HP	hydrostatic pressure
FIX	factor IX	HP_{BC}	hydrostatic pressure in Bowman's capsule
FIXa	active form of factor IX		
FRC	functional residual capacity	HR	heart rate
FSH	follicle-stimulating hormone	HSD	hydroxysteroid dehydrogenase
FV	factor V	HSEC	hepatic sinusoidal endothelial cell
FVa	active form of factor V		
FVII	factor VII	IBD	inflammatory bowel disease
FVIIa	active form of factor VII	ICF	intracellular fluid
FVIII	factor VIII	IF	intrinsic factor
FVIIIa	active form of factor VIIIa	IFN	interferon
FX	factor X	Ig	immunoglobulin
FXa	active form of factor Xa	IGF	insulin-like growth factor
FXI	factor XI	IL	interleukin
		IP_3	inositol triphosphate
G	guanine	IPSP	inhibitory post-synaptic potential
G0	quiescent phase of the cell cycle	IRS	insulin receptor substrate
G1	first growth phase of the cell cycle	IRV	inspiratory reserve volume
G2	second growth phase of the cell cycle	IV	intravenous
GABA	γ-aminobutyric acid		
GALT	gastrointestinal-associated lymphoid tissue	JGA	juxtaglomerular apparatus
GC	guanylate cyclase	LDL	low-density lipoprotein
GFR	glomerular filtration rate	LH	luteinising hormone
GH	growth hormone	LMN	lower motor neurone
GHRH	growth hormone–releasing hormone	LoH	loop of Henle
G_i	G protein α subunit i (inhibitory)	LOS	lower oesophageal sphincter
GI	gastrointestinal	LPL	lipoprotein lipase
GLP	glucagon-like peptide		
Glu	glutamate	M	mitosis phase of the cell cycle
GLUT	glucose transporter	M_3-AChR	muscarinic acetylcholine receptor subtype 3
GnRH	gonadotrophin-releasing hormone		
GORD	gastro-oesophageal reflux disease	mABP	mean arterial blood pressure
GP	general practitioner	MAC	membrane attack complex
Gp	glycoprotein	MELAS	myoclonic epilepsy, lactic acidosis and stroke-like episodes
GPCR	G-protein–coupled receptor		
G_q	G protein α subunit q	MG	monoglyceride
G_s	G protein α subunit s (stimulatory)	MHC	major histocompatibility complex

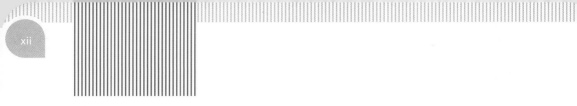

MIT	monoiodothyronine
MLCK	myosin light-chain kinase
MLCP	myosin light-chain phosphatase
MLH	MutL homologue
MMC	migrating motor complex
MR	mineralocorticoid receptor
mRNA	messenger ribonucleic acid
MSH	melanocyte-stimulating hormone
MSH	MutS homologue
MTC	medullary thyroid carcinoma
NA	noradrenaline (norepinephrine)
NAChR	nicotinic acetylcholine receptor
NAD^+	nicotinamide adenine dinucleotide
NADH	reduced form of nicotinamide adenine dinucleotide
NCC	Na^+-Cl^- cotransporter
NK cell	natural killer cell
NK	neurokinin
NKCC2 cotransporter	$Na^+/K^+/2Cl^-$ cotransporter
NMDA	N-methyl-D-aspartic acid
NO	nitric oxide
NP	natriuretic peptide
NPR	natriuretic peptide receptor
NSAID	non-steroidal anti-inflammatory drug
OAT	organic anion transporter
OCT	organic cation transporter
OVLT	organum vasculosum of the lamina terminalis
P_A	alveolar air pressure
P_ACO_2	partial pressure of alveolar carbon dioxide
P_aCO_2	partial pressure of arterial carbon dioxide
P_AO_2	partial pressure of alveolar oxygen
P_aO_2	partial pressure of arterial oxygen
P_{BS}	hydrostatic pressure in Bowman's space
PC	protein C
P_{cap}	hydrostatic pressure in the capillary
pCO_2	partial pressure of carbon dioxide
PCT	proximal convoluted tubule
PDE	phosphodiesterase
PG	prostaglandin
P-gp	permeability glycoprotein
π_{BC}	oncotic pressure in Bowman's capsule

π_{cap}	oncotic pressure in the capillary
π_{TS}	oncotic pressure in tissue space
P_i	inorganic phosphate
P_iO_2	partial pressure of inspired oxygen
PIP_2	phosphatidyl-inositol bisphosphate
PKA	protein kinase A
PKC	protein kinase C
PKG	protein kinase G
PLA_2	phospholipase A_2
PLC	phospholipase C
PNS	parasympathetic nervous system
PNS	peripheral nervous system
pO_2	partial pressure of oxygen
POMC	pro-opiomelanocortin
PRL	prolactin
PS	protein S
PTH	parathyroid hormone
p_{total}	total pressure in a system
P_{TS}	hydrostatic pressure in tissue space
PVN	paraventricular nucleus
PZ	pancreozymin
$\dot{Q}$	perfusion (the volume of blood per set weight of tissue per unit of time)
R	receptor
RAAS	renin–angiotensin–aldosterone system
RBC	red blood cell
RBF	renal blood flow
Re	Reynolds's number
RER	rough endoplasmic reticulum
RNA	ribonucleic acid
ROMK	renal outer medullary potassium channel
RQ	respiratory quotient
rT_3	reverse tri-iodothyronine
RV	residual volume
S	DNA synthesis phase of the cell cycle
SAN	sinoatrial node
S_aO_2	haemoglobin saturation
SBP	systolic blood pressure
SER	smooth endoplasmic reticulum
SERCA	sarcoplasmic reticulum calcium-transporting ATPase
SFO	subfornical organ
sGC	soluble guanylate cyclase

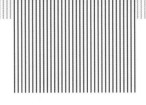

SGK	serum- and glucocorticoid-regulated kinase
SGLT	sodium–glucose transport protein
SGLUT	sodium–glucose transporter
SNS	sympathetic nervous system
SON	supraoptic nucleus
SSR	somatostatin receptor
SUR	sulphonylurea receptor
SV	stroke volume
T	thymine
T_3	tri-iodothyronine
T_4	thyroxine
TAL	thick ascending limb (of Loop of Henle)
TBBC	TATA box–binding complex
TCA	tricarboxylic acid
TCR	T-cell receptor
TF	tissue factor
TG	triglyceride
ThG	thyroglobulin
TM	thrombomodulin
T_M	transport maximum
TNF-α	tumour necrosis factor-α
tPA	tissue plasminogen activator
TPR	total peripheral resistance
TRH	thyrotrophin-releasing hormone

tRNA	transfer ribonucleic acid
TSH	thyroid-stimulating hormone
U	uracil
UGT	uridine diphosphate glucuronosyltransferase
UMN	upper motor neurone
UOS	upper oesophageal sphincter
$\dot{V}$	ventilation (the volume of air moving in and out of the lungs per unit of time)
$\dot{V}_A$	alveolar ventilation (the volume of air reaching the alveoli in a given time period)
VC	vital capacity
$V\text{CO}_2$	rate of metabolic carbon dioxide production
V_{dist}	volume of distribution
VLDL	very-low-density lipoprotein
$V\text{O}_2$	rate of oxygen use in cellular respiration
VSD	ventricular septal defect
V_T	tidal volume
V_{total}	total volume in a system
vWF	von Willebrand factor
WBC	white blood cell

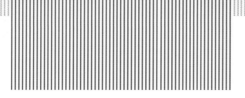

Acknowledgements

Thanks to the following medical students for their help reviewing chapters: Jessica Dunlop, Aliza Imam, Roxanne McVittie, Daniel Roberts and Joseph Suich.

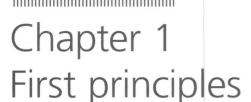

Chapter 1
First principles

Starter questions

Answers to the following questions are on page 37.

1. What is the central dogma of molecular biology and genetics?
2. If DNA is comprised of a sugar, phosphate and a base, why is it an acid?
3. Why is it thought that mitochondria were once separate organisms?
4. How do cells keep a different apical and basal membrane?
5. How does fish oil interfere with arachidonic acid signalling?
6. Why is it difficult to utilise adult stem cells to grow organs?

Introduction

Genetic material codes for the production of proteins, which go on to assemble the machinery and structures of cells. These cells associate with each other to form tissues, and multiple tissues interact and combine to form organs. Thus the body has layers of complexity that, in principle, can ultimately be reduced to cells and the molecules they contain. Human physiology – the normal functions and interactions of human tissues – is described in terms of cells and molecular reactions.

Levels of organisation

Cellular theory of life

Cells are membrane-bound units capable of self-replication. All living things are composed of cells, from humans, with about 10 trillion cells, to single-celled organisms such as amoebas.

Organisms are divided into two groups:

- Eukaryotes, which sequester their genetic material (DNA) within a membrane-bound structure (the nucleus) inside the cell
- Prokaryotes, which do not have a nucleus separating their DNA from the rest of the cell

There are a number of differences between the two (**Table 1.1**).

Mammals are eukaryotic organisms with a huge diversity of cell types, each specialised for a particular function. When cells with a particular function are grouped together, a tissue is formed. This is the basis for how the human body functions (**Figure 1.1**).

Macromolecules

Four elements comprise the majority of every biomolecule: oxygen, carbon, hydrogen and nitrogen. A large number of other elements (e.g. iron, magnesium, selenium and copper) are present in the human body in smaller amounts.

Biomolecules range from very small molecules such as metabolic intermediates (e.g. cyclic AMP) to large macromolecules such as proteins, lipids, carbohydrates and nucleic acids). Large macromolecules are formed by the assembly of smaller molecules that undergo activation to allow the formation of bonds. The principal macromolecules are:

- Proteins
- Lipids
- Carbohydrates and
- Nucleic acids

Proteins

Proteins are a diverse group of macromolecules with a range of functions (**Table 1.2**). Many are enzymes, proteins that control many of the body's processes, including production of the other macromolecules.

Each protein is composed of a number of amino acids, small molecules that each contain an amine group ($-NH_2$) and a carboxylic

Differences between eukaryotic and prokaryotic cells		
	Eukaryote	Prokaryote
Nucleus	Present: membrane bound with genetic material in chromosomes	Absent: genetic material free as plasmids
Size	10–100 μm	0.2–10 μm
Cell division	Mitosis	Binary fission
Recombination	Meiosis and gamete fusion	Asexual reproduction and plasmid exchange
Ribosomes	Larger	Smaller
Organelles	Present: mitochondria, endoplasmic reticulum, Golgi, lysosomes	Absent
Examples of organisms	Animals, plants – usually multicellular organisms	Bacteria – usually single celled organisms

Table 1.1 Differences between eukaryotic and prokaryotic cells

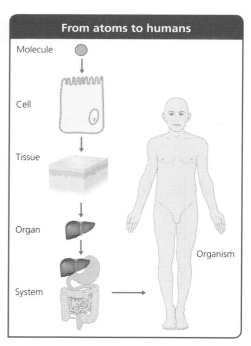

Figure 1.1 Organisms, systems, organs, tissues and cells are composed of atoms and the reactions between them.

Types of protein			
Type	Location	Function	Example
Enzymes	Cytosol, membranes, organelles, extracellular	Catalyse intra- and extracellular reactions	Adenylate cyclase
Channels and transporters	Plasma and intracellular membranes	Channels: pores for transmembrane passage of small molecules and ions.	Channel: voltage-gated Na⁺ channel in nerve cells
		Transporters: mechanically change shape to allow transmembrane transport of molecules	Transporter: GLUT-4, a glucose transporter
Structural	Cytosol	Form filaments and tubules that hold cell shape or facilitate movement	Actin of intracellular cytoskeleton

Table 1.2. Proteins grouped by function

acid group (–COOH). Peptide bonds form between the amine group of one amino acid and the carboxylic acid group of the next amino acid, to create form chains called peptides (short chains of 2–4 amino acids) or polypeptides (longer chains) . Each peptide folds into complex three-dimensional structures (**Figure 1.2**). In this way, there are four 'levels' of protein structure, summarised in **Table 1.3**. Some proteins comprise a single polypeptide chain and therefore have no quaternary structure.

There are hundreds of amino acids but only 22 are used by the body to make proteins. Four of them are made by the body (non-essential amino acids): alanine, asparagine, aspartic acid and glutamic acid. The rest are obtained from the diet and are termed essential amino acids because the diet must contain enough of each to maintain health.

Lipids

A lipid comprises a long hydrocarbon chain that ends with a carboxyl group; the hydrocarbon chain is insoluble in water, but the carboxyl group is water soluble. A phospholipid ends in a charged phosphate group instead of a carboxyl group. These are the archetypal amphipathic molecules: containing a hydrophobic region (hydrocarbon tail) and hydrophilic region (phosphate head).

Diglycerides are formed of several lipids united by a glycerol group: diglycerides comprise two hydrocarbon chains plus a glycerol group; triglycerides comprise three hydrocarbon chains plus a glycerol group. Other

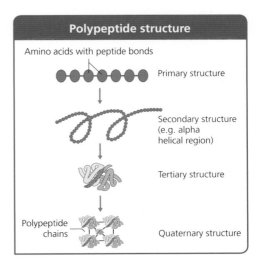

Polypeptide structure

Amino acids with peptide bonds

Primary structure

Secondary structure (e.g. alpha helical region)

Tertiary structure

Polypeptide chains

Quaternary structure

Figure 1.2 The amino acid sequence of a protein is its primary structure; this ultimately determines its secondary (α-helix or β-pleated sheet) and tertiary structure.

Protein structure	
Level of protein structure	Description
Primary	Amino acid sequence
Secondary	Local interactions between amino acids that leads them to take up structures such as β-sheets or α-helices
Tertiary	Interactions between secondary structures to create 3-dimensional structure
Quaternary	Formation of large proteins from several polypeptide chains

Table 1.3 The four levels of protein structure

lipids, such as cholesterol, have several carbon rings. The carbon rings in cholesterol are important for interrupting the bonds between adjacent hydrocarbon chains in phospholipid membranes. The principal roles of lipids are as:

■ the main component of cell and organelle membranes (see page 16)
■ amphipathic molecules at the body's water interfaces, due to the hydrophobic nature of lipids (e.g. pulmonary surfactant, bile acids)
■ high-energy storage molecules
■ intracellular signalling molecules

Carbohydrates

Simple sugars (monosaccharides) are linked together by glycosidic bonds to form polysaccharides, also called carbohydrates. These act as energy sources, structural molecules, signalling molecules and are a major component of nucleic acid.

Nucleic acids

A nucleic acid is a macromolecule comprised of a sugar and phosphate backbone and nitrogenous bases (also called nucleobases). Their structure is described in detail on page 5. The most abundant nucleic acids in human cells are deoxyribose nucleic acids, referred to as deoxyribonucleic acid (DNA), and ribose nucleic acids, referred to as ribonucleic acid (RNA). These form the genetic material that controls all cell processes and allows conservative replication of living organisms, i.e. formation of a new, daughter organism using the nucleic acid template of the parent organism.

> **Mucopolysaccharidosis is one of the rare diseases involving abnormal storage of macromolecules,** in this case, glycosaminoglycans. It is caused by a dysfunctional mutation of a catabolic enzyme and causes liver and heart failure.

The cell

Cell structure

Human cells are 10–100 μm structures bound by a phospholipid membrane. They contain an aqueous solution of chemicals, the cytosol. Lying within the cytosol are smaller, membrane-bound, functional units called organelles, each with their own specific role

(**Figure 1.3**). Together, the cytosol and organelles are referred to as cytoplasm.

Cytosol

Most of the cell's volume is cytosol, and over 80% of this is water. It also contains dissolved ions, signalling molecules, reaction substrates

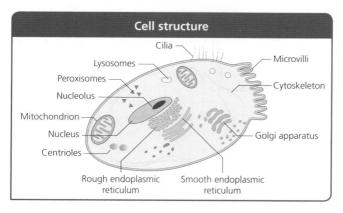

Cell structure

Cilia
Lysosomes
Peroxisomes
Nucleolus
Mitochondrion
Nucleus
Centrioles
Microvilli
Cytoskeleton
Golgi apparatus
Rough endoplasmic reticulum
Smooth endoplasmic reticulum

Figure 1.3 General cell structure. This generic cell shows multiple organelles that are not necessarily present in all cells. Most human cells have specialisations related to their function.

and macromolecules. However, only a minority of cell reactions occur in the cytosol itself, glycolysis being a major example; the majority occur on the surfaces of membranes.

Nucleus

The nucleus is the location of the cell's genetic material, its DNA, which controls the cellular processes. It is bounded by a double membrane with perforations to allow passage of macromolecules to and from the cytosol. As well as DNA, it contains nucleoli, which are condensed areas of RNA and protein and are the location of ribosome synthesis.

The essence of nuclear (and cellular) function is that DNA is used to make RNA, which then is used as a code to follow in constructing proteins. The process is controlled at multiple levels, especially during the transcription (copying) of DNA into RNA (**Figure 1.4**), which is the first step in moving from a permanent copy of genetic material (the DNA) to a temporary form (RNA). A further key feature of DNA is that it is replicated and transmitted through successive generations of cells. Together these are said to be the 'Central Dogma' of molecular biology and genetics.

Structure of DNA

DNA is made of two helical strands of nucleotides. Each nucleotide is formed from a deoxyribose sugar group, a phosphate and a nitrogenous base. The sugar and phosphate groups form the backbone of the strand, and the bases hang off the strand like the charms on a bracelet. There are four different bases, divided into two groups:

- **pyrimidines:** cytosine (C) and thymine (T)
- **purines:** adenine (A) and guanine (G)

In DNA, two strands are held together by hydrogen bonds between the bases. These bonds are formed only within two specific pairings: thymine–adenine and cytosine–guanine (**Figure 1.5**). Other pairings are not possible, for example cytosine does not pair with adenine. In this way, each strand is like a mirror image of its partner, which is an essential characteristic for replication (see below). Note that a purine always pairs with a pyrimidine.

The two ends of a DNA strand are different: one terminates in a phosphate group and is called the 5' end; the other terminates in a hydroxyl group and is called the 3' end. DNA strands have polarity, a 'direction', because new DNA is always synthesised in the 5'-to-3' direction. The polarity refers to the carbon atom in the ribose sugar on the free end of the DNA strand. The two DNA strands are anti-parallel: one strand is 5'-to-3', the other is 3'-to-5'.

Folding of DNA

The helical strands of DNA are packaged with a number of proteins in a form termed chromatin. The DNA is wrapped around small complexes of histone proteins (**Figure 1.6**) to form a nucleosome, with about 200 base pairs to each nucleosome. On high-power electron microscopy the nucleosomes look like beads on a string. There are then further levels of coiling and winding to produce densely packed chromosomes formed of chromatin.

This tightly packed inactive DNA, not undergoing replication or transcription, is termed heterochromatin. Active DNA is relatively unwound, as euchromatin.

Replication of DNA

The ability of DNA to be replicated exactly is fundamental to tissue function. Replication is called semi-conservative because the parent

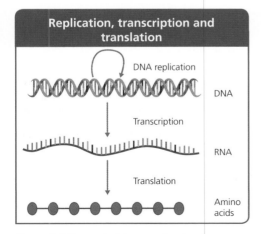

Figure 1.4 The central dogma of molecular biology and genetics: replication of DNA, transcription of DNA and translation of RNA.

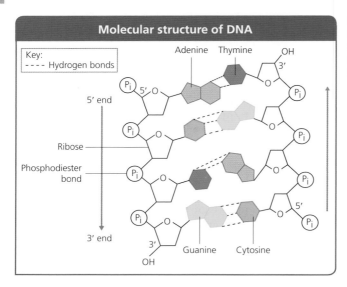

Molecular structure of DNA

Key:
- - - - Hydrogen bonds

Adenine   Thymine

5′ end

Ribose

Phosphodiester bond

3′ end

Guanine   Cytosine

Figure 1.5 The two anti-parallel strands of DNA. These entwine to form a helix, which must be opened or unwound to allow access to the DNA.

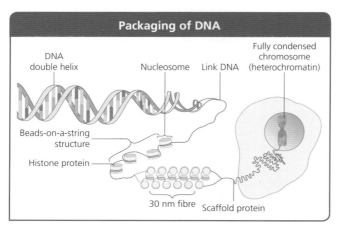

Packaging of DNA

DNA double helix

Nucleosome   Link DNA

Fully condensed chromosome (heterochromatin)

Beads-on-a-string structure

Histone protein

30 nm fibre   Scaffold protein

Figure 1.6 The DNA helix is wrapped around histone proteins, forming nucleosomes, in a 'beads on a string' appearance. It is further condensed to give chromosomes formed of chromatin.

DNA is split in half, with each strand 'directing' the formation of a new daughter strand. Because there are only two possible pairings of the bases in DNA, the resultant pairs of strands are exact copies of the original parents, for example:

Parent strands: TATAAT
                      ATATTA
                        ↓

Daughters (bold)   TATAAT   **TATAAT**
and parents: **ATATTA** + ATATTA

DNA replication is extremely accurate but occasional errors do occur. Mismatch repair proteins – for example, mutation S (MutS) and L homolog (MSH and MLH, respectively) proteins – help identify base pairing errors. Lynch syndrome is a hereditary disease of increased risk of non-polyposis colorectal cancer due to mutations in *MSH-2* and *MLH-3*.

The enzyme DNA helicase opens up the helix at a point called the replication fork, which is stabilised by topoisomerase, i.e. closure of the separated strands is prevented and DNA is kept relatively unwound (**Figure 1.7**). A new strand is synthesised in a 5'-to-3'direction on the leading strand as DNA polymerase moves along the parent 3'-to-5' strand. This enzyme uses new nucleotides to match corresponding base pairs. It does this with high accuracy. In addition there are a number of other

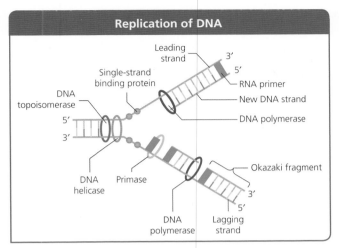

Figure 1.7 In semi-conservative replication there is formation of two new DNA strands, with half of each strand consisting of half of the parent strand.

Replication of DNA

Leading strand

Single-strand binding protein

DNA topoisomerase

RNA primer

New DNA strand

DNA polymerase

DNA helicase

Primase

Okazaki fragment

DNA polymerase

Lagging strand

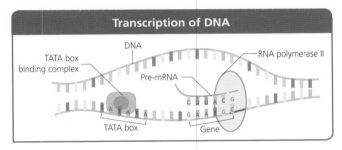

Figure 1.8 DNA is unwound and opened to allow transcription to take place. Pre-mRNA, a single-stranded molecule, is formed and then is moved from the nucleus to the cytosol.

Transcription of DNA

DNA

TATA box binding complex

RNA polymerase II

Pre-mRNA

TATA box

Gene

mechanisms that check for and repair errors during replication.

The daughter formed on the other ('lagging') strand is made in a 3'-to-5' direction and is formed in small sections known as Okazaki fragments, made by DNA polymerase moving in the 5'-to-3' direction. Each fragment is begun with a RNA primer (made by RNA polymerase), which allows DNA polymerase to add subsequent bases. The Okazaki fragments are joined together by DNA ligase. The RNA primer is cleared from DNA and recycled.

From DNA to RNA to protein

A gene is a section of DNA that contains a code for the production of a single protein, first by transcription to produce an RNA transcript, and then by translation of the RNA into an amino acid chain, i.e. a polypeptide or protein. This type of RNA is called

messenger RNA (mRNA) because it acts as a messenger between the gene and the cellular mechanism that builds proteins.

In a typical eukaryotic gene several stretches of DNA called exons code for the protein; these are interrupted by regions called introns. The introns are removed from ('spliced' out of) the RNA transcript before it is translated into a polypeptide. Some genes undergo alternative splicing, where different exons end up in the mRNA, thus resulting in a group of related protein products called splice variants.

Transcription

The first step in the formation of a protein is transcription (**Figure 1.8**): this is the process of turning a gene (DNA) into an mRNA template. Only one strand of the double-stranded DNA is copied and the product is a single-stranded mRNA molecule that detaches from the DNA. There are four stages:

1. **Initiation:** a complex of transcription factors and proteins bind to a promoter region of DNA 'upstream' of the gene (i.e. towards its 5′ end). The transcription factor complex causes separation of DNA strands and guides RNA polymerase to the site of the gene. RNA polymerase is guided into place by the TATA box, a region of DNA of alternating thymine and adenine bases.
2. **Elongation:** RNA polymerase II binds to the DNA and catalyses formation of a single-stranded mRNA chain that is complementary to the DNA (here are several RNA polymerases but only RNA polymerase II forms mRNA). The nucleotides used to synthesise the (m)RNA contain ribose sugar groups instead of deoxyribose sugars and include uracil instead of thymine.
3. **Termination:** specific codes and repetitive sequences in the DNA result in dissociation of RNA polymerase from DNA when copying has reached the end of the gene, and transcription ends
4. **Post-transcriptional modification:** the mRNA initially formed (pre-mRNA) undergoes a series of modifications in the nucleus, as outlined in **Table 1.4**, before it is translated into protein

Translation

In translation amino acids are matched to codons on the mRNA, and the amino acids are joined together in sequence to form a protein.

mRNA processing		
Name	Process	Reason
Guanine cap	A guanine residue is added to the 5′ end	Improved stability and recognition
Poly-A tail	Multiple adenines are added to the 5′ end	Improved stability and recognition
Intron removal	Introns (non-coding sections of genes) are spliced out	Only mRNA that contains coding is translated into protein

Table 1.4 Processing of pre-mRNA prior to translation

A codon is a trinucleotide. Each of the 22 amino acids has one or more RNA codons that correspond only to that amino acid. For example AUG is one codon for the amino acid methionine and GGA is one codon for glycine. The matching of amino acids to codons is performed by transfer RNAs (tRNAs). At one end of each tRNA molecule there is an anticodon, a trinucleotide that binds to a specific codon; at the other end there is a binding site for the corresponding amino acid.

Translation is mediated by ribosomes, specialist protein complexes (**Figure 1.9**). The ribosome binds to, and moves along the mRNA. As it does this it reveals each codon in sequence, and facilitates binding of the corresponding tRNA, thereby bringing into line the sequence of amino acids determined by the codon sequence of the mRNA. The ribosome catalyses the formation of peptide bonds between the adjacent amino acids, generating the polypeptide chain. This continues until a 'stop codon' (e.g. UAG) is reached; there is no corresponding tRNA for this codon (and no amino acid), and translation ends.

There tends to be only one ribosome translating upon each mRNA at any one time; however ribosomes are short-lived structures that may not even translate an entire mRNA molecule; they undergo frequent recycling. Occasionally several ribosomes join together as a polysome on a single mRNA, each ribosome translating it at the same time; this allows for formation of multiple polypeptide chains simultaneously.

Regulation of protein production

Cells produce some proteins constitutively, i.e. at a constant rate, whereas others are inducible, i.e. they are only produced in response to specific signals. Control for these processes exists both before and after transcription.

For example, in response to growth factor stimulation there is activation of a tyrosine-kinase pathway called the Ras-kinase pathway, which results in generation of the Fos and Jun family of transcription factors. These transcription factors bind to promoter regions on DNA; these regions are associated with growth-related genes. Binding of the transcription factors

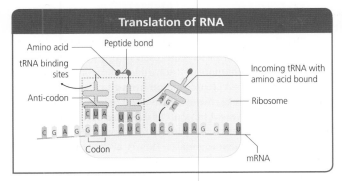

Figure 1.9 Translation is mediated by ribosomes. Each ribosome has two binding sites for tRNA. When a tRNA anti-codon binds the mRNA codon, a peptide bond can form between the amino acids attached to that tRNA and the adjacent tRNA.

promotes assembly of the TATA-box binding complex (TBBC), which recognises a T-A-T-A section of DNA downstream from the promoter region but upstream from the gene. Assembly of the TBBC guides RNA polymerase II to the site of the gene and increases transcription.

Another form of regulation is degradation and post-transcriptional modification of mRNA to reduce gene translation. A further mechanism that is still poorly understood is performed by micro-RNAs. These are small RNAs that are able to bind to and interfere with the function of mRNAs in a sequence-specific manner. Micro-RNAs are likely to be one of the major areas of scientific discovery and be potential therapeutics in the next 20 years.

> **Oncogenes are normal genes that promote growth or cell survival** (e.g. growth factors and anti-apoptotic factors). In carcinogenesis, function mutations occur in oncogenes disrupting normal regulation of gene production and culminating in increased synthesis of growth-related proteins and cell proliferation.

Mitochondria and energy production

Mitochondria

The mitochondrion is a structure that has its own double membrane, separating it from the rest of the cell, and its own DNA. Mitochondria are thought to have originated as separate organisms that developed a symbiotic relationship with early eukaryotic cells.

They are the sites of oxidative phosphorylation and generation of ATP (adenosine triphosphate), the final stage in aerobic respiration where all pathways of energy generation converge (**Figure 1.10**). Thus mitochondria are

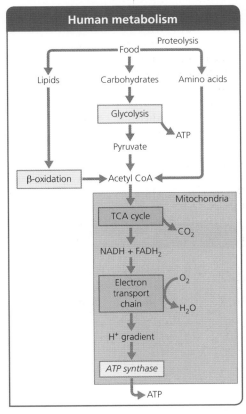

Figure 1.10 Outline of human metabolism showing energy generation from the three main macromolecules: protein, carbohydrate, and fat. All converge on the Krebs' cycle (i.e. the TCA cycle or citric acid cycle) for oxidative phosphorylation.

often described as the powerhouses of the cell and are more abundant in cells with high-energy demands, e.g. skeletal muscle cells.

> **Mitochondria contain their own genome coding for proteins involved in their function.** Rare inherited conditions caused by mutations in mitochondrial DNA usually affect tissues with high energy demand, such as brain, muscle and eyes, e.g. MELAS (myoclonic epilepsy, lactic acidosis, and stroke-like episodes). Mitochondrial DNA is inherited exclusively from the mother's ovum.

Overview of energy production

The cellular 'currency' for energy exists in the form of adenosine triphosphate (ATP). ATP is able to act as an energy store because when it is hydrolysed to ADP and phosphate (P_i) there is release of energy that drives other reactions, for example conformational change of a membrane channel for active transport (see page 18). Therefore, the aim of energy production is to generate ATP. This is the main function of macronutrients: carbohydrates, fats and, to a certain extent, protein.

Glycolysis

Many carbohydrates are broken down to glucose, the starting molecule for glycolysis.

The overall function of glycolysis is to convert glucose into pyruvate and generate two molecules of ATP. This process occurs independent of oxygen; therefore, in the absence of adequate oxygen, anaerobic respiration relies on ATP production from glycolysis alone.

Pyruvate is converted to acetyl CoA (co-enzyme A) in one of the main rate-determining steps in metabolism, regulated by pyruvate dehydrogenase. This is also the point where energy from fat, protein, or fructose enters the pathway for energy generation. Acetyl CoA is the breakdown product of fat, protein and fructose, so is an intermediate between macromolecules and the tricarboxylic acid cycle (see below).

Fat and protein metabolism

Fats are broken down by β-oxidation, a process of multiple oxidation reactions that occurs within the mitochondria. Protein is stripped of its nitrogen and then converted to pyruvate.

Tricarboxylic cycle

Acetyl CoA is the initial molecule in the tricarboxylic acid cycle (TCA cycle, citric acid cycle or Kreb's cycle). The TCA cycle takes place inside mitochondria (**Figure 1.11**). It is a series of reactions that result in the generation of reduced dinucleotide intermediates: nicotinamide adenine dinucleotide (NAD⁺) is converted to NADH (the reduced form

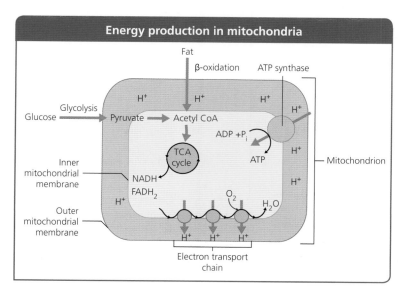

Figure 1.11 Glycolysis and β-oxidation of fat supply acetyl CoA to the TCA cycle inside mitochondria. The NADH and FADH₂ that are generated by this drive the electron transport chain, which provides a hydrogen ion gradient which ATP synthase uses (on the inner mitochondrial membrane), to make ATP.

of NAD⁺) and flavin adenine dinucleotide (FAD) is converted to $FADH_2$ (the reduced form of FAD).

Electron transport chain

The formation of NADH and $FADH_2$ is a crucial step in ATP generation. These molecules donate H⁺ to protein complexes on the inner mitochondrial membrane, in a process called the electron transport chain), which pumps H⁺ to the inter-membrane space. Oxygen is required for the final stage of the ETC and is reduced to H_2O.

The resulting H⁺ gradient across the inner mitochondrial membrane drives ATP synthase, an enzyme that uses the passage of H⁺ through its transporter domain to allow combination of ADP⁺ P_i to ATP. This form of ATP synthesis is known as oxidative phosphorylation; it is the most efficient method of energy production.

> Mitochondrial dysfunction can arise from congenital genetic conditions, acute toxicity, or chronic dysfunction. In iron poisoning, alterations in the balance of oxidation reactions within mitochondria cause cell death and liver failure. Chronic changes in mitochondrial β-oxidation of fat contribute to the inflammation seen in fatty liver disease.

Endoplasmic reticulum and Golgi apparatus

The endoplasmic reticulum is a series of interconnecting membrane laminae (sheets) and tubules that are the location of the synthesis and modification of many molecules.

Rough endoplasmic reticulum

Rough endoplasmic reticulum (RER) is covered with ribosomes, which dock to a protein complex called the translocon. The translocon is a group of proteins in the membrane of the RER that is used to transport polypeptides into the endoplasmic reticulum once they have been synthesised by ribosomes. Some ribosomes are free floating in the cytosol and then bind to the translocon, if they have a corresponding amino acid sequence in the synthesised polypeptide.

The main of the RER role is 'the production of secretory and intrinsic proteins. The proteins are synthesised by ribosomes and pass through the translocon into either the lumen or the membrane of the RER. Some proteins undergo post-translational modifications inside the RER, such as glycosylation, cleavage or adenylation, prior to being fully functional; enzymes in the RER mediate this.

Smooth endoplasmic reticulum

Smooth endoplasmic reticulum (SER) has several functions. It is the site of synthesis of steroid hormones in endocrine cells (e.g. in the cortex of the adrenal gland). It is a store

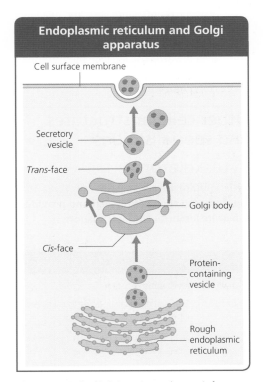

Endoplasmic reticulum and Golgi apparatus

Cell surface membrane

Secretory vesicle

Trans-face

Golgi body

Cis-face

Protein-containing vesicle

Rough endoplasmic reticulum

Figure 1.12 The Golgi apparatus has a *cis* face that receives proteins from the endoplasmic reticulum. The *trans* face produces secretory vesicles that travel to the cell surface membrane.

for calcium, which is released as a 'second messenger', i.e. an intracellular signal (see page 22). In its membranes, SER also has specialised calcium release channels that open in response to other second messenger signals such as inositol triphosphate (IP_3; see page 23).

The SER in muscle cells is specialised, and is known as the sarcoplasmic reticulum. It contains very high Ca^{2+} concentrations due to active uptake via a SERCA pump.

Golgi apparatus

The Golgi apparatus (or organ) consists of a stack of plate-like cisternae that are flattened balloons of membrane. Material enters the Golgi by endocytosis, travels between cisternae and departs for other regions of the cell, all by vesicular trafficking. After proteins (or large lipids) have been synthesised in the endoplasmic reticulum, they pass into the cis-Golgi network. Enzymes within the cisternae modify the proteins (for example by glycosylating them), and sort and package them for particular cellular targets. Secretory vesicles bud off the trans-Golgi network and travel towards the surface membrane of the cell before exocytosis, i.e. discharge out of the cell (**Figure 1.12**).

Other cellular structures and specialisations

Cytoskeleton

Cells contain three networks of fibres that maintain the shape of the cell and provide a substrate for intracellular transport.

Microfilaments

These are composed of actin and are particularly prominent near the periphery of cells. They form the core of microvilli and the pseudopodia of motile cells. They often anchor membrane proteins in particular domains and help cells attach to other body components.

Microtubules

These are composed of tubulin molecules. They are polar with a 'minus' end usually anchored in an area of cytosol that acts as an organising centre (see page 13), and a growing 'plus' end. Typically the plus ends radiate towards the periphery of the cell, though in epithelial cells they are often in an 'apical-to-basal' orientation. (The apical membrane of an epithelial cell faces outwards, for example towards the gastrointestinal lumen; the basal, or basolateral, membrane faces towards the basal membrane, underling capillaries, or further layers of epithelial cells.) The microtubule network is quite dynamic and has a major role in organising the distribution of other cellular components within the cell. Microtubules are particularly important in cell division (see page 14) when they are required for formation of the mitotic spindle and therefore are needed for progression through metaphase.

There are several cytoskeletal motor proteins that drive vesicle movement along microtubules and microfilaments (**Table 1.5**).

The intermediate filaments

These have a mainly structural role. Different cell types have intermediate filaments made

Cytoskeletal motor proteins		
Protein	Mechanism of action	Role
Dyneins	Transport retrogradely (towards minus end of microtubules)	In most cells: transport material towards centre of cell
		In cilia, ciliary dynein drives bending movement of cilia
Kinesins	Large family of motor proteins, most moving anterogradely on microtubules	Transport material towards periphery (in most cells), e.g. axonal transport of material towards synapse in nerve cells
Myosins	Myosin II forms thick filaments (crucial for muscle, see page 53)	Drive motility on actin
	Other myosins drive vesicle trafficking along microfilaments	Transport of neurotransmitter in neurones

Table 1.5 Cytoskeletal motor proteins and their function

up of different proteins for example, epithelial cell intermediate filaments are made of keratins.

Centrioles

The centrioles are a pair of small structures made up of microtubule triplets (usually 9 triplets arranged as a short hollow cylinder). During much of the cell cycle they appear quiescent, though they form the core of the microtubule organising centre. However during cell division (mitosis) they are responsible for production of the mitotic spindle, a network of filaments that is needed for separation of the chromosomes and for cytokinesis (see page 14).

Lysosomes

These vacuoles contain many hydrolytic enzymes, which are used for a variety of processes. For example, in granulocytes, lysosomes are used to produce toxic radicals (e.g. O_2^-) that kill bacteria. In thyroid follicular cells, lysosomal enzymes are used to cleave thyroglobulin into thyroxine and triiodothyronine. More generally, they degrade any proteinaceous material that needs to be removed from the cell.

Peroxisomes

These are small vacuoles that contain enzymes needed for β-oxidation breakdown of very-long chain fatty acids.

Motile cilia

These are thin projections from the apical membrane of some epithelial cells, for example into the bronchial airways. They drive movement of material over the surface of the cells. They are formed of an axoneme, a microtubule-based cytoskeleton, covered in plasma membrane. They beat rhythmically to assist movement of mucus in the respiratory system and flow through the Fallopian tubes.

Microvilli

These are multiple small fingers of the apical plasma membrane, with a core of microfilaments. Microvilli are a feature of absorptive epithelia because they greatly increase a cell's surface area. Basolateral membrane does not contain microvilli, but may have deep folds to increase surface area.

Cell cycle

The normal life cycle of a cell's quiescence, growth and division is termed the cell cycle (**Figure 1.13**). Mitosis, the process of division into daughter cells, represents only a very small fraction of the cell cycle, so in any one tissue relatively few cells are actively dividing at any one time. The duration of the cell cycle varies greatly between cell types. For example, intestinal epithelium renews itself every 3 days whereas the majority of cardiac muscle cells (myocytes) never divide.

> **Most cardiac myocytes never divide,** only doing so under certain conditions, e.g. after sublethal ischaemic injury followed by rapid reperfusion. Most of the (minimal) production of new cardiac myocytes occurs from stem cells residing within the myocardium.

The cycle is divided into five phases:

■ **G0** – a quiescent phase without growth, replication or division. This phase has a

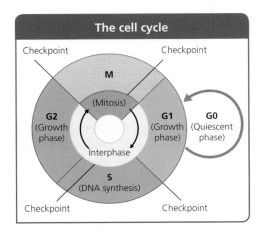

Figure 1.13 For much of the cell cycle, the cell is in interphase (G0, G1, S, G2), with mitosis (M) comprising only a minority of the time. Checkpoints must be passed to allow cycle progression.

highly variable duration and is when most normal cell processes take place.

- **G1** – the first phase of growth, with an increase in cytoplasm and organelle numbers
- **S** – synthesis of new set of DNA, by replication (as described above). This converts each chromosome from a single chromatid into two chromatids; the resulting chromosome appears as two strands, joined by a centromere at the centre; see **Figure 1.14**).
- **G2** – a further growth phase
- **M** – mitosis phase, with division of the cell into two daughter cells

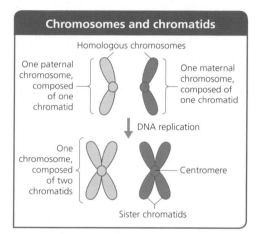

Chromosomes and chromatids

Homologous chromosomes

One paternal chromosome, composed of one chromatid

One maternal chromosome, composed of one chromatid

DNA replication

One chromosome, composed of two chromatids

Centromere

Sister chromatids

Figure 1.14 For most of the cell cycle chromosomes are formed of one chromatid, but after DNA replication chromosomes are comprised of two sister chromatids joined at the centromere. Maternal and paternal copies of the same chromosome are known as homologous chromosomes.

Mitosis

This is the process of symmetrical cell division into two identical daughter cells, each containing a complete set of genetic material (two copies of each of the 23 chromosomes). The term 'n' is used to describe the amount of genetic material; a full set (i.e. two copies of each of the 23 chromosomes) is 2n. Therefore n is one set of 23 chromosomes. Replication occurs in the S phase, before mitosis begins; therefore at the start of mitosis cells have 4n DNA and chromosomes are composed of sister chromatids (two exact copies of each chromosome, joined by the centromere). Mitosis is divided into four phases (**Figure 1.15**):

- **Prophase:** condensation of the chromosomes, breakdown of the nuclear membrane and synthesis of the mitotic spindle (using microtubules).
- **Metaphase:** aligning of sister chromatids on the mitotic spindle with crossing-over of chromosome sections for exchange of alleles between chromosomes.
- **Anaphase:** separation of chromatids as the spindle contracts, pulling one chromatid towards each pole of the cell, with separation through the centromere.
- **Telophase:** cytokinesis, i.e. division, of the cell into two, and re-formation of the nuclear membrane and re-establishment of normal cell function.

Cell cycle regulation

The cell cycle is carefully controlled. Excessive cycling results in aberrant growth and proliferation of cells (neoplasia), while a lack

Figure 1.15 Mitosis is divided into prophase, metaphase, anaphase, and telophase (which includes cytokinesis).

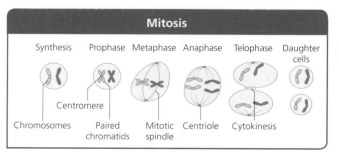

Mitosis

Synthesis   Prophase   Metaphase   Anaphase   Telophase   Daughter cells

Centromere

Chromosomes   Paired chromatids   Mitotic spindle   Centriole   Cytokinesis

of cycling causes atrophy (wasting). There are several checkpoints throughout the cell cycle, each requiring a specific signal to allow continued cycling. These signals result in a rise in cyclin proteins, which control progression through the cycle by activating cyclin-dependent kinases (CDK) that phosphorylate the proteins required for the cycle to continue. Mutation in the proteins that control the cell cycle checkpoints results in continued cycling in the absence of appropriate signals. This is one of the hallmarks of cancer (**Figure 1.16**).

Cancers are caused by dysregulation of cell cycle control. Mutations in genes controlling growth result in more frequent mitosis and increased generation of new cells. Conventional chemotherapy targets rapidly-cycling cells but, in consequence, also damages tissues with short cell cycles, e.g. hair, gut.

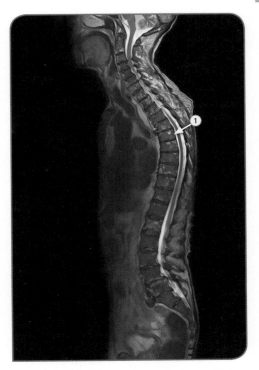

Figure 1.16 MRI of spine demonstrating multiple malignant metastases throughout the spine. The primary tumour was never found in this patient. ① Metastatic deposit.

Non-dysjunction, in which chromosomes or chromatids fail to separate during meiosis or mitosis, results in daughter cells with abnormal numbers of chromosomes. Down's syndrome (trisomy 21) occurs when an extra copy of chromosome 21 enters a gamete during meiosis. Upon fertilisation by a normal gamete, the resultant zygote has three copies of chromosome 21.

Meiosis

In contrast to mitosis, meiosis results in production of gametes, cells that have half the amount of genetic material of the parent cell. The process begins with DNA replication, which is then followed not by one division but by two divisions, resulting in only a single set of 23 chromosomes in each of the four daughter cells.

Cell membranes

Every eukaryote cell is enveloped by a semipermeable membrane. Most of the total surface area of a cell's membrane is intracellular and acts as a site for reactions and covering organelles.

The fluid mosaic model

The cell membrane is not a fixed, unchanging structure. It has the nature of a fluid mosaic, as originally postulated by Singer and

Nicholson in 1972. The membrane is a phospholipid bilayer, in which the hydrophobic lipid tails of the phospholipids face in towards each other and the polar (charged and therefore hydrophilic) phosphate group at the heads of the molecules interface with the fluid inside or outside the cell (**Figure 1.17**). Van de Waals forces hold the lipid tails together.

> **Congenital defects in cell membranes are extremely rare, as most are not compatible with life.** A few patients have been described with an inability to make phosphatidylcholine, the main glycophospholipid in cell membranes. This causes severe metabolic disturbance with a lack of peripheral adipose, fatty liver disease, and diabetes.

Embedded in the bilayer, or passing through it, are many proteins and other large molecules that add structure to the lipid membrane and allow the controlled transport of substances across the membrane. Many of these components diffuse freely around in the membrane, though some are anchored to the actin cytoskeleton.

The membrane is semi-permeable:

- **small non-polar molecules** (e.g. CO_2, free fatty acids, and usually water) are able to diffuse through the hydrophobic regions of the membrane
- **ions and large or polar molecules** cannot pass through the membrane except where there are specific channels in the membrane or specialised transporters (see page 19)

Cholesterol

Cholesterol molecules are embedded in the phospholipid bilayer, which disrupts the forces between phospholipids and stabilises the membrane. The rigid structure of cholesterol reduces the mobility of adjacent lipid molecules, thus reducing the permeability of the membrane. At low temperatures cholesterol prevents solidification by interrupting attractive forces. At high temperatures cholesterol acts to reduce phospholipid activity and maintains constant fluidity.

Membrane proteins

A huge variety of proteins are associated with the plasma membrane, including enzymes, channels, structural proteins and intracellular signalling proteins.

Intrinsic proteins are those that completely span the phospholipid membrane. Part of their protein structure lies within the hydrophobic region of the membrane, while hydrophilic domains interact with molecules inside and outside the cell. There are also extrinsic proteins that are closely associated with the membrane and are bound to it but do not traverse the hydrophobic region.

In addition, the membrane has polysaccharide residues and glycoproteins that act as external receptors or surface identity markers. These are either extensions of integral proteins or they are attached to lipids.

Membrane potential
Resting potential

Most cells have an electrical potential across their plasma membrane in a steady state, known as the resting membrane potential (E_m). This is usually negative (between −90mV and −30mV), as the inside of the cell has slightly more negatively charged ions than positive ones.

Figure 1.17 Two layers of opposing phospholipid with free-floating proteins form the cell membrane. Proteins that traverse the membrane have α helices on their external face.

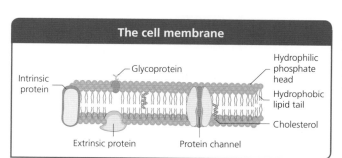

The cell membrane

Glycoprotein

Intrinsic protein

Hydrophilic phosphate head

Hydrophobic lipid tail

Cholesterol

Extrinsic protein   Protein channel

Ion permeability

The resting membrane potential is determined by the cell's permeability to different ions and the electrochemical gradient, from one side of the cell membrane to the other, for those ions. The resting permeability to an ion is dependent on the number of cell membrane 'leak channels' that are available for that ion. Leak channels are always open and allow ion movement in accordance with the electrochemical gradient.

The overall ion concentrations inside the cell are maintained by active transport, most importantly by the enzyme Na^+/K^+-ATPase, which keeps intracellular Na^+ concentration low, and K^+ concentration high. Because most cells have a much higher membrane permeability to K^+ than to Na^+, the diffusion of K^+ out of cells is not compensated by Na^+ entry, which leaves the inside of the cell with a net negative charge. However, each membrane has permeabilities for multiple different ions (e.g. sodium, chloride, potassium and calcium) and the overall resting potential is derived from the net balance of these. For example, a cell with higher sodium permeability will have a less negative E_m (e.g. –30 mV) than a cell with low sodium permeability (e.g. –90 mV).

Depolarisation and hyperpolarisation

A shift in membrane polarity away from the cell's resting potential is described as

- **depolarisation**, more positive, or
- **hyperpolarisation**, more negative

These are caused by ion movements across the membrane, driven by changes in ion permeability and electrochemical gradients. An influx of cations (positive ions, e.g. potassium) or efflux of anions (negative ions) causes depolarisation, with the converse causing hyperpolarisation. Equally, cessation of the efflux of cations causes depolarisation. These changes are crucial to the function of excitable cells, i.e. nerve and muscle, and are discussed in Chapter 2.

> Severe hyperkalaemia (plasma potassium level > 7 mmol/L) is a medical emergency causing potentially fatal cardiac arrhythmias including asystole. The change in K^+ gradient across cell membranes results in hyperpolarisation, slowed firing of action potentials, and increased refractory period.

Transport across membranes

Substances are transported across the plasma membrane either in a channel-dependent or channel-independent manner (**Table 1.6**). Membranes are described as semi-permeable or selectively permeable, i.e. some substances can pass through membranes whereas others cannot. This is determined by the mechanisms below.

Transport of substances across membranes				
	Diffusion	Facilitated diffusion	Active transport	Endocytosis
Substances transported	Small, uncharged molecules	Ions and molecules	Ions and molecules	Large molecules and complexes
Specific transporter	No	Yes	Yes	No, but activated by specific receptors
Uses ATP	No	No	Yes	Yes
Move against concentration gradient	No	No	Yes	Yes

Table 1.6 Comparison of major methods of transport across membranes

Channel-independent transport

Diffusion

Small, non-polar molecules are able to diffuse through the lipid membrane itself. Examples include carbon dioxide, free fatty acids, cholesterol and steroid hormones. The rate of diffusion is dependent upon the concentration gradient of the substance, the surface area and the permeability of the membrane – this is Fick's law.

Osmosis

Osmosis is diffusion of water and is dependent upon the osmolar gradient across the membrane, which is influenced by both water and solute content.

Water and ions can move across cell layers between cells (paracellularly) through occluding junctions (**Figure 1.18**). These occluding junctions can be described as 'leaky', being relatively permeable to water and ions, or 'tight', where they do not allow movement of across them. Water is also able to move into and out of cells by diffusion through the cell membrane.

Aquaporins

Cells that either need particularly high water permeability or have membranes that are particularly water impermeable, have specialised water channels called aquaporins. An aquaporin comprises a number of protein subunits that span the cell membrane. There are several forms of aquaporin channel. Some,

like AQP1 in erythrocytes, are constitutively expressed (i.e. always present within, or on the surface, of cells, without need for specific stimulation) in cells and give a high water permeability. Others, like AQP2 in the kidney collecting duct, are only made available (by movement from intracellular storage to incorporation in the apical membrane) in response to specific stimuli (in this case antidiuretic hormone), thus allowing the water permeability of the tissue to be regulated.

Endocytosis and phagocytosis

Endocytosis and phagocytosis are 'active' uptake processes that do not utilise protein channels. Targets, often proteins bound to a receptor on the membrane, are drawn into the cell as the membrane invaginates to form a vesicle in the process of endocytosis. This is the opposite of the secretory mechanism exocytosis. Phagocytosis is conceptually similar to endocytosis in that a large substance is drawn into the cell intact, but involves a more active rearrangement of the cytoskeleton to produce cell processes that reach out to engulf large targets, e.g. invading organisms or damaged cells.

Channel- or transporter-dependent processes

Primary active transport

Membrane transport molecules or transporters are proteins that provide a channel for movement of substances across a membrane.

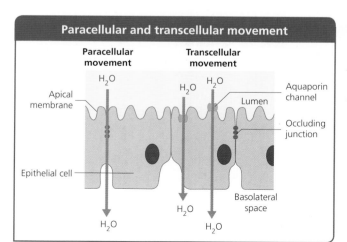

Paracellular and transcellular movement

Figure 1.18 Paracellular movement involves passage of small molecules through occluding junctions between cells. Transcellular movement sometimes utilises a specific transport channel (and other times does not).

Some transporters require energy to change shape in a way that facilitates transport of substances across the membrane; this is termed primary active transport. The energy is obtained by the hydrolysis of ATP (adenosine triphosphate), producing the lower energy ADP (adenosine diphosphate). Transporters that allow substance movement against the electrochemical gradient are described as primary active transporters or pumps. One example is the sodium–potassium pump, which maintains the relatively low sodium and high potassium concentration in cells (**Figure 1.19**).

Secondary active transport

In secondary active transport the energy to drive the process comes from an ionic concentration gradient set up by a pump; the transport channel does not hydrolyse ATP itself. For example, the sodium–glucose cotransporter uses the sodium gradient created by the sodium–potassium pump to pump glucose into cells (**Figure 1.20**).

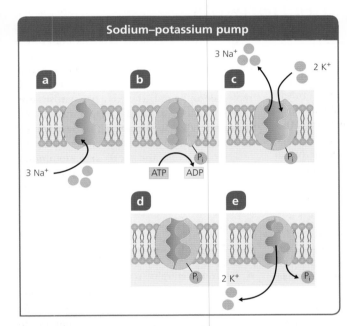

Figure 1.19 The sodium–potassium pump exports sodium from cells and imports potassium. Hydrolysis of ATP is required for the initial step of sodium export. Three Na^+ ions bind intracellularly (a). ATP binds to the transporter and is hydrolysed producing ADP and releasing energy (b) that causes a conformational change in the transporter such that sodium exits the cell (c). K^+ ions bind extracellularly, whilst inorganic phosphate (P_i) remains bound to the channel (d). P_i dissociates from the intracellular domain, which causes the transporter to revert back to its original confirmation (e). K^+ enters the cytosol, then ATP and sodium can re-bind.

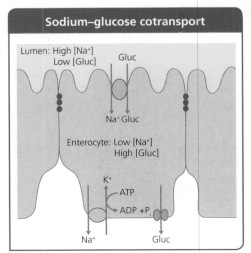

Figure 1.20 The sodium–glucose cotransporter exploits the sodium concentration gradient that is set up by the sodium–potassium pump using ATP. This allows co-transport of glucose with sodium over the apical membrane. Gluc, glucose.

Facilitated diffusion

Substances transported by facilitated diffusion pass through a transmembrane channel or transporter that does not consume ATP. Because it is not an 'active' process, substances move only in the direction of their electrochemical gradient, but the presence of a protein channel or transporter increases the rate of transport compared to diffusion alone.

Potassium and hydrogen are small, monovalent cations capable of binding to the Na$^+$/K$^+$-ATPase. When hydrogen levels are high (acidosis), H$^+$ competes for K$^+$ binding sites, so less K$^+$ is exported from the blood and excreted in the kidney, building up in the blood (hyperkalaemia). Conversely alkalosis can cause hypokalaemia.

Cell signalling mechanisms

Principles of signalling

Tissue function is dependent on the ability of cells to interact with each other and this is mediated by a number of signalling methods (**Figure 1.21**). All begin with an intracellular event that causes release of an extracellular signalling molecule. This then binds to a receptor on the 'effector' cell (a cell that responds to stimulus) and causes intracellular changes.

Receptors

Proteins with the ability to bind a signalling molecule and cause a downstream response (the intracellular cascade that carries out the effect) are receptors. Almost all receptors follow a similar pattern of phases. After the receptor is activated by the binding of a signal molecule (or ligand), there is a phase when the receptor is unresponsive ('refractory') to further stimulation, before it eventually becomes active again. Some signalling molecules (such as steroids) cross the target cell membrane and interact with receptors in the cytoplasm.

Types of receptor

There are four types of receptor (**Figure 1.22**):

- ion channels
- enzyme-associated receptors
- G-protein coupled receptors
- intracellular receptors

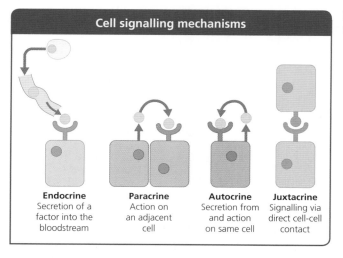

Cell signalling mechanisms

| **Endocrine** | **Paracrine** | **Autocrine** | **Juxtacrine** |
| Secretion of a factor into the bloodstream | Action on an adjacent cell | Secretion from and action on same cell | Signalling via direct cell-cell contact |

Figure 1.21 Cell signalling mechanisms.

Cell signalling receptors

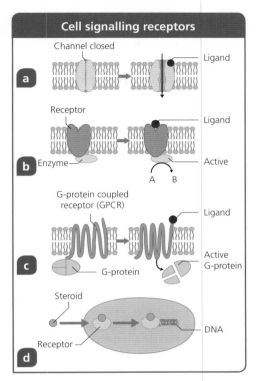

a Channel closed — Ligand, Receptor

b Enzyme — Ligand, Active, A B

c G-protein coupled receptor (GPCR) — Ligand, Active G-protein, G-protein

d Steroid, Receptor — DNA

Figure 1.22 Receptors for cell–cell signals. (a) Ion channels. (b) Enzyme-associated receptors. (c) G-protein coupled receptors. (d) Intracellular receptors.

Ion channels

When activated these receptors form a channel to allow passage of ions across the cell membrane (**Figure 1.22a**). For example nicotinic acetylcholine receptors allow the movement of cations when acetylcholine binds to the receptor, resulting in depolarisation of the membrane potential. These are called ionotropic receptors.

Enzyme-associated receptors

Following binding of their ligand, these receptors activate an intracellular enzyme (**Figure 1.22b**). This may be a domain (functional area) of the receptor itself or a separate enzymatic closely associated with the receptor.

One example of this is the insulin receptor, tyrosine kinase. When insulin binds, the enzymatic domain becomes active and phosphorylates tyrosine residues (areas on the protein where tyrosine is exposed on its external surface) on intracellular proteins. Tyrosine-kinase

receptors often have an intrinsic domain that initiates a phosphorylation cascade whereby each successive enzyme in the pathway is activated by phosphorylation and then performs tyrosine phosphorylation on the subsequent protein. In contrast, the growth hormone receptor does not have an intrinsic domain capable of triggering the cascade but activates a separate tyrosine kinase. Another subtype of enzymatic receptor is represented by the ANP (atrial natriuretic peptide) receptor, which is itself a guanylate cyclase (an enzyme that catalyses the formation of cyclic guanine monophosphate (cGMP)), and produces cGMP (an important intracellular signalling molecule) (see page 22).

G-protein coupled receptors

G-protein coupled receptors (GPCRs) are associated with GTP-activated proteins – G-proteins. These are heterotrimeric proteins composed of α, β and γ subunits. They become active when the GPCR is ligated, i.e. bound by a signalling molecule (**Figure 1.22c**).

Activated G-proteins stimulate intracellular cascades that have a wide variety of intracellular effects, including metabolic processes, growth and formation of ion channels. The stages of activation are shown in **Figure 1.23**. Their separated subunits mediate intracellular effector functions. Typically the α subunit activates an enzyme that results in the production of a second messenger: an intracellular signalling molecule, which leads to the final effects. Examples of these second messengers include cyclic adenosine monophosphate (cAMP, see page 22), Ca^{2+}, and inositol trisphosphate (IP_3; see page 23).

> **McCune Albright syndrome is a congenital syndrome caused by a mutation in the α subunit of G-proteins (G_s).** It causes skin pigmentation, early-onset puberty (sometimes by 2 years of age), polyostotic fibrous dysplasia causing bone fractures and abnormalities and endocrine disorders including thyrotoxicosis.

Intracellular receptors

All the receptor types discussed above are present in the plasma membrane of the cell,

GPCR activation of G proteins

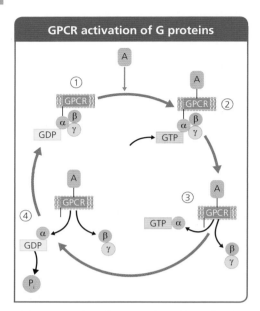

Figure 1.23 When there is no ligand bound to the GPCR, the three G-protein subunits are bound to each other, with GDP bound to the α subunit ①. Ligation of the GPCR (by a theoretical compound, 'A') causes GTP to be exchanged for GDP ②, which results in dissociation of the α subunit away from the β and γ subunits ③. The α subunit has intrinsic GTPase activity, which hydrolyses GTP to GDP. This causes the subunits to re-associate ④, terminating G-protein activity.

but some receptors are intracellular and respond to molecules that are able to diffuse through the cell membrane, for example steroid hormones, or the thyroid hormones. Once the ligand has bound to the receptor in the cytosol, some receptor–ligand complexes enter the nucleus (others first interact with further proteins in the cytosol) and acts as a transcription factor (**Figure 1.22d**). In this way intracellular receptors influence protein synthesis for a wide variety of processes. As the action is via changes in transcription the effects are slow, typically taking several hours to develop and lasting for days.

Other intracellular receptors include the ionotropic IP_3 receptors found on the endoplasmic reticulum, which release calcium ions.

Intracellular signalling pathways

There are many intracellular signalling pathways or cascades, controlling wide variety of cellular processes. However, there are several which are particularly significant in transducing the effects of receptors (transmitting the signal from activation of a receptor to the functional effect on the cell) and these are the ones described below. These pathways interact and it is possible for several to be active simultaneously within one cell. This allows the cells to integrate their response to multiple signals about their surrounding environment.

cAMP and cGMP pathways

Activation of GPCRs linked to G proteins, either G_s or G_i, alters the activity of adenylate cyclase, an enzyme that converts ATP to cyclic adenosine monophosphate (cAMP), a second messenger. This in turn activates protein kinase A (PKA), which phosphorylates target proteins, altering their activity. These targets may themselves be kinases, initiating a cascade of changes in cellular activity.

G_s stimulates the activity of adenylate cyclase, while G_i inhibits it. Activation of G_s to increase cAMP is the method of signalling used by adrenaline (through β-adrenoreceptors – a type of GPCR), which results in an increase in intracellular cAMP, activating PKA. Cyclic AMP is broken down by phosphodiesterases (PDEs) to 5' AMP, which prevent the signal persisting for too long (**Figure 1.24**).

The cGMP (cyclic guanine monophosphate) pathway (**Figure 1.25**) is similar in principle to the cAMP pathway. Guanylate cyclase (GC) catalyses the formation of cGMP from GTP (guanine triphosphate). cGMP leads to activation of protein kinase G (PKG), though PKA has quite different actions to PKA. A different isoform of phosphodiesterase (PDE) degrades cGMP.

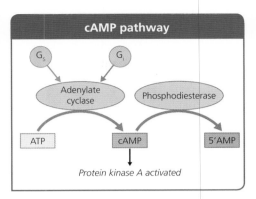

Figure 1.24 In the cAMP pathway, adenylate cyclase converts ATP to cyclic AMP (cAMP). cAMP is degraded to 5' AMP by phosphodiesterase. G-proteins, G_s and G_i, activate and inhibit adenylate cyclase, respectively.

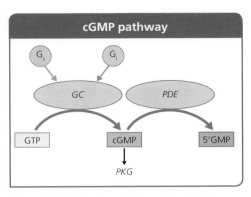

Figure 1.25 Similar in principle to the cAMP pathway, the cyclic guanine monophosphate (cGMP) pathway results in activation of protein kinase G (PKG).

> **Sildenafil (Viagra) is a phosphodiesterase inhibitor,** which increases the level of cGMP causing relaxation of vascular smooth muscle and vasodilatation in the corpora cavernosa resulting in an erection. Viagra's side-effects due to vasodilatation in other tissues include headaches, flushing and hypotension.

Phosphatidyl–inositol pathway

This pathway is activated by signalling through GPCRs linked to G_q (a G-protein). These include the α-adrenoreceptor, which is the main receptor to which noradrenaline binds to cause an increase in blood vessel constriction – this process is crucial in maintaining normal blood pressure. G_q causes an increase in the activity of phospholipase C (PLC), which cleaves phosphatidyl-inositol bisphosphate (PIP$_2$, a phospholipid) into inositol trisphosphate (IP$_3$) and diacyl glycerol. IP$_3$ binds to receptors on the endoplasmic reticulum causing them to open and calcium to be released. DAG causes activation of protein kinase C (PKC), which is also activated by the rising calcium concentrations. PKC has many intracellular effects especially relating to growth and proliferation (**Figure 1.26**).

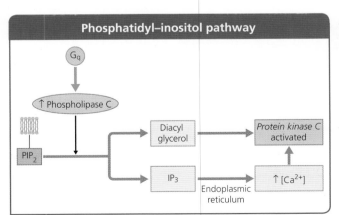

Figure 1.26 In the phosphatidyl–inositol pathway membrane-bound phosphatidyl-inositol bisphosphate (PIP$_2$) is cleaved by phospholipase C. Inositol trisphosphate (IP$_3$) causes calcium release from the endoplasmic reticulum. Calcium and diacyl glycerol both cause activation of protein kinase C.

Protein kinase C-Ca²⁺ pathway

Protein kinase C can also be activated by direct entry of Ca^{2+} into the cell, for example via ionotropic receptors or voltage-gated Ca^{2+} channels. Direct entry of Ca^{2+} also activates pathways that are regulated by calmodulin (an intracellular calcium-binding protein), which has a role in multiple cellular processes, for example inflammation and immune responses. Ca^{2+}–calmodulin complex also causes further Ca^{2+} to be released from the endoplasmic reticulum, for example via ryanodine receptors (a specific type of calcium channels) in muscle cells. This process is called calcium-induced calcium release (CICR).

Non-steroidal anti-inflammatory drugs (NSAIDs), such as ibuprofen are reversible inhibitors of cyclo-oxygenase. Reduction in COX-2 prostanoid level mediates analgesic, antipyretic and anti-inflammatory actions. As they also limit synthesis of COX-1 prostanoids, side effects include renal impairment, fluid overload, gastritis and peptic ulcers.

Arachidonic acid pathway

Arachidonic acid is a component of some membrane phospholipids. It is an omega-6 polyunsaturated fatty acid and is the starting molecule for the synthesis of eicosanoids (lipid-derived signalling molecules derived from arachidonic acid e.g. prostacyclin). As long as it is membrane-bound it is inactive, so the first step in the pathway is cleavage from the membrane by phospholipase A_2 (PLA_2) or phospholipase C (PLC). These enzymes are activated by a rise in intracellular calcium or by signalling from inflammatory mediators such as interferon.

One of two enzymes acts on free arachidonic acid: cyclo-oxygenase (COX) or 5-lipoxygenase (5-LO) (**Figure 1.27**). There are two isozymes of COX:

- COX-1 is constitutive and is needed for normal tissue homeostasis.
- COX-2 is inducible and is involved in inflammation.

Arachidonic acid metabolites	
Metabolite*	Function
PGE₂	Vasoconstriction; gastric mucus production; bronchoconstriction
PGI₂	Inhibition of platelet aggregation; vasodilatation
PGF₂α	Uterine myometrial contraction
TXA₂	Vasoconstriction; platelet aggregation
Leukotrienes	Bronchoconstriction; leukocyte chemotaxis

*PGE₂, prostaglandin E2; PGI₂, prostacyclin; PGF₂α, prostaglandin F₂α; TXA₂, thromboxane.

Table 1.7 Functions of the arachidonic acid metabolites

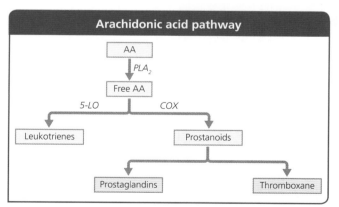

Figure 1.27 Membrane-bound arachidonic acid is freed from the membrane by PLA_2. It is then metabolised by either cyclo-oxygenase (COX) or 5-lipoxygenase (5-LO) to prostanoids or leukotrienes (LT), respectively. Prostanoids are then converted to either prostaglandins (PG) or thromboxanes.

All metabolites of the COX pathway are known as prostanoids, which are acted upon by further enzymes to produce prostaglandins or thromboxanes. The effect of prostanoids is dependent on their concentration, the tissue and whether they are formed by COX-1 or COX-2 (**Table 1.7**).

Tissues

A tissue is a group of specialised cells that have a similar function. There are four major tissue types:

- epithelium
- neural tissue
- muscular tissue
- connective tissue

The features of neural and muscular tissue are described in Chapter 2.

Cell junctions

Almost all cells in the body are held in place by a combination of cell-cell and cell-matrix junctions, only cells of the haematogenous system are free to move. Cell junctions are a broad group of structurally and functionally diverse mechanisms that connect cells together. **Table 1.8** outlines the main forms of cell junctions. Not all tissues express all forms of cell junction and there can be variation within a tissue (for example, only basal layer of epidermal keratinocytes have hemidesmosomes to connect to the underlying basal lamina).

Epithelium

An epithelium forms a boundary between different environments or regions and has two sides, apical and basolateral, which face different environments:

- the apical side typically faces an open space, for example the outside world in the case of the skin, the lumen of the gut or a blood vessel, or the acini and ducts of a gland
- the basolateral surface sits on a basement membrane (basal lamina) of connective tissue, within and below which run blood vessels, nerves, and lymphatics.

The apical and basolateral faces of epithelium are separated by occluding junctions between adjacent epithelial cells. These junctions prevent large substances (e.g. proteins

Intercellular junctions		
Junction	Composition	Function
Occluding	Protein complexes that fasten together the plasma membranes of two adjacent cells. Described as 'leaky' or 'tight' depending on permeability to small ions and water	Separate apical and basolateral membrane compartments
Adherens	Link cellular actin cytoskeletons using β-catenin and cadherin	Adhesion belt in epithelial tissues, for structural support
Desmosomes	Link intermediate fibres between cells using desmoplankins and cadherins	Structural support in epithelia: like 'spot-welds' between cells
Hemi-desmosomes	Join basal cell intermediate fibres to basement membrane integrins	Bind epithelium to basement membrane (e.g. epidermis to dermis)
Gap junctions (see Figure 2.4)	Made of connexin proteins, arranged around a central pore	Provide a route for electrical signals and small ions and molecules to pass between cells

Table 1.8 Intercellular junctions. Adherens, desmosomes and hemi-desmosome junctions are all types of anchoring junction (i.e. junctions with a primarily structural role hold cells together or hold cells to connective tissue)

or lipids) from travelling from one side of the epithelium to the other through the paracellular space between adjacent cells. For this reason, occluding junctions are also called 'tight' (occluding) junctions because they form a barrier. The presence of this barrier between the apical and basolateral sides of layer of cells makes possible the expression of different proteins, channels and receptors on the two sides of the layer. This confers a polarity on each of the epithelial cells. For example in gut epithelial cells (enterocytes) glucose is pumped out of the lumen of the gut across the apical surface by sodium-linked glucose transporters, but on the basolateral surface glucose can leave the cells passively via a glucose transporter, to enter the bloodstream.

In some types of epithelium the tight junctions are leaky, i.e. they permit the passage of certain molecules through the paracellular space (the intercellular space adjacent to the basolateral membrane of two epithelial cells). For example, they allow resorption of water in the kidney (see **Figure 5.5**).

Epithelia can be grouped in different ways. Morphologically, they are classified by histological appearance based on the shape of the cells and their layering (**Table 1.9**). Functionally, they can be classified as:

- Absorptive, for example the gut and kidney tubules
- Secretory for example glandular acinar cells or
- Occluding, i.e. having a barrier function, for example the skin or the endothelium lining blood vessels

Stem cells

Stem cells are cells that are able to undergo asymmetrical mitosis, i.e. they form one daughter cell that differentiates into a specialised cell type and one other stem cell. Most adult stem cells only produce one cell type whereas embryonic stem cells have the potential to produce almost any cell type, depending on the stage of embryonic development. This is termed plasticity (**Table 1.10**).

> **'Stem cell therapy' includes all treatments exploiting stem cells,** ranging from bone marrow transplant in which donor multipotent hematopoietic stem cells populate the recipient's marrow, to experimental processes such as the growth of new organs (e.g. bladder) using induced-pluripotent stem cells and an extracellular matrix.

Connective tissue

Connective tissues provide structure and support for other specialised tissues. They include adipose tissue (fat), cartilage, bone and other fibrous or elastic structures. All connective tissues have cellular and extracellular components: the cells produce and remodel the extracellular matrix.

Extracellular matrix

The extracellular matrix (ECM) is the acellular connective component that surrounds

Types of epithelium		
Type	Appearance	Examples
Simple columnar/ cuboid	Single layer of cuboidal or columnar (tall) cells	Gastric mucosa, renal tubules
Stratified squamous	Multiple layers of flat polyhedral cells	Epidermis
Pseudostratified columnar	Single layer of cells, but nuclei at different heights gives appearance of stratification, often due to presence of smaller precursor cells that don't extend as far as the apical surface	Respiratory tract
Transitional	Multiple layers of cuboidal cells that slide over each other to allow stretch of the organ	Bladder mucosa

Table 1.9 Types of epithelium, classified by histological appearance

Plasticity of stem cells	
Type of stem cell	Plasticity
Totipotent	Able to form any tissue, including placenta, and a whole organism, e.g. zygote (fertilised ovum) or cell from a morula (first 16-cell ball of cells)
Pluripotent	Able to form any tissue except placenta and cannot make a whole organism, e.g. cell from the inner cell mass of a blastocyst (after the first division into placenta and embryo)
Multipotent	May differentiate into several cell types within one tissue, e.g. hematopoietic stem cell
Adult stem cell/unipotent	Resident in differentiated adult tissues; able to divide to give new cells of one type, e.g. intestinal epithelial stem cells
Induced-pluripotent	A laboratory-generated pluripotent stem cell formed by 'de-differentiating' an adult cell

Table 1.10 The plasticity of stem cells

cells and tissues. It includes fibrous proteins (collagen, elastic fibres, reticular fibres) and ground substance.

- **fibrous proteins** provide tensile strength (collagen), elastic properties (elastic fibres) and support for cells (reticular fibres)
- **ground substance** is composed of highly hydrated non-fibrous proteins (glycosaminoglycans and hyaluronic acid) that surround other cells, filling in spaces and providing resistance to compression

Ehlers–Danlos syndrome is an inherited condition caused by a defect in type 1 collagen. Patients have extremely stretchy skin, hypermobile joints, bruise easily and have poor wound healing. They are at risk of pneumothoraces, aortic root dilatation and aortic dissection.

Adipose tissue

Adipocytes are connective tissue cells specialised for storing fat in large intracellular vacuoles. They are present in small numbers in most connective tissues, but adipose tissue is characterised by a high density of adipocytes. The fat they store is used for energy and thermal insulation but also acts as a cushion around some organs, such as the kidneys.

Cartilage

There are four forms of this strong connective tissue, each with slightly different composition and function. All cartilage is formed by chondroblasts, cells which ultimately mature into chondrocytes, the cells that maintain cartilage. It is an avascular tissue, so all nutrients and waste products exchange with the bloodstream by passive diffusion through the matrix.

Hyaline cartilage This form of cartilage is made of type II collagen. It is firm and clear in colour. In children, most bones are comprised of hyaline cartilage; these are referred to as unossified bones. The cartilage is replaced by bone, i.e. ossified, in a process that continues from early childhood through adolescence, until growth stops. In adults it also provides support in the form of cartilaginous rings around the trachea and the nasal septum.

Articular cartilage This is a specialised form of hyaline cartilage that lines the surfaces of bones at synovial joints. Its fibres are regularly arranged to keep friction to a minimum.

Fibrocartilage The collagen fibres in fibrocartilage are irregularly arranged but it has high tensile strength; it forms the cranial sutures, intervertebral discs and pubic symphysis.

Elastic cartilage This is the most pliable of all types of cartilage because it has a relatively higher density of elastic fibres. It is found in the larynx, ear and epiglottis.

Bone

Bones have both a structural and a physiological role. Structurally, they allow movement; physiologically, they are needed for blood cell production and calcium regulation. To understand these processes, it is necessary to know about the formation of bone, the structure of bone and its turnover on a cellular level.

Formation and resorption of bone

Bone is produced by osteoblasts. These cells form osteoid, a collagenous extracellular matrix, which then undergoes mineralisation with hydroxyapatite (calcium and phosphate). This process is countered by the action of osteoclasts, large multinucleate cells that cause resorption of bone. The balance of activity of these two cell types determines whether there is net formation or resorption of bone. Specialised cells – osteocytes – are needed for maintenance of bone. Bone stem cells are found in the periosteum, a connective tissue layer covering the bone.

Development of bones

Most bone is formed by a process called endochondral ossification. Bones are initially formed entirely from hyaline cartilage, which then undergoes ossification through secretion of osteoid by osteoblasts and calcification by chondrocytes. This process forms most of the body's long bones. However skull bones, for example, are formed in a different manner. These bones are formed by secretion of osteoid (without a cartilaginous base) by osteoblasts, which then become mineralised; a process known as intramembranous ossification. This is also the method by which fractures heal.

Osteopetrosis is a rare condition in which thickened dense bones are caused by lack of osteoclast function and continued deposition of osteoid by the unchecked bone-forming osteoblasts. The normal differentiation between cortex and medulla is lost and the resulting loss of marrow space causes bone marrow failure (i.e. anaemia, thrombocytopenia).

The multiple roles of bones

The skeleton is more than just a rigid frame for support and attachment of muscles. It is the main store of calcium and phosphate and therefore is involved in their homeostasis (see below). In addition, most haematopoiesis (blood cell production) occurs in the medullary cavity of bones.

Structure of adult bone

Adult long bones comprise several layers: outer compact bone, inner cancellous or 'spongy' bone, and marrow core (**Figure 1.28**).

Compact bone is comprised of Haversian systems; these are concentric rings (lamellae) of collagen fibres around a central canal that carries blood vessels. This concentric arrangement gives bone its strength and resistance to deformation (**Figure 1.29**).

The inner spongy bone that lies inside is much less regularly organised than compact

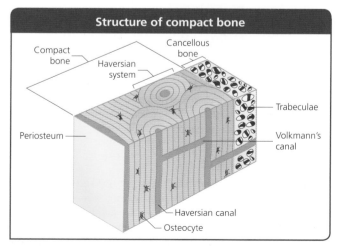

Structure of compact bone

Compact bone
Haversian system
Cancellous bone
Periosteum
Trabeculae
Volkmann's canal
Haversian canal
Osteocyte

Figure 1.28 Compact bone is formed of Haversian systems, which are made of concentric lamellae of bone. Horizontal Volkmann canals connect the vertical Haversian canals. Trabeculae of spongy bone are inside.

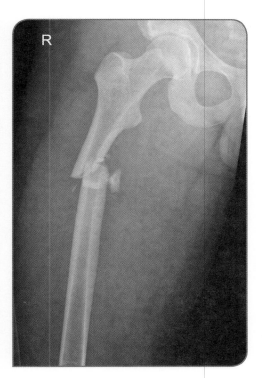

Figure 1.29 X-ray showing a right femoral shaft fracture. Note the very thin and pale bones. This patient had osteogenesis imperfect, a genetic condition where impaired collagen cross-linking causes a propensity for fractures with minimal trauma.

bone; it is made of interconnecting cavities with traversing bony trabeculae. This makes it strong but relatively light. The trabeculae can restructure in response to stress, to strengthen the bone in response to regular challenges.

Homeostasis

Homeostasis is the processes of maintaining a constant internal environment despite changes in environmental influences. The term is often used to describe one particular variable, e.g. blood pressure homeostasis, and it almost always involves interaction of several body systems. An example is maintenance of intravascular volume, which is dependent on hormones, the kidneys, cardiac function and hepatic function.

Feedback principles

The concept of negative feedback underpins homeostasis and many physiological processes (**Figure 1.30**). Key components of a negative feedback system are:

- **a set point**: this is the ideal state for the system to remain in (perhaps a mean arterial pressure of 100 mmHg).
- **a sensor**: this detects any deviation from that set point (for example, baroreceptors sensing a change in blood pressure)
- **a controller or integrating centre**: this uses input from the sensor(s) and controls the effector(s) accordingly (for example, centres within the brain stem)
- **one or more effectors**: these will act to move the system back towards the set point, for example a fall in blood pressure might lead to vasoconstriction, increased cardiac output and reduced urine production, while a rise might have the opposite effects

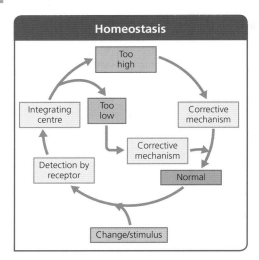

Figure 1.30 In homeostasis an integrating centre determines whether the physiological parameter is too high or low. It provides a correcting response, which is continuously measured.

Whenever a parameter of the system moves too far away from its set point, an effector will be activated to oppose that change. Once the system has returned to the set point, the effector will be switched off. There may be a small degree of overshoot; such systems are said to hunt around their set point. It is common to have two effector systems, one to act when the parameter is too high and one when it is too low.

> **Blood pressure is tightly controlled by a homeostatic mechanism, the baroreflex (page 92).** This is sometimes over-ridden; raised core temperature causes vasodilatation in the skin, irrespective of blood pressure, exacerbating the hypotension that arises with dehydration due to sweating in a hot environment. Conversely, certain emotional–neural reflexes (e.g. alerting response) cause a rise in blood pressure bypassing normal control.

Body fluids and their compartments

Water makes up more than half of the body's volume: 60% in men and 55% in women (women have a higher percentage of body fat). It is divided between physiological fluid compartments that contain fluids of different composition.

> **Disturbances in the volume or composition of fluid compartments cause serious clinical conditions,** e.g. hypertension caused by excessive salt ingestion (which increases fluid volume within the extracellular fluid, including the plasma).

The fluid compartments

Body water is distributed between a number of compartments (**Figure 1.31**). Each compartment has different constituents reflecting different metabolic needs and functions. It is essential to homeostasis that the compartments are maintained at constant volume and composition. These characteristics are controlled by two mechanisms, including:

■ Selective permeability of cell membranes (see page 16)
■ Active transport of substances (see page 18)

Constituents of body fluid compartments

Extracellular and intracellular fluids (ECF and ICF) have significantly different concentrations of nutrients, proteins, ions (dissolved electrolytes), waste products and dissolved gases (**Table 1.10**).

Water

Water is the universal solvent, facilitating transport of proteins, ions, respiratory gases,

Fluid compartments

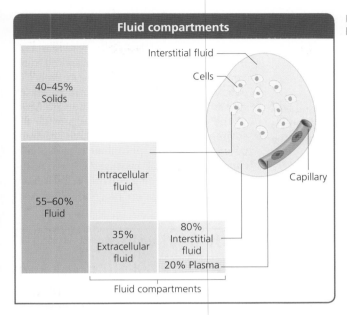

40–45% Solids

55–60% Fluid

Interstitial fluid

Cells

Intracellular fluid

Capillary

35% Extracellular fluid

80% Interstitial fluid

20% Plasma

Fluid compartments

Figure 1.31 Fluid compartments, by volume.

Composition of intra- and extracellular fluid

	Extracellular fluid	Intracellular fluid
pH	7.4	7.2
Osmolality (mOsm/kg H_2O)	285–290	28–290
Na^+ (mmol/L)	140	15
K^+ (mmol/L)	4.5	140
Cl^- (mmol/L)	105	20
HCO_3^- (mmol/L)	22	16
PO_4^{3-} (mmol/L)	1	100
Ca^{2+} (mmol/L)	1.2	<0.01
Protein (g/L)	0.7	3.0
Glucose (mmol/L)	5.5	<0.1

Table 1.10 The composition of intracellular and extracellular fluid

Polarity

Because the shape of the water molecule is a shallow V, with the slightly negatively charged oxygen atom at the base of the V and the slightly positively charged hydrogen atoms as its arms, the molecule has a slight electrical gradient. It is this polarity that allows other polar or ionic substances (e.g. Na^+ ions) to interact with water to dissolve in it.

Hydrogen bonding

Hydrogen bonds are temporary weak bonds that form due to this polarity. Hydrogen bonding between the oxygen and hydrogen atoms of adjacent water molecules gives water the property of cohesion: the tendency of water molecules to stick together. This explains why water is a liquid at body temperature, when most similarly sized molecules are gases. Surface tension represents this cohesion at gas–water interfaces.

Extracellular fluid

The extracellular fluid (ECF) contains large amounts of sodium, chloride, and bicarbonate ions, plus smaller amounts of nutrients for the cells, including oxygen, glucose, amino acids, and fatty acids. It also contains

mobile cells and metabolites, such as glucose. It also forms the basis of a controlled environment conducive to biochemical reactions. Two aspects of its unique structure underlie its essential biological properties: polarity and hydrogen bonding.

carbon dioxide that is being transported to the lungs to be excreted, plus other waste products that are being transported to the kidneys for excretion.

Blood

Blood is roughly 50% fluid (plasma) and 50% cells by volume. The total volume of blood is about 80 ml/kg, i.e. 5 litres in an adult. The principle blood cells are

- red blood cells (RBCs), which carry oxygen, and
- white blood cells (WBCs), which fight infection and regulate inflammation

There are also platelets, fragments of cells integral to blood clotting (**Table 1.11**; see page 92).

Plasma

Plasma is the fluid component of blood. It has a similar ionic composition to tissue fluid (fluid that surrounds all cells, excluding the blood), except that it contains many proteins that are unable to escape from the blood vessels. In contrast, water and other solutes (dissolved substances), are constantly moving between plasma and the ICF. The plasma proteins have a variety of functions, including binding some solutes, immune defence, and coagulation.

Intracellular fluid

In contrast to the ECF, the ICF contains higher concentrations of potassium, magnesium and phosphate ions. Thus there are ionic gradients between the compartments. These gradients require a lot of energy to maintain them but they are crucial for many cell functions. One example is their role as a store of potential energy that cells use to transport substances against a concentration gradient.

The constituents of ICF also provide the environment in which the cellular reactions occur. For example, phosphate is particularly concentrated in ICF because ADP and ATP – essential for the energy driving cellular reactions (see page 10) – are predominantly intracellular molecules.

Body fluid volume

Regulation of fluid volume

Maintaining the normal volume and composition of the body fluids is crucial to cellular function. This autoregulation, or homeostasis, of body fluid volume is largely a function of the kidney (see Chapter 5),

The principle regulators of total body fluid volume are:

- the renin–angiotensin–aldosterone system (RAAS; page 152), which controls the amount of salt and fluid in the body
- atrial natriuretic peptide (ANP), which control the amount of salt in the body (page 154),
- anti-diuretic hormone (ADH), which controls the amount of water (page 151).

These factors work together to maintain plasma at a constant volume and concentration. Consequently, they also maintain interstitial fluid, given that solutes (other than plasma proteins) freely diffuse across the capillary endothelium.

Exchange between interstitial fluid and the ICF is more tightly regulated. Small, uncharged molecules (O_2, H_2O) can pass through the plasma membrane. Ions (Na^+, Ca^{2+}) and larger molecules (glucose, amino acids) move through specific channels or transporter proteins. In most cases the exchange is governed by the rules of diffusion, i.e. is proportional and in the same direction as a substance's concentration gradient, but active transport may allow some substances

Composition of blood		
Constituent	Percentage of total	Function
Plasma	50	Contains H_2O, CO_2, glucose, ions, proteins; exchange with interstitial fluid
Red blood cells	49	Carriage of O_2
White blood cells	<1	Defence against infection
Platelets	<1	Haemostasis

Table 1.11 Blood constituents, their proportions and functions

to move against their concentration gradients, establishing the differences in composition described earlier.

> **Intravenous fluid replacement is often used to increase blood pressure and rehydrate patients, for example:**
>
> - 0.9% sodium chloride ('normal saline'), isotonic with plasma and expands the volume of the ECF, including plasma as sodium chloride is found mainly in the ECF
>
> - 5% dextrose (5%) also isotonic with plasma, but swiftly taken up by cells and metabolised, so like water, it distributes itself through all fluid compartments

Measurements of fluid volumes

The volumes of fluid compartments are rarely measured in clinical practice. Predominately measurements are used for research purposes, for example in drug development.

Measurement exploits the dilution principle: that the different concentrations of an injected substance in a compartment reflects their volumes. The main measurements are for total body water, plasma and extracellular fluid volumes, with the remainder calculated by inference.

Dilution principle, or volume of distribution (V_{dist})

A known amount of a substance X is injected intravenously and allowed to fully equilibrate between compartments. The concentration of the X in a venous blood sample is then measured. This allows calculation of the volume that X is distributed in when at equilibrium:

$$\text{volume of compartment (s) or volume of distribution } (V_{dist}) = \frac{\text{amount of } X \text{ administered}}{\text{concentration of } X}$$

As long as it is known how substance X distributes between compartments, compartment volumes can thus be calculated.

A correction may be needed to compensate for the amount of the X excreted in the urine during the equilibration.

Total body water

Total body water is estimated as $0.6 \times$ body mass. Accurate measurement is done by injecting a known amount of deuterated water ('heavy water'), which equilibrates with all body water. The fraction of deuterated water in exhaled breath (relative to normal water) is measured to calculate total body water.

Extracellular fluid volume

ECF volume is approximately one-third of total body water. It is measured using a substance that disperses throughout the compartment, such as inulin, an exogenous polysaccharide.

Total plasma and blood volumes

Total blood volume is estimated to be approximately 80 mL/kg. Plasma volume can be measured with a substance that remains trapped within the circulation; an example is Evan's blue, a dye that binds to albumin. Once plasma volume is known, blood volume can be calculated from the haematocrit (the percentage of blood comprised of red cells).

Interstitial and intracellular fluid volumes

Interstitial fluid volume is calculated by the subtraction of plasma volume from extracellular fluid volume. ICF volume is total body water minus the ECF.

Solute concentrations

The individual and collective concentrations of solutes in a fluid affect whether a solute or water moves across cell membranes, and in which direction. On a larger scale, this affects how they move between the different fluid compartments.

The key measures of solute concentration are osmolarity, osmolality, and tonicity, as discussed below. The key unit used for the first two is the osmole. An osmole is one mole of osmotically active particles in solution. For example,

1 mole of glucose dissolved in water gives it 1 osmole, whereas 1 mole of sodium chloride (NaCl) dissolves as sodium ions and chloride ions and therefore generates 2 osmoles.

- Osmolarity is a measure of solute concentration as the number of osmoles of solute per litre of solution.
- Osmolality is a measure of solute concentration as the number of osmoles of solute per kilogram of solvent. This is used in clinical practice, for example normal serum osmolality is 285 mosmol/kg H_2O, as it is independent of temperature (because water changes its volume with temperature, which affects osmolarity but not osmolality).

Note that both of these measures are independent of the solute's ability or inability to move across membranes.

Osmotic pressure and tonicity

If two solutions are separated by a semi-permeable membrane, i.e. a membrane that is permeable to water and some solutes (e.g. small ions), and if the concentration of water is higher in one of the solutions, water moves across the membrane towards the more concentrated solution to equalise the water concentrations. This movement is termed osmosis. Osmotic pressure is the physical pressure that would have to be applied to prevent it; in other words, the pressure with which water is drawn into the less concentrated solution.

Tonicity (also called osmolar concentration) is a measure of the difference in osmotic pressure between two solutions separated by a semi-permeable membrane, for example a cell membrane. Thus, only solutes that do not cross the membrane contribute to tonicity:

- A hypertonic solution has a higher concentration of these solutes than does the solution on the other side of the membrane
- A hypotonic solution has a lower concentration: water is drawn from it to the other side of the membrane
- An isotonic solution is one in which the tonicity is the same both sides of the membrane

Movement of solutes and water

Water and its solutes enter the body through the gastrointestinal tract (**Table 1.12**). Internally, water moves fairly freely between compartments because it crosses cell membranes, but membranes control the movement of most solutes. The movement of solutes determines the movement of water by osmosis, as described above. Ultimately the solutes and water are excreted via the lungs, skin, gut and kidneys. Any change in a fluid compartment's solute concentration will also change the net water movement.

Movement across cell membranes

The selective permeability of cell membranes governs the movement of water and solutes. Small amounts of water pass straight through plasma membranes, but in some membranes, for example the tubular cells of

Sites of water and solute exchange		
Organ/location	Barrier	Function
Lungs	Alveolar membrane, basement membrane, capillary endothelium	Exchange of respiratory gases, e.g. oxygen, carbon dioxide
Skin	Water-resistant epidermis and dermis	Water and salt loss through sweat
Gastrointestinal tract	Enterocytes and the internal lumen	Absorption of substances from the lumen
Kidneys	Glomerulus, tubular cells, and collecting duct	Blood levels of salts and water is regulated

Table 1.12 Key sites of water and solute exchange in body fluids

the kidney, water also crosses membranes via aquaporin channels (see page 152).

As discussed earlier (page 16), small, non-polar molecules diffuse freely across membranes, whereas polar and/or larger molecules require dedicated transmembrane protein channels (see page 18).

Passive diffusion versus active transport

Passive diffusion is the movement of a substance from an area of high concentration to an area of lower concentration by random molecular motion through plasma membranes or via carrier proteins. Active transport uses specific protein transporters [that form channels] to move a substance in an energy-dependent way, including against their concentration gradient.

Filtration pressures

Filtration pressures (**Figure 1.32**) are the forces that drive the movement of fluid across a semi-permeable membrane. Starling's forces (see page 18) are these pressures acting across a capillary membrane. They are most often used to describe the movement of fluid in/out of blood, but apply to any other body fluid. Filtration pressures include:

■ **Hydrostatic pressure**: this is the force exerted by a fluid on the walls of its container, for example the force of blood

against vessel walls. Blood pressure is measured as the hydrostatic pressure in the large arteries of the body. Hydrostatic pressure forces fluid out of the vasculature into the tissues (see page 86)
■ **Osmotic pressure**: this is the pressure at which water is drawn towards the more concentrated solution when an osmotic gradient exists between two fluids
■ **Oncotic pressure**: this is osmotic pressure relating to colloids in solution. In the circulation it is the osmotic pressure caused by plasma proteins, which are too large to leave the vasculature and therefore draw water into it. This is the main force that counterbalances hydrostatic pressure in controlling fluid movement in and out of the vasculature.

> **Albumin is a major plasma protein produced by the liver which contributes to the oncotic pressure of plasma.** In chronic liver disease, a decrease in plasma albumin causes water to leave blood vessels and collect in interstitial fluid causing peripheral oedema (leg swelling) and in the abdominal cavity causing ascites.

Fluid absorption from the external environment

The gastrointestinal tract is the main site for fluid intake from the external environment. Passive absorption of water occur secondary to active solute uptake.

As well as fluid movement in the GI tract, fluid is lost in the formation of urine; there is loss of fluid from the lungs (as exhaled water vapour) and through the skin (as sweat). There can be significant loss of salt as well as water in sweating.

Hypovolaemia is a lack of total or compartmental fluid volume and can be caused by:

■ insufficient intake
■ excess loss (bleeding, vomiting, diarrhoea, polyuria),
■ distributive losses, e.g. the opening of extra capillary beds during an inflammatory response

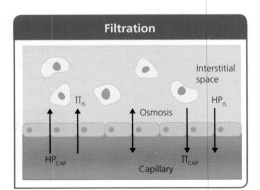

Figure 1.32 Filtration pressures. Π_{CAP} and Π_{IS} represent oncotic pressure in the capillary (CAP) and interstitial space (IS), respectively; HP_{CAP} and HP_{IS} represent hydrostatic pressure.

Hypervolaemia is caused by an excess of fluid intake relative to fluid loss, with or without pathology causing fluid retention (e.g. renal failure with an inability to excrete fluid).

Movement of fluid between body compartments

Fluid must move between body compartments in a regulated manner to keep the normal fluid composition of each area constant.

Lungs and blood

There is minimal movement of fluid between the lungs and blood, however it the main site for gaseous exchange therefore O_2 passes from alveoli to blood and CO_2 moves in the opposite direction.

Blood and interstitial fluid

Substances including ions, glucose, small lipids and water move by diffusion across capillary endothelial cells (and through the paracellular space between cells). This allows equilibration of the interstitial fluid with the blood. There is also bulk movement of fluid into the interstitial space at the arterial-end

of the capillary, where hydrostatic pressure exceeds oncotic pressure. At the venous end of the capillary hydrostatic pressure is lower, and plasma oncotic pressure causes reabsorption of interstitial fluid back into the vascular space.

Interstitial fluid and cells

As described above, the majority of movement of substances into cells is through a combination of transcellular passage (H_2O, CO_2), facilitated diffusion (Na^+, glucose), and active transport (K^+).

Interstitial fluid and lymph

Lymphatics are a system of vessels that uptake interstitial fluid, small proteins, large lipids, and immune cells from the tissue space and transport them back to the venous circulation, via lymph nodes. Uptake is passive by diffusion.

Regulation of the constituents of body fluid

The constituents of the different compartments are regulated by a variety of physiological processes (**Table 1.13**). Intracellular fluid

Regulation of constituents of body fluid		
Constituent	Membrane transport	Regulation
pH	Proton pumps	Ventilation rate and renal excretion (page 155)
Osmolality (mOsm/kg H_2O)	Various	Anti-diuretic hormone (page 151)
Na^+ (mmol/L)	Epithelial sodium channels, Na^+–H^+ exchange, Na^+/K^+ pump	Gastrointestinal uptake, renal losses, hormones (e.g. angiotensin) (page 152)
K^+ (mmol/L)	K^+-ATPase, K^+-H^+ exchange, Na^+/K^+ pump	Gastrointestinal uptake, renal losses, hormones (e.g. insulin) (page 143)
Cl^- (mmol/L)	Paracellular, Cl^-–HCO_3^- exchange, γ-Aminobutyric acid* channels	Gastrointestinal uptake, renal losses (page 144)
HCO_3^- (mmol/L)	Cl^-–HCO_3^- exchange, Na^+–HCO_3^- exchange	Gastrointestinal uptake, renal losses (page 155)
Ca^{2+} (mmol/L)	Na^+–Ca^{2+} exchange, Ca^{2+}-ATPase,	Bone turnover, gastrointestinal uptake, renal losses (page 180)
Glucose (mmol/L)	GLUT-2, GLUT-4 (glucose transporters)	Insulin, glucagon, adrenaline, cortisol, growth hormone (page 173)

*A neurotransmitter.

Table 1.13 Regulation of the constituents of body fluid

is more closely regulated than other compartments, in order to maintain an optimum environment for all intracellular biochemical reactions.

For example, regulation of potassium and pH are particularly essential for the function of every cell, especially the heart:

■ Potassium is controlled at the cellular level by the Na^+/K^+-ATPase and leak channels (see page 19).

■ Total body potassium is regulated by the renin–angiotensin–aldosterone system.
■ pH (see page 155) is controlled at the cellular level by a number of transporters.
■ Plasma pH is controlled through a complex interaction through the respiratory and renal systems; pH disturbance can occur due to abnormalities in many body systems.

Answers to starter questions

1. The central dogma describes how DNA controls life through the production of proteins, which then mediate all other bodily processes. The ability of DNA to be replicated and transmitted without error is crucial the to propagation of proteins, cells, tissues, and therefore organisms.

2. The nitrogenous base of DNA faces inwards and is bound to an opposing base by hydrogen bonds; therefore they aren't available to bind external protons, which is the main property of a base. However, the phosphate groups which form the phosphodiester bonds of the double helix's backbone are acidic because they release protons. These face outwards and interact with the surrounding environment.

3. Mitochondria are double-membrane bound organelles with their own DNA. They are capable of self-replication and producing energy, which would have allowed them to exist as separate organisms. Furthermore, their double membrane (the inner of which has prokaryotic features) suggests an origin as a prokaryote, phagocytosed by a eukaryote, and developing into a symbiotic relationship. By existing within our cells their substrate supply would be increased while human cells benefit from their ATP production. Over time some of their genes have migrated to the human cell nucleus meaning they are no longer capable of independent life.

4. Epithelial cells have different channels, receptors and transporters on their apical and basal membranes. This allows specialisation of two different parts of the cell's membrane, for example, an apical surface for absorption from a lumen, and a basal membrane for secretion into the bloodstream. Occluding junctions separate the two by forming a barrier, which prevents free movement of proteins from one part to the other.

5. Fish oil, e.g. cod liver oil, can act as an alternative substrate for cyclooxygenase enzymes. The molecules formed from this are similar to arachidonic acid prostanoids but have some key differences. For example, those derived from cod liver oil are stronger inhibitors of platelet aggregation; therefore they reduce the risk of heart attacks by lowering the risk of clots forming.

6. Organs are composed of many cell types: epithelial cells, vascular cells and cells of the extracellular matrix. Most adult stem cells can only differentiate into one (or two) cell types within one tissue. Therefore you would need a combination of different adult stem cells, with complex combination of multiple cell types, to produce a whole organ.

Chapter 2
Neuromuscular systems

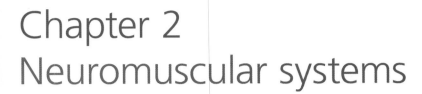

Starter questions

Answers to the following questions are on page 66.

1. How can an electrical impulse convey complex information about movements?
2. Can ions pass directly from one cell to another?
3. How do our muscles allow us to lift objects heavier than ourselves?
4. Why are some people 'born sprinters'?
5. Why do we sweat when we are nervous?

Introduction

Muscles are used in a huge range of conscious and unconscious processes, from body movement and interaction with the external environment to internal activity, such as propelling food through the gut or altering blood vessel diameter. Muscle function is largely driven by the nervous system, which provides control and feedback via reflexes.

> Nerves carrying information from the CNS, or relaying it onwards from the CNS via the PNS, are termed **efferent** (they have an effect). Nerves conveying information towards the CNS are termed **afferent**.

The nervous system comprises the central and peripheral nervous systems, the CNS and PNS (**Figure 2.1**). The PNS has two 'divisions':

■ The autonomic nervous system (ANS) regulates the body's internal environment and controls involuntary muscles, e.g. in the gut, as discussed in this chapter (see pages 62–64); it has two components, the sympathetic and parasympathetic nervous systems

■ The somatic nervous system directs movement (somatic motor function, controlling voluntary muscles, see page 40) and receives sensory information; this sensory input to the CNS (via the PNS) is covered in chapter 8

The ANS itself has two divisions, the sympathetic and parasympathetic nervous systems (PNS and SNS).

This chapter focuses on the physiology of the peripheral nervous system. However, the general principles of neurophysiology – neuronal physiology, activity at synapses, and reflexes, etc. – also apply to the physiology of the central nervous system (see Chapter 8) and enteric nervous system (see Chapter 7).

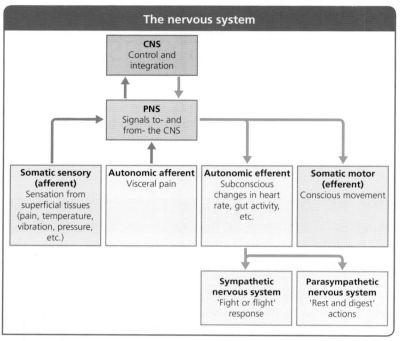

Figure 2.1 The central nervous system (CNS, the brain and spinal cord) controls the remainder of the body via the peripheral nervous system (PNS). The somatic motor (efferent) and sensory (afferent) nerves control voluntary action, whilst the autonomic nervous system is subconscious.

Case 1 Two days of leg weakness

Presentation

John, a 47-year-old plumber, presents complaining of 2 days of leg weakness. Apart from a cold 10 days ago, he has otherwise been fit and well and has no history of neurological disease. He is finding it difficult to climb stairs or stand from a seated position. He has no family history of note. On examination, John has markedly reduced lower-limb tone and power bilaterally, with absent reflexes at the ankle and knee. He has reduced sensation to all modalities (pain, soft touch, temperature, and vibration) over his legs.

Analysis

John has presented with a bilateral mixed motor–sensory neuropathy without prior neurological disease. The onset has been rapid and has a history of a recent viral upper respiratory tract infection. In addition, his neuropathy shows lower motor neurone (LMN) signs on examination: absent reflexes and reduced tone. This combination of features is suggestive of Guillain–Barré syndrome, a post-infectious peripheral demyelinating neuropathy. Guillain–Barré often occurs following a gastrointestinal or genitourinary infections.

Case 1 *continued*

Guillain-Barré syndrome: diagnosis

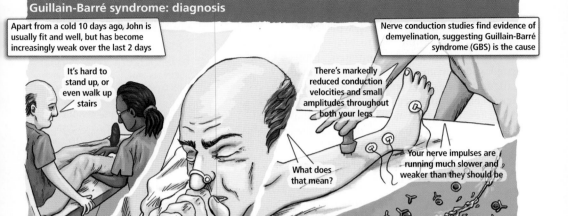

Apart from a cold 10 days ago, John is usually fit and well, but has become increasingly weak over the last 2 days

Nerve conduction studies find evidence of demyelination, suggesting Guillain-Barré syndrome (GBS) is the cause

It's hard to stand up, or even walk up stairs

There's markedly reduced conduction velocities and small amplitudes throughout both your legs

What does that mean?

Your nerve impulses are running much slower and weaker than they should be

Myelin sheath

Antibody-mediated attack

I'm afraid the condition is starting to affect your breathing. We need to treat you quickly, and you may need help with your breathing

Neuromuscular junction

John's leg weakness is ascending and is now limiting his ventilation. His FEV$_1$ is monitored; if it deteriorates further he may require mechanical ventilation

GBS is a post-infectious autoimmune disease that usually presents with acute or subacute onset limb weakness after an infection. It is a potentially fatal medical emergency

Had there been a family history of a hereditary sensory–motor neuropathy this might have been considered but a slower onset would have been expected. There are also many toxins and poisons that can cause peripheral neuropathies, which should also be considered.

Further case

John is referred to the neurologist at the local hospital but begins to deteriorate. He starts to find it difficult to walk and tests demonstrate loss of expiratory capacity. Nerve conduction studies show slowed conduction velocities with small amplitudes.

He is treated with steroids and immunoglobulin; over a few days he starts to show signs of recovery. Over the next week he regains all his strength and he does not suffer any further episodes.

Further analysis

Guillain–Barré syndrome is a progressive, ascending neuropathy and John displays the typical pattern of disease. Symptoms begin in the lower limbs but ascend to affect the upper limbs, cranial nerves and respiratory function. Functional vital capacity is measured to monitor respiratory function and some patients require ventilation to support their breathing.

Guillain–Barré syndrome is an autoimmune condition directed against the myelin within Schwann cells. Nerve conduction studies show evidence of slowed conduction and smaller potentials due to the absence of myelin.

Treatment is with steroids, to reduce the autoimmune inflammatory activity, and immunoglobulin, to bind and remove pathogenic antibodies. Most patients make a full recovery and do not suffer further episodes.

Neurones and action potentials

All information in the nervous system is carried by electrical impulses, which function in a similar manner to Morse code. Electrical impulses are initiated, propagated and transmitting by specialised cells called neurones (**Figure 2.2**). A neurone, or nerve cell, comprises a cell body, axons and dendrites that end in synaptic terminals (synaptic bouton); the functions of these components are described in **Table 2.1**.

Action potentials

Electrical impulses are transmitted as action potentials. An action potential is a wave of depolarisation of a cell membrane (loss of its normal electrical potential) that spreads along the membrane in one direction. Action potentials obey certain principles:

- They are 'all-or-nothing' events (there is no such thing as a large or small action potential)
- They propagate without decay (they do not decline with distance)
- They are governed by the ion permeabilities (or conductances) of membranes
- There is a step-wise sequence of events, as shown in **Figure 2.3** and described below.

Functional microanatomy of neurones		
Structure	Composition	Function
Cell body (perikaryon)	Contains nucleus, ribosomes and mitochondria	Protein production, energy generation and neurotransmitter synthesis
Axon	Extends away from cell body without changing diameter; divides into ≥ 2 parts in some neurones	Transmits action potentials
Dendrites	Extend away from cell body, reducing in diameter as they divide	Collect incoming stimuli from other neurones; often the location of initiation of an action potential
Synaptic terminals	Contain mitochondria, neurotransmitter secretory granules and calcium channels	Release neurotransmitters to spread excitation to other cells

Table 2.1 Features common to all neurones and their function

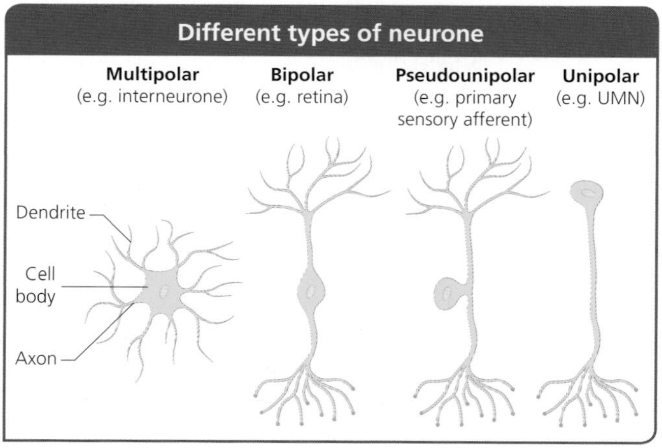

Different types of neurone			
Multipolar (e.g. interneurone)	Bipolar (e.g. retina)	Pseudounipolar (e.g. primary sensory afferent)	Unipolar (e.g. UMN)

Dendrite

Cell body

Axon

Figure 2.2 Each type of neurone has a nucleus in a cell body and axonic and dendritic projections. The number of axons determines whether a neurone is multipolar, bipolar, pseudounipolar, or unipolar.

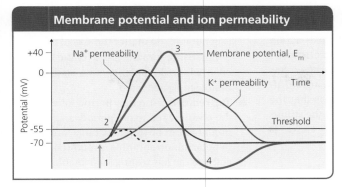

Membrane potential and ion permeability

Figure 2.3 Changes in membrane potential and ion permeability during an action potential (not to scale). Sodium permeability rises and falls sharply whereas potassium permeability rises late and is more sustained. A stimulus that has failed to pass threshold is illustrated by the dotted line.

Resting membrane potential

The plasma membrane of the neurone has a resting potential (E_m) of approximately –70 mV (see page 16). Although membrane potential is determined by the cell's permeability to many ions, by far the major contributor is the high intracellular concentration and high membrane permeability to K^+. Membrane permeability is determined by the presence of 'leak' channels. These are membrane transporters that allow passive movement (facilitated diffusion) of ions (e.g. K^+) through a membrane. The more leak channels a membrane has for a specific ion, the more permeable a membrane is to that ion. The combination of a high intracellular concentration of K^+ with high membrane permeability allows potassium movement out of cells (efflux), against the action of the Na^+/K^+-ATPase pump (see page 19). As a positive ion (cation) leaves the interior of the cell, membrane potential is negative relative to its exterior.

In contrast with K^+, the intracellular Na^+ concentration is low and resting membrane permeability to Na^+ is relatively low (i.e. there are few leak channels). The balance of concentrations and permeabilities for Na^+ and K^+ determine the resting E_m of –70 mV in neurones.

Depolarisation and hyperpolarisation

When a membrane becomes more positive (e.g. -30 mV) it is referred to as depolarisation. Whereas, hyperpolarisation is when a membrane becomes more negatively charged (e.g. -90 mV).

Initiation

To begin the membrane depolarisation that leads to an action potential, a stimulus is required ('1' on **Figure 2.3**). The type of stimulus varies, but most commonly it is

- Another action potential arriving from further along the cell or
- The opening of ion channels in response to an external stimulus (e.g. from another nerve cell).

Unlike action potentials, stimuli are graded in size, i.e. some cause large and some cause small changes in E_m, and they do decay.

Threshold

Neurones have a 'threshold': a membrane potential above which they spontaneously depolarise further or 'fire', leading to an action potential that propagates along the entire length of the cell. Once depolarisation caused by a stimulus reaches this threshold ('2' on **Figure 2.3**), neighbouring voltage-gated Na^+ channels open. This raising the membrane's permeability to sodium and Na^+ ions enter the cell carrying positive charge. This further depolarises the cell and activates adjacent Na^+ channels, which in turn activate their adjacent channels and so on, which causes rapid depolarisation of the membrane until it reaches around +40 mV. It is the existence of the threshold and propagation without diminishing which gives action potentials their all-or-none characteristic.

If the threshold is not reached, then a few Na^+ channels may open, but not enough to affect adjacent channels. The result is that the depolarisation originally caused by the stimulus decays back towards resting E_m as Na^+ is pumped back out of the cell.

Repolarisation

Voltage-gated K^+ channels are activated by depolarisation at the same time as Na^+ channels. However, K^+ channels are slower to open, and so K^+ permeability rises towards the end of the depolarisation spike ('3' on **Figure 2.3**). The faster Na^+ channels close soon after opening, therefore the net ion movement results in a shift towards cation efflux. Thus E_m reaches a peak then becomes more negative again, repolarising the membrane. The K^+ channels are slow to close, so K^+ efflux continues past resting membrane potential to give an E_m of less than −70 mV known as 'overshoot' or 'after-hyperpolarisation' ('4' on **Figure 2.3**).

Refractory period

The refractory period is the time after an action potential when a stimulus that would usually pass threshold is unable to trigger a further action potential:

- **The absolute refractory period** is the early stage in which no action potential is generated, no matter the size of the depolarising stimulus; most of the fast Na^+ channels are in their 'inactive' state so are unable to be activated
- **The relative refractory period** follows the absolute refractory period: an action potential can be initiated, but a larger depolarisation stimulus is required to activate the few resting (activatable) Na^+ channels and overcome after-hyperpolarisation. Most Na^+ channels remain refractory (not activatable).

Propagation

Because cells are filled with a conducting solution, in effect salty water, the transmembrane voltage change caused by the action potential spreads electrically to neighbouring parts of the cell, depolarising them in turn. This allows the action potential to travel along the surface of the nerve cell.

Non-myelinated neurones

Depolarisation spreads to all adjacent areas of the neuronal membrane, but membrane that has just conveyed an action potential will be in the absolute refractory period, which prevents movement backwards (**Figure 2.4**). Therefore an action potential propagates in only one direction of travel and spreads progressively along the nerve.

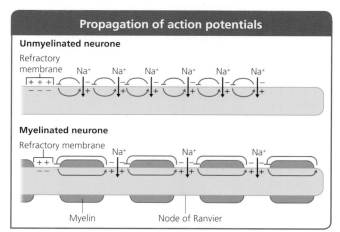

Propagation of action potentials

Unmyelinated neurone

Refractory membrane

Na^+ Na^+ Na^+ Na^+ Na^+ Na^+

Myelinated neurone

Refractory membrane

Na^+ Na^+ Na^+

Myelin   Node of Ranvier

Figure 2.4 Action potential propagation in unmyelinated and myelinated neurones. Adjacent membrane is depolarised but the AP cannot travel backwards because those areas of the membrane are in the refractory period. This process occurs only at nodes of Ranvier in a myelinated neurone.

Myelinated neurones

Some axons are wrapped in myelin sheath (a phospholipid), which is produced by Schwann cells in the peripheral nervous system and oligodendrocytes in the central nervous system. This forms an insulated area of membrane where transmembrane movement of ions cannot occur. There are segments of unmyelinated membrane between areas of myelin. These are the nodes of Ranvier and are the only place where ion movement and hence depolarisation occurs.

In an action potential the electrical current flowing through the cell from one node of Ranvier depolarises the next, causing it to reach threshold and trigger the action potential afresh. Thus the action potential jumps between nodes. This is termed saltatory conduction. Since the electrical current within the neurone travels much faster than the progressive membrane depolarisation along unmyelinated neurones, this greatly increases the speed of transmission (**Figure 2.4**).

Factors influencing speed

The factors increasing the speed of transmission of action potentials are:

- Myelination (see above and **Table 2.2**)
- Larger diameter, which leads to a lower electrical resistance, therefore less loss of current

Larger diameter also allows an action potential to can propagate between more widely spaced nodes of Ranvier.

Processing of information: coding

Action potentials and synapses do not convey information by themselves; it must be coded and integrated to give meaning.

Each neurone conveys a certain modality of afferent (inward, i.e. towards the brain) or efferent (outward, i.e. from the brain) information, known as the 'line code'. For example,

Types of nerve fibre and transmission speeds

Fibre type	Structure	Function	Speed
A-α	Large and thick myelin	A-α sensory fibres (1a and 1b sensory fibres): proprioception Efferent: motor fibres	Fastest
A-β	Medium and thick myelin	Afferent: proprioception and sensation Efferent: muscle spindles	Fast
A-γ	Medium and thick myelin	Efferent: muscle spindles	Fast
A-δ	Medium and thin myelin	Afferent: sensation and pain	Medium
C	Small and unmyelinated	Afferent: pain	Slowest

Table 2.2 Examples of types of neurones (and their axons) categorised by their speed of transmission

one afferent neurone might only transmit information regarding proprioception (i.e. position of the body and movements).

Each action potential is of equal intensity, therefore to code for magnitude the frequency of action potential is altered: a higher frequency codes for higher stimulus intensity.

Demyelination is loss of myelin from neurons resulting in markedly reduced transmission speeds in affected nerves. Multiple sclerosis is a demyelination disorder in which symptoms depend on the location of demyelination; in the central nervous system it causes stroke-like features with weakness and numbness.

Synapses

A synapse is a connection or communication between two cells. There are two different kinds of synapses:

- **Chemical**, between two neurones or between a motor neurone and muscle fibre: a neurotransmitter is released from one neurone, which binds to receptors on the membrane of the next one and results in a change in this membrane's potential
- **Electrical**: these are gap junctions, channels which link two cells and allow the passage of ions between them, carrying a current (**Figure 2.5**); they are rare between neurones but are important in allowing the spread of depolarisation across several myocytes (muscle cells), facilitating the spread of waves of contraction in cardiac muscle and in smooth muscle (e.g. in the gastrointestinal tract)

Sequence of events at a chemical synapse

The events that take place at a chemical synapse are summarised in **Figure 2.6**.

Initiation

Transmission at a synapse begins with an action potential arriving at the pre-synaptic neurone's synaptic bouton. The depolarisation spreads into the synaptic terminal and activates voltage-gated Ca^{2+} channels ('1' on **Figure 2.6**).

Neurotransmitter is stored in secretory vesicles (or 'granules') in the presynaptic terminal. As Ca^{2+} floods into the cell, it causes the vesicles to fuse with the presynaptic membrane, releasing neurotransmitter into the

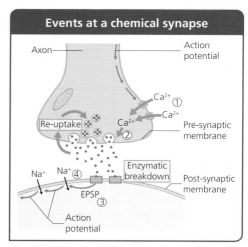

Figure 2.6 At a chemical synapse voltage-gated calcium channels are activated by the arriving action potential ①. Calcium causes fusion of neurotransmitter-containing synaptic vesicles with the pre-synaptic membrane ②. After binding a receptor on the post-synaptic membrane an excitatory post-synaptic potential (EPSP) ③ stimulates an action potential if threshold is passed ④.

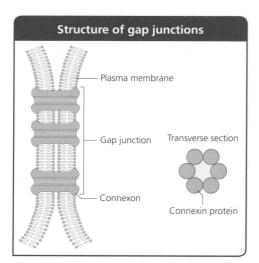

Figure 2.5 Gap junctions are small pores linking the cytoplasm of two adjacent cells and is composed of 6 connexin proteins linked together in a format called that make one channel, a connexon.

synaptic cleft, the space between two neurones or between a neurone and a muscle cell ('2' on **Figure 2.6**).

Post-synaptic activation

Neurotransmitter diffuses across the synaptic cleft and binds to specific receptors on the post-synaptic membrane. The post-synaptic response is dependent upon both the neurotransmitter and the receptor. The neurotransmitter causes a change in membrane potential either by opening ion channels directly or by activation of an intracellular signalling cascade ('3' on **Figure 2.6**). The mechanism by which the neurotransmitter functions is determined by the transmitter (e.g. GABA, glutamate, substance P) and the receptor (e.g. NMDA-receptor, AMPA-receptor, NK-1-receptor).

Excitatory and inhibitory potentials

A change in post-synaptic membrane potential is not the same as an action potential: it is transient and decays. An excitatory post-synaptic potential (EPSP) causes depolarisation, whilst an inhibitory post-synaptic potential (IPSP) causes hyperpolarisation. An action potential will only fire in the post-synaptic cell only if its threshold depolarisation is reached ('4' on **Figure 2.6**).

Termination

Several mechanisms contribute to the termination of the synaptic transmission:

- Spontaneous dissociation of the receptor–neurotransmitter bond
- Enzymatic breakdown of the neurotransmitter in the cleft, e.g. acetylcholinesterase destroys the neurotransmitter acetylcholine

- Re-uptake of the neurotransmitter into the pre-synaptic terminal, followed by re-packaging into secretory vesicles
- Uptake into the post-synaptic terminal, followed by enzymatic breakdown

Integration of synapses

Many individual neurones receive synaptic input from multiple neurones, each generating an EPSP or an IPSP. The probability of generating an action potential in the output neurone is dependent on summation of the synaptic inputs (**Figure 2.7**). The same principle applies to initiation of an action potential through other graded stimuli; for example, activation of both a temperature receptor and a pressure receptor in activating a sensory neurone in the skin that signals pain.

A 56-year-old woman is referred to the neurology clinic with fatigue and weakness. She has bilateral symmetrical weakness that is worst towards the end of the day.

Myasthenia gravis is an autoimmune condition caused by antibodies that block nicotinic acetylcholine receptors at the neuromuscular junction (NMJ), impairing acetylcholine binding and muscular contraction. Treatment with acetylcholinesterase inhibitors, which prevent acetylcholine breakdown in the synaptic cleft increases the concentration of acetylcholine which competes with the autoantibodies and increases the effect at the remaining receptors.

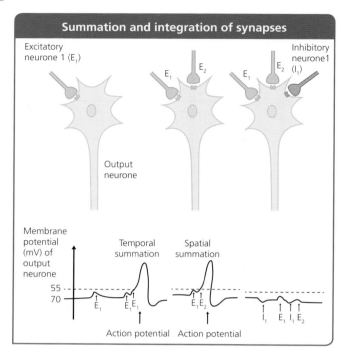

Summation and integration of synapses

Excitatory neurone 1 (E_1)

Inhibitory neurone1 (I_1)

Output neurone

Membrane potential (mV) of output neurone

Temporal summation

Spatial summation

55
70

E_1 $E_1 E_1$ $E_1 E_2$ I_1 E_1 I_1 E_2

Action potential   Action potential

Figure 2.7 Summation and integration of synapses. In (a) two excitatory post-synaptic potentials (EPSPs) occurring in quick succession from the same neurone together cause threshold to be passed. In contrast, in (b) two simultaneous EPSP are enough to reach threshold. If an inhibitory post-synaptic potential is also stimulated (c) then this may summate to prevent an action potential.

Motor control

Motor control refers to the way that movements are generated. Beginning in the central nervous system (CNS), signals pass through peripheral nerves and result in skeletal muscle contraction to produce an effect.

There are always two neurones in a motor pathway: an upper and lower motor neurone (UMN and LMN). The upper neurone originates in the CNS and synapses with a LMN that terminates on a group of muscle fibres where it causes contraction. Such a group, innervated by a single LMN, is called a motor unit.

Pathways

A pathway is the term given to the route taken by a group of neurones with similar function. An example is the descending pathways from the brain down the spinal cord, before individual groups of neurones split off to supply their individual muscles.

Cerebral cortex

The cerebral cortex is the site of the primary motor cortex, which is located on the pre-central gyrus in the frontal lobe of the brain. The primary motor cortex is the region that initiates voluntary movements and serves as the origin of the main descending motor pathways. However, many other brain areas modify its activity. For example, there are supplementary and accessory motor areas in the frontal lobe that are involved in the planning and sequencing of movement. These connect with the pre-central gyrus and provide input affecting its descending output to the muscles.

Lesions to the CNS, such as strokes, tend to cause contralateral deficits as the part of the primary motor cortex that controls the left side of the body lies on the right side of the brain, and vice versa. A right-sided cerebral infarction therefore causes left-sided weakness.

Somatotopic mapping

This describes a spatial correlation of areas in the CNS with specific regions of the body. For example, the lateral part of the primary motor cortex controls the face, whereas the medial part controls the legs. This principle of a spatial mapping holds true throughout almost all of the CNS, including the spinal cord.

A drawing representing this mapping is called a homunculus, which is a distorted view of the body in which the size of the body region is related to the size of area of CNS attributed to it. For example, a larger area is devoted to control of hand movements than to those of the leg. The motor homunculus and somatotopic mapping are shown in **Figure 2.8**.

Association areas in the CNS

In addition to cortical areas, there are other regions that play an important part in modifying movements. The basal ganglia are nuclei (collections of neuronal cell bodies within the CNS) lying deep in the cortex, which are important for the timing and initiation of movement. They control the amount of motor activity through connections with the cerebral cortex.

The cerebellum has several roles in relation to movement. It is vital for postural control and balance by giving output to axial muscles. It also plays important roles in co-ordination of complex movements and for motor learning.

Feedback

Throughout the motor system feedback signals help to ensure accurate, smooth movements. Sensory organs (collections of cells providing specific sensory information, e.g. Golgi tendon organ, muscle spindles) in muscles, joints and tendons convey proprioceptive information – information on what position the body is in and how it has moved. This information passes via a reflex arc (a rapid, repeatable connection between two or more neurones, where a specific input always gives the same specific output) to influence muscle contraction. These processes occur continuously and may be obvious (e.g. tendon jerk reflex) or more subtle, such as head control (e.g. movement of the head towards a loud sound).

Corticospinal tract

The corticospinal tract (or pathway) is the main descending motor pathway and is illustrated in **Figure 2.9**. It is particularly important for control of fine, flexor movements of the peripheries. It originates in the primary motor cortex, where the cell body of the UMN is located. The UMN axon passes down to the brainstem, where 80% of the fibres decussate – i.e. cross over to the opposite side of the body – in the pyramids of the medulla:

- **the lateral corticospinal tract** comprises the fibres that decussate in the spinal cord.
- **the ventral corticospinal tract** comprises the fibres that remain ipsilateral as they descend; these decussate at the level where they synapse.

The UMN synapses with the LMN in the ventral horn of the spinal cord (**Figure 2.9**).

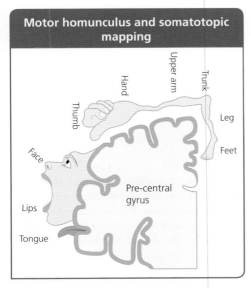

Motor homunculus and somatotopic mapping

Hand · Upper arm · Trunk · Thumb · Leg · Face · Feet · Lips · Pre-central gyrus · Tongue

Figure 2.8 Each part of the pre-central gyrus is responsible for movement of one part of the body: this is somatotopic mapping. The size of the area is related to the level of control required, shown by the motor homunculus. (This is a sagittal hemisection of the brain i.e. looking from the back of the head forwards.).

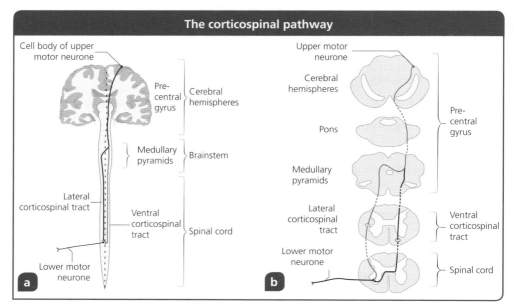

Figure 2.9 The corticospinal pathway: simplified (a) and classic (b) depictions. The cell body of the upper motor neurone lies in the pre-central gyrus; 80% of these neurones decussate (cross the midline) in the medulla to form the lateral corticospinal tract. The remaining 20% decussate at the level of the lower motor neurone and synapse in the ventral horn of the spinal cord.

LMNs exits the spinal canal via the anterior (ventral) ramus or branch of the cord and pass to the peripheral muscles.

There are many other motor pathways that have different anatomy and functions, for example the rubrospinal pathway and tectospinal pathway. In general, they act on the cell bodies of LMN to modify the effects of UMN activity.

> **Fasciculation is a visible spontaneous contraction seen in denervated muscle,** caused by passive acetylcholine release from injured neurones. **Fibrillation is** spontaneous membrane depolarisation from increased sensitivity seen on electromyography.

Spinal cord

Structure and function

The spinal cord is considered to be an extension of the brainstem because of its ability to integrate afferent signals and produce a coordinated output.

The cord is composed of grey and white matter. Grey matter is the location of neuronal cell bodies and many interneurones (the neurones that connect an input (afferent) and output (efferent) neurone). White matter contains the myelinated axons in the tracts, as shown in **Figure 2.10**.

Blood supply

Three arteries supply the spinal cord. One anterior spinal artery provides blood to the anterior two-thirds of the cord, in particular the ventral horns. Two posterior spinal arteries supply the dorsal horns and posterior columns (sensory pathways conveying proprioception and vibration, which lie medial to the dorsal horns).

Ventral horn

The ventral horn is the location of the cell bodies of lower motor neurones. It also

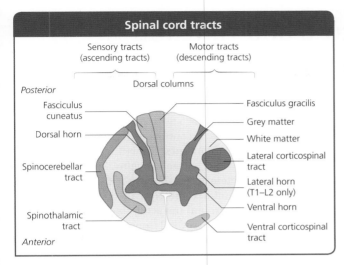

Spinal cord tracts

Sensory tracts
(ascending tracts)

Motor tracts
(descending tracts)

Dorsal columns

Posterior

Fasciculus
cuneatus

Dorsal horn

Spinocerebellar
tract

Spinothalamic
tract

Anterior

Fasciculus gracilis

Grey matter

White matter

Lateral corticospinal
tract

Lateral horn
(T1–L2 only)

Ventral horn

Ventral corticospinal
tract

Figure 2.10 All tracts in the spinal cord are bilateral, but for simplicity the main motor tracts are shown here on one side and the main sensory tracts on the other.

demonstrates somatotopic mapping: the medial part is concerned with axial and proximal muscles whilst the lateral part is concerned with distal muscles. The dorsal part of the ventral horn controls extensor muscles, while the ventral part of the ventral horn controls flexors.

Pattern generators

Central pattern generators are areas in the spinal cord and brainstem where complex motor functions can be controlled without conscious influence, for example locomotion. Higher centres (i.e. more complex parts of the CNS, e.g. cerebral cortex) are involved in initiation of walking but central pattern generators control its perpetuation. Neuronal networks in the spinal cord integrate proprioceptive and stretch receptor (e.g. muscle spindles, see page 58) inputs to influence the output. For example, increasing stride length with one leg whilst walking can be detected, which then causes a match in stride length by the other leg. This is one case of a complex cross-side reflex that can be modulated by sensory input.

Upper and lower motor neurone lesions can be differentiated by their clinical signs (Table 2.3). An UMN lesion increases activity in the LMN within its distribution, causing increased muscle tone and brisk reflexes. LMN lesions present with decreased tone, absent tone and muscle wasting.

Comparison of motor neurone lesions

	UMN lesion	LMN lesion
Power	Reduced (weakness)	Reduced (weakness)
Tone	Increased	Reduced
Reflexes	Exaggerated	Reduced or absent
Babinski response	Up-going	Down-going
Muscle bulk	Normal (except in disuse atrophy)	Reduced (wasting)
Fasciculations	Not present	Visible
Fibrillations	Not present	Seen on electromyography

Table 2.3 Features of an upper motor neurone (UMN) or lower motor neurone (LMN) lesions

Muscle structure and function

There are three types of muscle (**Table 2.4**):

- Skeletal
- Smooth and
- Cardiac

Skeletal muscle and cardiac muscle are both striated muscle, having a striped histological appearance that reflects their microstructure (see below). Smooth muscle lacks striation. The function of muscle is to contract, causing shortening. The degree of contraction of a muscle at rest is termed the tone.

Skeletal muscle

Structure

Skeletal muscle is made up of long fibres called myofibres (**Table 2.5**), which are myocytes. A myocyte is a syncytium of muscle cells, i.e. several cells' cytoplasm and organelles are contained within a single plasma membrane and the resulting syncytial cell is multinucleate.

Most of the volume of the myofibre is taken up by bundles of myofilaments. These are the contractile units and are arranged parallel to each other within the myofibre.

Myofilaments

Myofibril comprises a number of thick and thin myofilaments, and it is the movement of these filaments past each other that causes muscle to shorten, i.e. contract (see below). This process is driven by cyclic shape changes in the myosin molecules of the thick filaments, which hydrolyse ATP to release energy for muscle contraction (see **Figure 2.14**).

Thin filaments Each thin filament is composed of several proteins. Actin, a long thin protein, forms the core of the filament. A thin strand-like protein called tropomyosin spirals around the actin core (see **Figure 2.14**). There are several troponin proteins (C, T and I) that bind to tropomyosin and to actin.

Structure of skeletal muscle	
Structure	Definition
Muscle	Composed of multiple fascicles separated by loose connective tissue
Muscle fasciculus	A group of myofibres acting together
Myofibre	A syncytium of myocytes.
Myocyte	Skeletal muscle cells containing many myofibrils
Myofibril	A long group of myofilaments divided into sarcomeres
Myofilament	Any contractile filament (thick or thin)

Table 2.5 The structural organisation of skeletal muscle, from macro- to microscopic

Types of muscle		
Muscle type	Structural features	Functional features
Skeletal	Inserts into bone via tendons Long myocytes with multiple nuclei Contractile filaments arranged in fixed position (giving striations)	Voluntary contraction to produce movement
Smooth	Single cells linked via gap junctions No striations Contractile filaments insert into dense bodies	Involuntary contraction in gut and blood vessels Highly influenced by autonomic and metabolic stimuli Spread of contraction through tissue
Cardiac	Long striated myocytes but with branching and fused plasma membranes Intercalated discs between cells containing gap junctions	No anaerobic metabolism Rhythmical contraction with spread throughout the tissue

Table 2.4 Differences and similarities between the three types of muscle

Thick filaments These are made almost entirely of the protein myosin. This forms a thick strand with bulbous projection, called myosin heads (see **Figure 2.14**). The heads connect to the strand via a hinge region that makes possible a change in angle of the myosin head with respect to the strand. The angle of this hinge and the affinity of the heads for actin depend on whether ADP + Pi (phosphate), or ATP is bound to the myosin (see page 56).

Sarcomeres

Thick and thin filaments are organised parallel to each other in a systematic fashion. The fundamental unit of this organisation is the sarcomere (**Figure 2.11**). Within the sarcomere there is overlap of the thick and thin filaments. It is the facility to decrease and increase the amount of overlap that allows muscle to contract and relax. A degree of overlap exists even when the muscle is not contracted, which is what gives muscle its striated appearance.

A sarcomere is the distance between two Z-lines, which are the site of attachment for thin filaments to the sarcolemma. The regions in a sarcomere and their functional relationships are:

- **Z-line**: insertion of thin filaments into the sarcolemma
- **I-band**: a section either side of the Z-line that contains only thin filaments. During

contraction, the I-band shortens and the Z-lines are pulled together
- **M-line**: centre of sarcomere where thick filaments insert into the sarcolemma
- **A-band**: the region of thick filaments either side of the M-line
- **H-band**: the central region of the A-band, in which there are no thin filaments. This gets smaller during contraction, as thin filaments move in between the thick filaments

Myocyte specialisations

Myocytes have a number of unique features. Their multiple nuclei are at their periphery, allowing maximum room for myofibrils. Between the myofibrils in their cytosol there is a complex web of sarcoplasmic reticulum for storing and releasing Ca^{2+} into the cytosol and there are numerous mitochondria to supply the energy needed for muscle contraction. The sarcoplasmic reticulum contains high concentrations of Ca^{2+} due to active calcium uptake by the SERCA – sarco-/endo-plasmic reticulum Ca^{2+} ATPase) pump. The high sarcoplasmic reticulum Ca^{2+} concentration is needed for excitation-contraction coupling (see below).

The myocyte cell membrane, the sarcolemma, is able to convey an action potential in the same way as a neurone, and it has invaginations called T-tubules, which can carry this

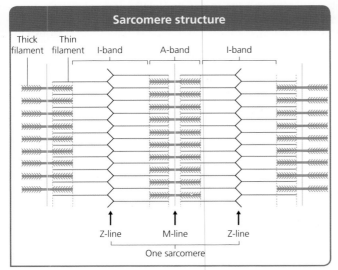

Figure 2.11 Within the sarcomere, thick and thin fibres interdigitate. They are shown in the relaxed state here, i.e. with minimal overlap. During contraction the I-band shortens as myofilaments pull past each other.

action potential deep into the cell. At T-tubules the sarcolemma comes into close proximity with the sarcoplasmic reticulum and influx of Ca^{2+} from the extracellular medium through voltage-gated channels induces additional Ca^{2+} release from the sarcoplasmic reticulum into the cytosol, triggering contraction.

The neuromuscular junction

The neuromuscular junction (**Figure 2.12**) is the synapse between a lower motor neurone and a muscle fibre. In principle it functions the same as any other chemical synapse, with some additional specialisations.

> **Hypocalcaemia (low serum Ca^{2+}) causes a shift in the electrochemical gradient across cell membranes,** increasing the propensity for spontaneous depolarisation and shortening the refractory period causing spontaneous muscle contraction. This is demonstrated clinically in Chvostek's sign in which tapping over the facial nerve causes contraction of the facial muscles.

Activation of voltage-gated Ca^{2+} channels in the pre-presynaptic terminal of the lower motor neurone causes Ca^{2+} entry [1] that stimulates exocytosis of vesicles containing acetylcholine (ACh) [2]. Acetylcholine diffuses across the synaptic cleft [3] and binds nicotinic acetylcholine receptors (NAChRs) on the motor end plate [4], a specialised area of sarcolemma with a high density of NAChRs. When acetylcholine binds, NAChRs function as cation channels increasing permeability to Na^+ and K^+ [5].

Sodium entry causes depolarisation and generates the end-plate potential, a form of excitatory post-synaptic potential but with a larger amplitude. The end-plate potential causes activation of voltage-gated Na^+ channels that then propagate an action potential along the full length of the myocyte [6].

> **Muscle relaxants** are used to cause flaccid paralysis during anaesthesia. They all bind and block NAChR on the motor end plate.
>
> They are divided into two groups:
>
> - depolarising (e.g. suxamethonium), initially causing activation of NAChR and initial muscle twitching prior to paralysis
>
> - non-depolarising (e.g. rocuronium), true antagonists at NAChR which work more slowly but without initial twitching

Figure 2.12 Events at the neuromuscular junction.

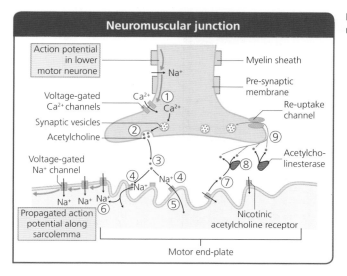

Acetylcholine esterase

The binding of acetylcholine to NACh receptors is transient; it then dissociates [7], with potential to re-bind. Once it has dissociated back into the synaptic cleft, acetylcholine is cleaved by acetylcholine esterase (AChE), an enzyme present in the cleft [8]. The cleavage products are acetate and choline, which undergo re-uptake into the pre-synaptic terminal for recycling [9].

Excitation–contraction coupling

Excitation–contraction coupling is the process that turns the arrival of an action potential into a muscle contraction.

The action potential spreads along the sarcolemma (away from the motor end plate) and passes down T-tubules. In these areas there are voltage-gated Ca^{2+} channels of the dihydropyridine type. These channels are physically associated with ryanodine receptors that sit on the membrane of the sarcoplasmic reticulum (**Figure 2.13**). Activation of the dihydropyridine receptors (that also function as Ca^{2+} channels), and the consequent influx of Ca^{2+} from outside the cell, causes a conformational change in ryanodine receptors that allows Ca^{2+} to exit from the sarcoplasmic reticulum. The result is a rapid rise in cytosolic calcium concentration, which activates the contractile mechanisms.

> **Hypokalaemia (low serum potassium)** affects the electrochemical gradient across the membrane of all excitable tissues. Clinical symptoms may not be evident but in significant hypokalaemia, cardiac arrhythmias, marked muscle weakness and constipation occur.

Mechanism of contraction

Sliding filament hypothesis

The sliding filament hypothesis describes how thick and thin myofilaments interact to cause sarcomere shortening, which results in muscle contraction (**Figure 2.14**):

1. Ca^{2+} binds troponin C, which causes movement in troponin I and then in troponin T, which is bound to tropomyosin.
2. Tropomyosin moves, revealing the myosin-binding sites on actin.
3. The myosin heads bind to actin – this is known as cross-bridge formation. Hydrolysed ATP is present on myosin heads at this stage, as ADP plus phosphate (P_i).
4. P_i is lost from myosin, which causes a change in the hinge region of myosin. The myosin heads pull actin past, increasing filament overlap and shortening the I-band.
5. ADP is then lost and fresh ATP binds to the myosin heads, which allows cross-bridges to break.
6. ATP is hydrolysed to ADP + P_i on myosin – this causes a change in the hinge region to revert back to the starting position, ready to form cross-bridges again.

Steps 3–6 continue in a cycle whilst intracellular Ca^{2+} concentration is high.

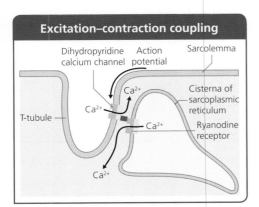

Excitation–contraction coupling

Dihydropyridine calcium channel — Action potential — Sarcolemma

Ca^{2+}

Ca^{2+}

T-tubule

Ca^{2+}

Ca^{2+}

Cisterna of sarcoplasmic reticulum

Ryanodine receptor

Figure 2.13 Excitation–contraction coupling. As the action potential passes along the membrane it activates dihydropyridine (DHP) calcium channels, which allows calcium entry into the myocyte. The DHP channels are connected to ryanodine receptors that open to let calcium out of the sarcoplasmic reticulum.

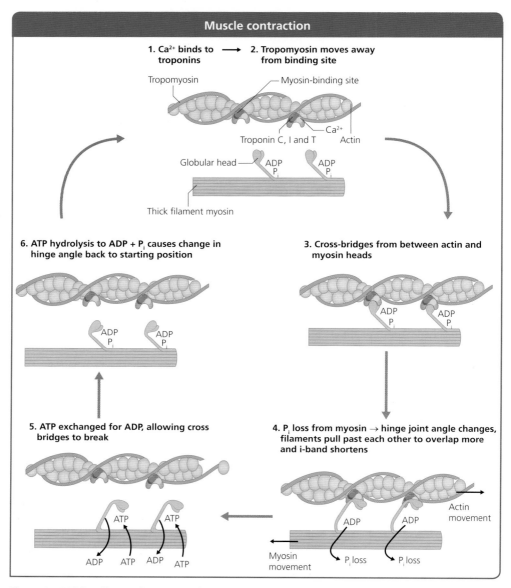

Muscle contraction

1. Ca²⁺ binds to troponins ⟶ 2. Tropomyosin moves away from binding site

Tropomyosin

Myosin-binding site

Ca²⁺

Troponin C, I and T   Actin

Globular head — ADP Pᵢ   ADP Pᵢ

Thick filament myosin

6. ATP hydrolysis to ADP + Pᵢ causes change in hinge angle back to starting position

ADP Pᵢ   ADP Pᵢ

3. Cross-bridges from between actin and myosin heads

ADP Pᵢ   ADP Pᵢ

5. ATP exchanged for ADP, allowing cross bridges to break

ATP   ATP

ADP ATP ADP ATP

4. Pᵢ loss from myosin → hinge joint angle changes, filaments pull past each other to overlap more and i-band shortens

Actin movement

ADP   ADP

Myosin movement   Pᵢ loss   Pᵢ loss

Figure 2.14 Sliding filament hypothesis of muscle contraction.

Rigor mortis is the stiffening of muscles that occurs soon after death, fixing them in position. This rigidity is caused by the discontinuation of ATP production, therefore actin–myosin cross-bridges cannot be broken and so can no longer slide past each other. 24 hours after death the muscles begin to degrade and the stiffness subsides.

Length–tension relationship

Maximum contraction force depends on the pre-contraction length of the muscle fibre, i.e. it depends on the length of the sarcomeres (**Figure 2.15**). Peak contraction force occurs when fibres are mid-length. In this state:

■ There is plenty of overlap between thick and thin filaments so a high number of actin–myosin cross-bridges can form

Length–tension relationship for muscle fibres

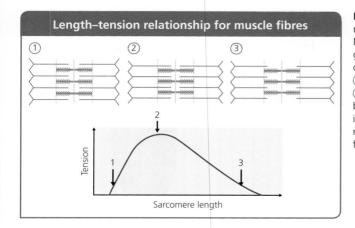

Figure 2.15 Length–tension relationship for muscle fibres. Maximum tension can be generated when there is optimum overlap of thick and thin filaments ②. When sarcomeres are too long ③ there is insufficient overlap between the filaments for them to interact. Shortened sarcomeres ① result in interference between the filaments.

Subtypes of skeletal myofibre

Fibre and LMN type	Contraction	Metabolism	Capillary density and density of myoglobin	Myosin ATPase activity
I	Slow and low power	Aerobic: high oxidative and low glycolytic	High	Low
IIA	Moderately fast and medium power	Anaerobic: intermediate oxidative and high glycolytic	Moderate	Moderate
IIB	Very fast and high power	Anaerobic: glycolytic only	Low	High
LMN, lower motor neurone.				

Table 2.6 Properties of the three myofibre types in skeletal muscle

■ There is space between the end of the thick filament and the Z-line, allowing contraction to take place (once the thick filaments meet the Z-lines, no further contraction is possible)

If the fibre is longer before contraction, there is little overlap between thick and thin filaments and therefore fewer cross-bridges can form. Conversely, when fibres are very short there is excessive overlap which causes interaction between opposing myofilaments reducing efficiency and force of contraction.

Fibre types

Table 2.6 summarises the properties of the different types of fibre in skeletal muscle. The lower motor neurone type determines the type of the skeletal muscle fibre, for example all muscle fibres innervated by a IIA neurone are type IIA.

Type I fibres are used for low-intensity, long duration activity; they use fats and glycogen as energy substrates in aerobic metabolism. Type IIB generate the highest contraction force and respond the most rapidly, using creatine phosphate and ATP as energy substrates. This means that type IIB fibres do not use aerobic respiration to generate energy for contraction. This allows these fibres to contract, even in the absence of O_2 (anaerobic metabolism), such as in situations of very high intensity exercise or at the very start of exercise, before blood flow has increased. The lower motor neurones that innervate fast twitch fibres (IIA and IIB) are of larger diameter than type I neurones, to facilitate faster conduction.

'Muscle fibre-type grouping' sometimes occurs when lower motor neurones are damaged and is seen in motor neurone disease. Adjacent neurones take over innervation of the muscle fibres the injured fibre was supplying. In response the muscle fibre type changes to become that of the new supplying neurone, reducing the variation of muscle fibre type, with large groups of adjacent fibres all of the same type.

Control of skeletal muscle length

Involuntary and voluntary processes interact to control the length of skeletal muscles. Innervation from the corticospinal tract allows conscious contraction of muscles and other pathways originating in the CNS facilitate the contraction at a subconscious level, for example the rubrospinal and tectospinal tracts (see Chapter 8, page 264).

Short-range reflexes are superimposed on top of descending CNS influences. Muscle spindles and Golgi tendon organs are the most important sensory organs involved in this short-range reflex control of muscle length, as described below.

Muscle spindles

A muscle spindle is a group of modified muscle fibres contained within a capsule of connective tissue and having axons of 1α sensory (afferent) neurones (form of an A-α neurone, see **Table 2.2**) wrapped around the capsule (**Figure 2.16**). The muscle fibres within the spindle are called intrafusal fibres; the 'ordinary' muscle fibres that surround and are external to the spindle are termed extrafusal fibres.

Muscle spindles lie in parallel with extrafusal fibres, so they are subjected to the same changes in length. A sudden increase in length of intrafusal fibres causes stretch of the spindle's sensory 1α neurone, which stimulates an action potential. This travels via a monosynaptic reflex (see page 61) to activate the lower motor neurone that provides efferent supply to the extrafusal fibres of the same muscle,

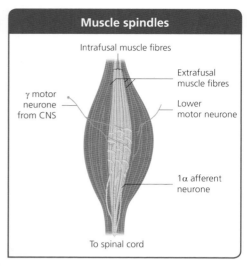

Muscle spindles

Intrafusal muscle fibres

Extrafusal muscle fibres

γ motor neurone from CNS

Lower motor neurone

1α afferent neurone

To spinal cord

Figure 2.16 Muscle spindles have axons of 1α sensory (afferent) neurones wrapped around intrafusal muscle fibres, which are innervated by γ motor neurones. Outside the spindle are extrafusal fibres, supplied by the main lower motor neurone.

causing them to contract. Therefore rapid muscle stretch causes reflex muscle contraction. Muscle spindles mediate the tendon jerk reflex used in neurological examination.

Gamma neurones

The response of muscle spindles is modulated by contraction of intrafusal muscle fibres. Gamma (γ) motor neurones innervate intrafusal fibres. Activation of γ motor neurone reduces the output of the sensory afferent 1α neurone for any specific amount of muscle stretch. This allows for anticipated (voluntary) muscle stretch (e.g. antagonist contraction of biceps to pick up a shopping bag causes anticipated (voluntary) stretch of triceps) without activation of the monosynaptic reflex arc.

Golgi tendon organs

Golgi tendon organs are composed of free nerve endings that lie in the tendons of skeletal muscle (nerve endings that do not synapse with other cells). When a muscle is relaxed the collagen fibres in its tendon are loosely spaced. However when tension is put through a tendon, i.e. during muscle contraction, the collagen fibres oppose each other closely.

This exerts a compressive force on the free nerve endings of the Golgi tendon organs, activating their afferent fibres.

The afferent nerves stimulate an inhibitory interneurone in the spinal cord. This is a neurone that runs from the sensory (afferent) to the motor (efferent) and inhibits the motor (efferent) neurone, stopping muscle contraction. Therefore forceful contraction and high tendon tension causes inhibition of muscle contraction. In this way, Golgi tendon organs give control when lifting heavy objects and they may serve a protective role against muscle damage in response to large forces from outside the body.

Cardiac muscle

Cardiac muscle is a striated muscle; like skeletal muscle it has sarcomeres with thick and filaments. Most of its characteristics, such as the length–tension relationship and control of muscle length (see page 57), are the same as for skeletal muscle. However, it has some significant differences from skeletal muscle, principally in the types of junctions between myocytes, in capacity for anaerobic metabolism, and in mitochondrial density.

The cardiac myofibres typically contain only a few nuclei and demonstrate branching and interconnection with other fibres at specialised cell junctions called intercalated discs. Intercalated discs contain:

- Gap junctions
- Adherens junctions (connected to the actin cytoskeleton)
- Desmosomes (connected to intermediate filaments)

In no other tissue are these three cell junctions found on every cell. The gap junctions facilitate spread of contraction throughout the myocardium, providing a coordinated and progressive contraction.

Cardiac muscle has high mitochondrial density and large glycogen and myoglobin (a molecule that allows storage of oxygen) stores, because, unlike skeletal muscle, cardiac myocytes can only use aerobic metabolism. There are also minor differences from skeletal muscle in T-tubules, troponin proteins and the appearance of sarcomeres.

Smooth muscle

Smooth muscle is present in blood vessels, the walls of the gastrointestinal tract, the uterus, the bladder, and the eye, as well as in other organs. It is sometimes called involuntary muscle because it is not under conscious control.

Structure

Smooth muscle contains thick filaments, made of myosin, and thin filaments, made of actin and tropomyosin. There is no troponin in smooth muscle, unlike skeletal muscle.

The thick and thin filaments are attached to the cell membrane at areas called dense bodies. The cells lack the striated 'sarcomere' structure of skeletal muscle. Instead they are elliptically-shaped and have irregularly arrange contractile fibres that traverse the cell. Contraction of smooth muscle is typically slower and weaker than contraction in skeletal muscle; however, the degree of shortening can be greater, contractions can be more prolonged and they require less energy because they do not have to generate large forces to move bones and joints.

Mechanism of contraction

Formation of cross bridges occurs when an enzyme, myosin light-chain kinase (MLCK), phosphorylates myosin, which allows binding of myosin to actin (**Figure 2.17**). Contraction continues to occur while MLCK is active. Myosin light-chain phosphatase (MLCP) reverses this process and causes relaxation.

MLCK is activated by the presence together of calcium (from voltage-gated calcium-channels and the sarcoplasmic reticulum) and calmodulin (an association protein).

Control of contraction and nitric oxide

An increase in intracellular cGMP (or cAMP) results in smooth muscle relaxation by activation of kinase proteins (PKG and PKA). The kinases cause opening of potassium channels, which hyperpolarises the cell and prevents contraction. There is also activation myosin

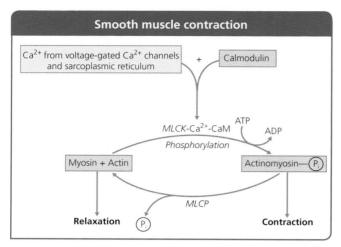

Figure 2.17 Smooth muscle contraction. Myofilaments interact causing contraction when myosin becomes phosphorylated by myosin light-chain kinase (MLCK). This enzyme requires the presence of calcium and its binding protein calmodulin. Myosin light-chain phosphatase (MLCP) reverses the reaction causing relaxation.

light chain phosphatase, which dephosphorylates myosin, preventing it binding to actin.

Nitric oxide (NO) is a potent smooth muscle relaxant that originates from endothelial cells, neurones and inflammatory cells. NO activates soluble guanylate cyclase (sGC), which increases conversion of GTP to cGMP, increasing activity in the above pathways.

Autonomic and hormonal control

The sympathetic nervous system has a major role in controlling smooth muscle contraction.

Vascular smooth muscle is able to contract or relax in response to sympathetic stimulation. Nerves release noradrenaline that bind α-adrenoreceptors, which signal through G_q to cause a rise in calcium. Alternatively, binding of noradrenaline or adrenaline to β-adrenoreceptors causes a rise in cAMP levels, which then promotes relaxation of vascular smooth muscle. This allows increased sympathetic drive to increase blood flow to muscles while reducing it to other organs such as the gut and kidney.

Enteric smooth muscle activity is decreased following sympathetic stimulation because catecholamines bind β-adrenoreceptors that cause a rise in cAMP and hyperpolarisation. Conversely, parasympathetic post-ganglionic neurones release acetylcholine. Vascular smooth muscle and enteric smooth muscle are both also controlled by the autonomic nervous system. This is described in more detail on page 198.

Reflexes

A reflex is a rapid, involuntary, patterned response of the CNS with a specific input and rapid output that is consistent and repeatable. Therefore, all reflexes:

■ Have an afferent and an efferent neurone
■ Have a receptor which transduces the specific input (turns a stimulus into an action potential)
■ Must pass through the CNS but not necessarily to the brain
■ Are subconscious processes that we become aware of after they have completed

There are two types of reflex: monosynaptic and polysynaptic.

A key component of neurological examination is testing of the reflexes; specifically looking for whether they are increased (brisk) or depressed (slowed). These useful physical signs allow localisation of the lesion. A depressed reflex usually indicates a peripheral nerve lesion because the afferent or efferent limb of the muscle spindle reflex arc has been damaged. A brisk reflex suggests an upper motor neurone lesion and pathology in the brain or spinal cord.

Monosynaptic reflex

This is a reflex arc in which there is only one synapse: the afferent neurone synapses directly onto the efferent neurone (**Figure 2.18a**). The muscle spindle stretch reflex is an example where afferent activation causes an action potential in the efferent and muscle contraction.

Polysynaptic reflex

More complex reflexes are termed polysynaptic because they include an interneurone or branching of the afferent neurone (**Figure 2.18b**). The Golgi tendon organ reflex arc (**Table 2.7**) is an example because the afferent neurone first synapses with an inhibitory interneurone that then causes a reduction in the activity of the efferent neurone.

Polysynaptic reflexes often have an ascending branch that passes to the brain; however, this is slower than the efferent impulse so we only become aware of the output after it has occurred.

Cross-side polysynaptic reflex   This is a complex form of a polysynaptic reflex that involves multiple branching interneurones with decussation (neurones passing from one side of the CNS to the other). One example is the withdrawal reflex that takes place when standing on a painful object when walking, from which the output is to move away and stand on the other foot (**Figure 2.18b**).

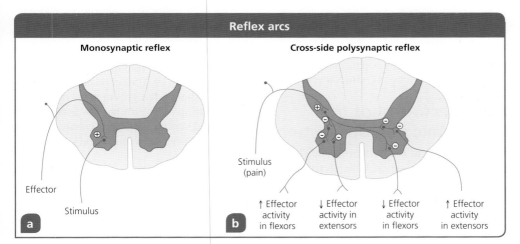

Figure 2.18 Reflex arcs. (a) In a monosynaptic reflexes involve only an afferent (sensory) neurone stimulates the efferent neurone. (b) Polysynaptic reflexes are more complex, for example this cross-side withdrawal reflex which has multiple interneurones to facilitate selective activation and inhibition of muscle groups.

	Golgi tendon organ	Muscle spindles
Control of muscle length		
Structure	Free nerve endings in tendons	Axons wrapped around specialised myocytes
Synapses in reflex pathway	2	1
Effect of muscle	Inhibits muscle contraction	Stimulates muscle contraction
Function	Fine control of movement	Opposes unexpected stretch (tendon jerk reflex)

Table 2.7 Comparison of two receptors involved in the control of muscle length, the Golgi tendon organ and muscle spindles

Autonomic nervous system

The peripheral nervous system includes all neurones outside the brain and spinal cord. It has a role in movement and sensation but a further component of the PNS controls the internal environment. The autonomic nervous system (ANS) is concerned with maintenance of internal homeostasis by sub-conscious processes, such as the control of blood pressure, gut motility and body temperature. The ANS has two components (or divisions):

■ Parasympathetic nervous system, with a role often summarised as having a 'rest and digest' role in homeostasis
■ Sympathetic nervous system, with a role summarised as the stimulation of a 'fight or flight' response

These differ in anatomy and physiology, often having opposing actions on the same organ.

Central control of the autonomic nervous system

Central control of the ANS originates in the medulla of the brainstem, which is the origin of efferent autonomic pathways. In both the parasympathetic and sympathetic nervous systems, each efferent pathway has two neurones:

■ A pre-ganglionic (myelinated) neurone and
■ A post-ganglionic (unmyelinated) neurone (a ganglion is a collection of cell bodies outside the CNS)

The physiology and anatomy of these differs in the parasympathetic and sympathetic divisions of the ANS. At the synapse between pre- and post-ganglionic neurones in both divisions the neurotransmitter is acetylcholine, which binds the nicotinic acetylcholine receptor (NAChR). However the post-ganglionic neurones release different neurotransmitters:

■ postganglionic sympathetic neurones release noradrenaline

■ parasympathetic neurones release acetylcholine in the

Autonomic afferent nerves (carrying signals from the periphery to the brain) travel in the same pathways as somatic afferent nerves, though they terminate in the hypothalamus or medulla.

Sympathetic nervous system

Pathway anatomy

An efferent pathway comprises a short pre-ganglionic neurone and a long post-ganglionic neurone (**Figure 2.19**). Descending neurones from the medulla activate the pre-ganglionic neurones, the cell bodies of which lie in the lateral horn of the spinal cord (**Figure 2.10**) between T1 and L2. The lateral horn is a collection of cell bodies (i.e. grey matter – the central part of the spinal cord) that lies between the dorsal and ventral horns, but is only found at spinal cord levels between T1 and L2.

Sympathetic chain

Pre-ganglionic neurones exit the spinal cord via the ventral horn and then pass into an interconnected set of ganglia called the sympathetic chain or trunk. The sympathetic chain is bilateral and lies just lateral to the spinal column in the paravertebral space on the posterior body cavity wall (**Figure 2.20**), extending up to the level of C4–5 and down to the sacrum.

Within the sympathetic chain, the majority of pre-ganglionic neurones synapse with their corresponding post-ganglionic neurone. The post-ganglionic neurone then exits the sympathetic chain to join the ventral ramus of the spinal cord and to be distributed with peripheral nerves to their target organ. Some pre-ganglionic neurones ascend or descend within the chain before synapsing as shown in **Figure 2.19**. Some pass straight through the chain to synapse in peripheral sympathetic ganglia such as the coeliac ganglion.

One exception is the adrenal medulla, which is innervated solely by a sympathetic pre-ganglionic neurone. This part of the adrenal gland can be thought of as an extension of the SNS because when activated it releases adrenaline and noradrenaline, together known as the catecholamines that augment sympathetic activity: in effect, the adrenal cells themselves function as postganglionic 'neurones'.

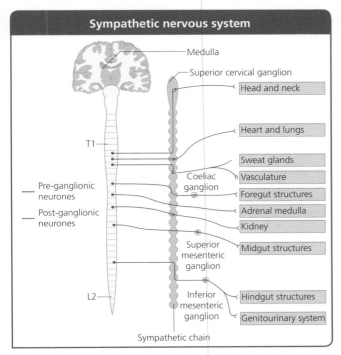

Figure 2.19 Sympathetic nervous system. All pre-ganglionic neurones originate from T1–L2 in the spinal cord before passing to the sympathetic chain. Some synapse with a corresponding post-ganglionic neurone, at the level at which they exit the spinal cord, some ascend or descend in the sympathetic chain before synapsing and some pass straight through the chain before synapsing. The abdominal viscera are supplied via three peripheral ganglia: coeliac, superior mesenteric and inferior mesenteric ganglia.

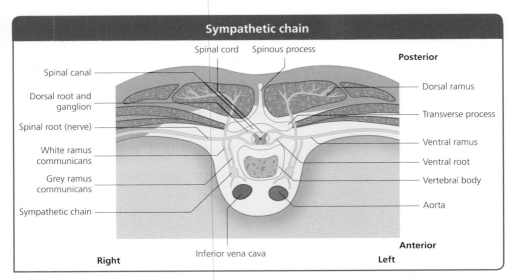

Figure 2.20 Anatomy of the sympathetic chain, showing its relation to the vertebrae, posterior wall of body, aorta, and inferior vena cava.

A 37-year-old woman presents with severe hypertension and episodes of sweating, severe anxiety and a 'sense of impending doom'. She is found to have a phaeochromocytoma growing from the adrenal medulla.

A **phaeochromocytoma** is a tumour of chromaffin cells, most of which are located in the adrenal medulla. The neoplastic cells produce catecholamines (adrenaline and noradrenaline) in surges that stimulate a massive sympathetic response.

Functions

Post-ganglionic sympathetic neurones release noradrenaline and a small amount of adrenaline. In contrast the adrenal medulla, acting like a neurone, releases mainly adrenaline. These catecholamines bind to α- and β-adrenoreceptors on the target organs to exert the actions of the sympathetic nervous system (**Table 2.8**). α-Adrenoreceptors are more responsive to noradrenaline than adrenaline, while β-adrenoreceptors have a higher affinity for adrenaline.

The post-ganglionic sympathetic neurones that supply sweat glands are an exception in that they do not release noradrenaline or adrenaline. Instead they stimulate increased in sweat production by releasing acetylcholine, which binds muscarinic acetylcholine receptors. Muscarinic acetylcholine receptors are a different form of acetylcholine receptor, mostly used by the parasympathetic nervous system, compared to the nicotinic acetylcholine receptor found at the neuromuscular junction.

Horner's syndrome is caused by an interruption to the sympathetic supply to one side of the face. The result is a small pupil (loss of dilator pupillae function), partial ptosis (drooping of the eyelid) lack of sweating and vasodilatation. It arises from damage to the sympathetic pathway at any point (e.g. apical lung tumour or a brainstem lesion).

Sympathetic nervous system		
Tissue	Receptor type	Effect
Vascular smooth muscle	α_1-adrenoreceptor	Vasoconstriction of arteries and veins
	β_2-adrenoreceptor (heart and skeletal muscle arterioles only)	Vasodilatation
Heart	β_1-adrenoreceptor	Increased heart rate at SAN
		Reduced AVN delay
		Increased ventricular contractility
Erector pili muscle	α-adrenoreceptor	Hair stands on end
Enteric smooth muscle	α-adrenoreceptor	Relaxation of intermittently contracting muscle
		Contraction of sphincters
Dilator pupillae	α-adrenoreceptor	Pupil dilation
Juxtaglomerular apparatus (kidney)	β-adrenoreceptor	Increased renin release
Salivary glands	β-adrenoreceptor	Thickened secretions
Bronchioles	β_2-adrenoreceptor	Bronchodilatation
Internal urethral sphincter (bladder neck)	α-adrenoreceptor	Retention of urine
Sweat glands	Muscarinic acetylcholine receptor	Increased sweat production

Table 2.8 Functions of the sympathetic nervous system and the receptors that mediate each effect

Parasympathetic system

Pathway anatomy

Parasympathetic pre-ganglionic neurones are relatively long and travel to ganglia close to the structure that they are innervating before synapsing. The pre-ganglionic neurones originate from the nuclei (collections of neuronal cell bodies within the CNS) of cranial nerves III, VII, IX and X and from the sacral outflow, where their cell bodies are in the conus medullaris (**Figure 2.21**).

Parasympathetic branches meet the motor and sensory fibres of the cranial nerves and closely follow the course of the latter to target organs. The vagus innervates the viscera of the thorax and the gut derived from foregut and midgut. The hindgut is innervated by the sacral outflow, which exits the spinal column with nerves S2–S4. These nerves also supply the pelvic structures.

Functions

All parasympathetic post-ganglionic neurones release acetylcholine, which binds to muscarinic acetylcholine receptors on effectors (the target organs, (**Table 2.9**). There are a number of different subtypes of muscarinic receptor but they all act through G-proteins.

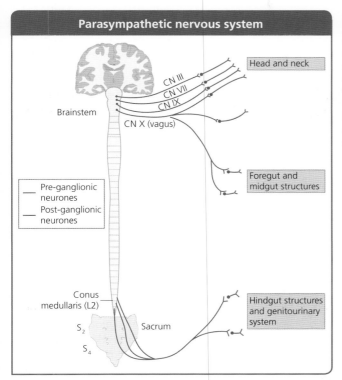

Parasympathetic nervous system

Head and neck

CN III
CN VII
CN IX

Brainstem

CN X (vagus)

Pre-ganglionic neurones
Post-ganglionic neurones

Foregut and midgut structures

Conus medullaris (L2)

S_2

S_4

Sacrum

Hindgut structures and genitourinary system

Figure 2.21 Parasympathetic nervous system. The efferent fibres originate in either the nuclei of cranial nerves III, VII, IX and X, or in the conus medullaris then exiting at the level of S2–4. The vagus innervates internal viscera including the intestine but all bowel distal to the transverse colon is supplied by the sacral outflow.

Parasympathetic nervous system		
Tissue (effector)	Efferent neurone	Effect
Constrictor pupillae	Occulomotor nerve (CN III)	Pupil constriction
Salivary gland	Facial nerve (CN VII)	Increased submandibular and submental gland production
	Glossopharyngeal nerve (CN IX)	Increased parotid gland production
Lacrimal gland	Facial nerve (CN VII)	Increased tear production
Heart	Vagus nerve (CN X)	Reduced heart rate at sinoatrial node
		Increased atrioventricular node delay
Enteric smooth muscle	Vagus: foregut and midgut	Increased activity of intermittently contracting muscle
	S2–4: hindgut	Relaxation of sphincters
Urinary system	S2–4	Detrusor contraction
		Relaxation of internal urethral sphincter

Table 2.9 Functions of the parasympathetic nervous system. The receptor that mediates the effect is a muscarinic acetylcholine receptor, usually subtype 3 (M_3-AChR)

Answers to starter questions

1. An impulse (or action potential) is a single all-or-nothing event that does not provide meaning on its own. However, several action potentials in succession are a 'code' to give information on the stimulus intensity. For example, a higher frequency of action potentials codes for a higher stimulus intensity. On the other hand a change in the frequency of action potentials (slow to fast) indicates a change in the intensity of the stimulus. Each neurone is coded to only confer one type of information (e.g. pain, or temperature, or muscle contraction); therefore its action potentials are given meaning and context.

2. Cell membranes are impermeable to charged molecules due to their phospholipid structure. However, gap junctions create pores between adjacent cells that allow the passage of small molecules, including ions. This facilitates the spread of depolarisation through a tissue, e.g. enteric smooth muscle, which is needed for simultaneous contraction of large sheets of myocytes to move food through the gut (by peristalsis, see chapter 7).

3. Muscles are able to shorten by overlapping their intracellular structural proteins. These thick and thin filaments have very little overlap when a muscle is relaxed, but energy is used to move the filaments past each other, shortening each muscle fibre and causing the muscle to contract. There is no reason why the force generated by muscle shortening should be limited by our own body weight. The main determinants of strength are the size of muscle fibres, types of fibres and number of contractile filaments, because our bones and tendons are able to withstand forces much greater than our muscles can exert.

4. Sprinting requires rapid exertion of a large force but does not need to be sustained. Some muscle fibres are better adapted to quick, powerful movements (e.g. type IIB) and some to longer, less powerful movements. The proportion of fibre types present is mostly genetically predetermined, meaning some people have more muscles that are naturally better for sprinting.

5. Nervousness and anxiety are both psychological and physical states. A large component of the physical symptoms is hyperactivation of the sympathetic nervous system. This increases heart rate, breathing rate and blood pressure, and also innervates sweat glands causing increased sweat production.

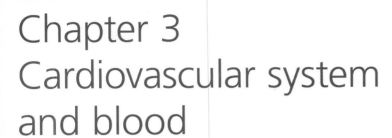

Chapter 3
Cardiovascular system and blood

Starter questions

Answers to the following questions are on page 104.

1. What causes the heart to beat rhythmically?
2. Why is blood pressure tightly regulated?
3. Why is the heart so susceptible to ischaemia?
4. How is blood flow matched to the activity of a tissue?
5. What happens when someone faints?

Introduction

The role of the cardiovascular system is to carry substances such as oxygen, energy sources and hormones to different tissues, and to carry other substances such as carbon dioxide and waste products away from tissues. To achieve this, the heart pumps blood rhythmically through the arterial tree until capillary vessels are reached. These thin-walled vessels allow exchange of substances between the blood and the tissues. Flow through capillaries is carefully controlled by regulating the contraction of the heart and vasculature.

The cardiovascular system acts in close cooperation with the respiratory system to achieve their shared gas exchange functions.

Case 2 Chest pain on exertion

Presentation

A 72-year-old retired teacher, Hannah, presents to her GP with episodes of chest pain. The pain tends to occur when she walks quickly up stairs or a hill. She experiences it in the centre of her chest and describes it as a sensation of 'heaviness'. However, as soon as Hannah stops walking and rests the pain subsides. Her GP has been treating her for high blood pressure and she has smoked for 45 years.

Analysis

Hannah has presented with a history typical of cardiac chest pain. The pain occurs with an increase in cardiac work, i.e. tachycardia and an increase in stroke volume caused by a rise in physical activity.

The pain is relieved by rest, a sign demonstrating reversibility, making her presentation typical of angina.

Further case

Hannah is referred to the local cardiac clinic, which has arranged for her to undergo percutaneous coronary angiography. This demonstrates atherosclerotic narrowing in her anterior interventricular artery, reducing the lumen diameter by 80%; all her other vessels are patent. She is started on regular bisoprolol (a beta-blocker), simvastatin (a cholesterol-lowering agent), aspirin (as an antiplatelet) and glyceryl trinitrate (GTN) spray, to use when the pain occurs. Over the next year this combination of medical therapy is sufficient to control her symptoms.

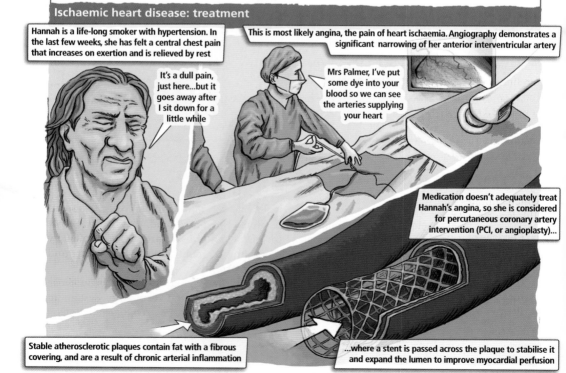

Ischaemic heart disease: treatment

Hannah is a life-long smoker with hypertension. In the last few weeks, she has felt a central chest pain that increases on exertion and is relieved by rest

This is most likely angina, the pain of heart ischaemia. Angiography demonstrates a significant narrowing of her anterior interventricular artery

It's a dull pain, just here...but it goes away after I sit down for a little while

Mrs Palmer, I've put some dye into your blood so we can see the arteries supplying your heart

Medication doesn't adequately treat Hannah's angina, so she is considered for percutaneous coronary artery intervention (PCI, or angioplasty)...

Stable atherosclerotic plaques contain fat with a fibrous covering, and are a result of chronic arterial inflammation

...where a stent is passed across the plaque to stabilise it and expand the lumen to improve myocardial perfusion

Case 2 *continued*

Further analysis

Coronary artery disease is the most common cause of angina, and of death, in the UK. It is due to formation of atherosclerotic plaques in coronary vessels, which, when the lumen is narrowed by over 70%, limit cardiac blood flow. As cardiac work increases, the oxygen demand exceeds supply even when the arterioles are maximally vasodilated.

Acute treatment This is aimed at reducing the heart's workload: GTN releases nitric oxide (NO), a potent vasodilator. Nitric oxide causes some vasodilatation of the coronary arterioles, increasing downstream flow. However its main action is systemic vasodilatation, which reduces central venous pressure and therefore end-diastolic volume. This causes stroke volume to fall (according to the Frank–Starling law of the heart) and limits cardiac work (heart rate and contractility). Beta-blockers also limit cardiac work, which helps prevent the onset of symptoms. By slowing the heart rate, there is more time for blood to supply the muscle before the next contraction begins.

Long-term medical treatment This is aimed at controlling hypertension (sustained pathologically high blood pressure) and hypercholesterolaemia (raised blood cholesterol levels), both of which promote atherosclerosis. Smoking cessation is vital to slow progression of atherosclerosis. In coronary artery disease, aspirin reduces the propensity of platelets to aggregate and form a thrombus (a blood clot in an intact vessel). Some patients benefit from surgical treatment such as stenting or bypass grafting, depending on the location of the atherosclerotic plaques.

Principles of circulation

The cardiovascular system operates as two circulations in series: the systemic and pulmonary circulations, united by the heart (**Figure 3.1**). Consequently, a change in pressure or resistance in one of these circulations results in changes in the other by feed-forward and feed-back mechanisms.

The overall function of the cardiovascular system is to perfuse the tissues with blood, which supplies and removes various factors. This is achieved by:

■ Carriage of substances in the blood
■ Maintenance of effective circulating pressure and flow in capillary beds (networks of small, narrow blood vessels that supply tissues)
■ Formation and reabsorption of tissue fluid

All of the pulmonary vessels, including the arteries, are structurally similar to the veins of the systemic circulation. They operate under a low-pressure system, are influenced by gravity and respiration, and their pressure

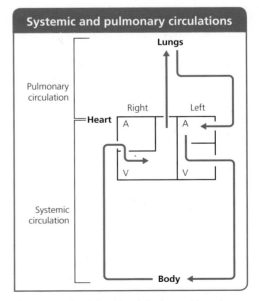

Figure 3.1 The right side of the heart drives the pulmonary circulation and the left side drives the systemic circulation. A, atrium; V, ventricle.

is important for cardiac filling. They function to link cardiac output on the right side of the heart with that on the left side, in accordance with the Frank–Starling law.

Flow dynamics

Movement of fluid through a tube occurs according to a number of principles that hold true whether applied to air in the bronchial tree or blood in vessels.

Pressure and flow

The flow of a fluid is the volume transported per unit time (e.g. litres/minute). Flow is driven by the pressure of the fluid, which is the force it exerts against the walls of the tube. Fluid will always travel from areas of high pressure to low pressure. Flow is reduced by the resistance the fluid meets as it passes through the blood vessels (influenced by a number of variables, described later). Therefore, blood flow is increased by either raising the pressure gradient or reducing the resistance to flow:

$$\text{Flow} = \frac{\text{arterial pressure} - \text{venous pressure}}{\text{resistance}}$$

In the vascular system, the pressure gradient is the difference between arterial and venous pressure either side of a capillary bed.

Tissues rely on a given flow for their activity. For example adult normal brain function requires about 3.5 mL of oxygen and 5.5 mg of glucose per 100 g of brain tissue per minute. This necessitates a blood flow to the brain of about 250 mL/min in an adult.

Cross-sectional area and flow

In a branching system of tubes, such as the vascular tree, the term cross-sectional area refers to the total area at a given level of branching. Typically, as the system divides into smaller but more numerous branches, the total area at that level increases. For example, the total cross-sectional area of the adult aorta is about 4.5 cm², whereas the total cross-sectional area of all the arterioles in the adult body is about 400 cm². The effect

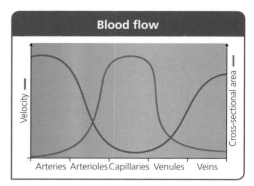

Figure 3.2 As the vascular tree divides, from arteries to arterioles to capillaries, the total cross-sectional area increases. As total flow throughout the system is constant, the velocity of blood decreases as cross-sectional area increases. Veins have a larger area and lower velocity than arteries.

is an exponential increase in total cross-sectional area as vessels divide (**Figure 3.2**).

Given that the vascular system is a closed system, flow is maintained across divisions of the vascular tree. Therefore the flow in the aorta is equal to the sum of the flow in all arterioles and equal to the sum of the flow in all capillary beds. If the same flow is occurring across a larger area, it follows that the actual velocity of the fluid will be lower:

$$\text{Flow} = \text{velocity} \times \text{cross-sectional area}$$

Consequently, as total cross sectional area increases, velocity decreases to maintain the same flow. This is shown in **Figure 3.2**: velocity is highest in the vessels closest to the heart and slowest in the microcirculation.

Resistance and flow

The movement of a fluid through a tube generates resistance, i.e. the force opposing that flow. The resistance arises from the shear of the fluid against the wall of the tube and of the fluid against itself.

If resistance is increased at one point in a closed system, this has downstream and upstream effects (**Figure 3.3**):

- Pressure is increased upstream
- Pressure and flow are reduced downstream

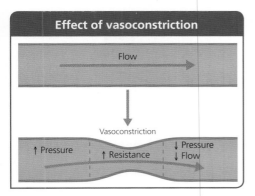

Effect of vasoconstriction

Flow

Vasoconstriction

↑ Pressure   ↑ Resistance   ↓ Pressure
↓ Flow

Figure 3.3 Vasoconstriction reduces vessel diameter and increases the resistance to flow. Consequently, pressure increases upstream and falls downstream with the reduction in flow.

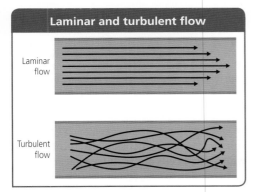

Laminar and turbulent flow

Laminar flow

Turbulent flow

Figure 3.4 Laminar flow occurs when all fluid movement is in the direction of the vessel, with the highest velocity at the centre. Turbulent flow is more chaotic and causes increased resistance.

Imagine how a dam causes water levels to rise upstream of it, while reducing the flow downstream. This is the basis of control of blood pressure and of flow in capillary beds by constriction or dilatation of arterioles (discussed in more detail on page 82).

Laminar and turbulent flow

There are two general descriptions for the flow of fluid through a tube: laminar or turbulent (**Figure 3.4**):

- **Laminar flow** involves all of the fluid moving parallel to the tube: the fluid at the centre has the highest velocity because it is least subject to resistance from the walls of the vessel

- **Turbulent flow** is more chaotic: whilst all the fluid is moving in a single direction of travel, flow is irregular and there are local currents ('eddies'). Turbulent flow generates much more resistance than laminar flow therefore requires more energy

The Reynolds's number of a fluid (Re) describes the likelihood that its flow will be turbulent: a fluid with a higher value has a higher chance of turbulent flow. A simplified definition of Re is:

$$Re = (velocity \times diameter) / viscosity$$

Therefore, turbulent flow is most likely in large tubes where fluid moves very quickly, for example in the aorta or trachea (air flow being like fluid flow). This is one of the reasons why most of the air resistance in the respiratory system is from the large airways.

Because blood is viscous, for example much more viscous than water, the Reynolds number for vascular systems tends to be low, and we regard most blood flow as laminar.

> **Turbulent flow at the branching of arteries has a role in precipitating formation of atherosclerotic plaques.** For example there is significant turbulent flow where the common carotid artery bifurcates to form the internal and external carotid arteries. This is a frequent site for atherosclerotic plaques, which cause strokes when they rupture.

Hagen–Poiseuille equation

A number of factors influence resistance to laminar flow through a tube:

$$Resistance = \frac{(8 \times viscosity \times length \times flow\ rate)}{(\pi \times radius^4)}$$

where π is the numerical constant 3.14159.

From this we can see that radius is the most important variable: a small decrease in radius greatly decreases the denominator and so is associated with a large increase in resistance.

In the vascular system, the radius of vessels is changed by the vasodilatation and vasoconstriction that takes place in order to regulate resistance and therefore pressure and, in turn, flow. This is a very powerful effect: reducing the radius of an arteriole by only 20% reduces the blood flow through it by about 60%.

Compliance

Compliance is the distensibility of a hollow structure when pressure on its walls changes:

$$\text{Compliance} = \Delta V/\Delta P$$

where ΔV is change in volume and ΔP is change in pressure. When a vessel, tube or other structure (e.g. the chest wall) is subject to a transmural pressure it will change volume. A positive transmural pressure exerts a distending force causing an increase in volume. A highly compliant structure will undergo a larger increase in volume than a less compliant structure, given the same distending pressure.

Compliance is determined by the intrinsic nature of the tissue comprising the structure, though it is also affected by muscular contraction and pathological changes. It can also change depending on the starting volume of the structure (**Figure 3.5**), i.e. there is a non-linear relationship between pressure and volume. At low volumes veins are highly compliant, but once the fibrous tissue in their walls becomes taught their compliance falls rapidly.

Elasticity

Elasticity is the tendency of the structure to return to its original shape:

$$\text{Elasticity} = 1 / \text{compliance}$$
$$= \Delta P / \Delta V$$

Like compliance, elasticity is determined by the tissue that makes the structure in question. It is most useful when describing the internal pressure of a structure (e.g. arteriole) at a given volume. Elasticity is discussed further in Chapter 4.

Blood flow

Approximately 54% of blood is plasma, 45% is red blood cells and 1% white blood cells and platelets (see pages 93–104). Plasma is a water-based solution of many dissolved

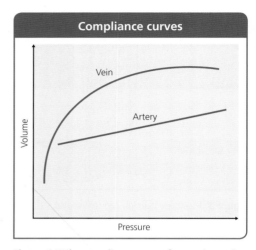

Figure 3.5 The compliance curves for arteries and veins differ. Elastic tissue in arterial walls makes their compliance low and causes a linear relationship between pressure and volume; the result is that there is a relatively small change in volume for a large change in pressure. Veins are highly compliant at low volumes: their volume increases rapidly with relatively small increases in pressure, until their fibrous tissue becomes taut and limits volume increase and hence further filling.

substances (e.g. glucose, salts, proteins) in which these cells circulate (see page 93).

In relation to flow dynamics, two characteristics of blood are particularly relevant:

- **Plasma proteins** are crucial to maintenance of intravascular volume and tissue fluid formation (see page 87)
- **Viscosity of blood**, which affects resistance (see above), is determined mainly by the percentage of red cells in the blood, i.e. the haematocrit. Under physiological conditions, the viscosity of blood is relatively constant.

Blood viscosity increases when the percentage of red cells (haematocrit) within it rises, as in extreme dehydration. Endurance athletes occasionally suffer strokes when dehydrated during competition after erythropoietin abuse (which promotes synthesis of red cells). The raised blood viscosity increases resistance, reducing cerebral blood flow, resulting in ischaemia.

The heart

Structure and function

The heart lies in the mediastinum, relatively anteriorly in the thorax and just above the diaphragm. It is surrounded by two layers of pericardium:

- The outer (parietal) layer: forms the pericardial sac
- The inner (visceral) layer or epicardium: forms the outer surface of the heart itself

A small volume of pericardial fluid fills the space between these two layers, which allows movement of the beating heart to be low friction. Inside the pericardium is the myocardium (the cardiac muscle). The innermost layer is the endocardium, a layer of tissue that separates the chambers of the heart from the myocardium.

Cardiac myocytes (cardiac muscle cells)

Cardiac muscle is a specialised form of striated muscle (see page 52). The gap junctions between cardiac myocytes facilitate low-resistance spread of ions through the myocardium, allowing action potentials to spread between the cells and therefore lead to co-ordinated contraction.

The cardiac chambers and fibrous skeleton

The heart comprises four chambers: the right atrium, right ventricle, left atrium and left ventricle (**Figure 3.6**). The atria are separated from each other by the interatrial septum, a layer of tissue between the left and right atria; the ventricles are separated by an equivalent interventricular septum. The interventricular septum contains large myocytes known as Purkinje cells, which specialise in the rapid conduction of action potentials. They are larger than other myocytes and have minimal glycogen stores, which reduces their resistance to the flow of electrical charge. Purkinje cells are grouped together into bundles (known as the bundle of His) which facilitate co-ordinated contraction down the interventricular septum.

Though the majority of the heart is composed of muscular tissue, it is supported by a fibrous skeleton that sits between the atria and ventricles. The fibrous skeleton is made of tough collagen, which holds its shape as the heart beats. It lies between the atria and ventricles so that the atria are superior and ventricles are inferior. The skeleton forms a complete layer of the heart at this level, except for gaps where the atrioventricular

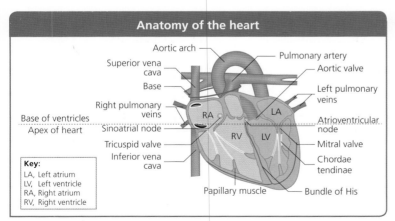

Anatomy of the heart

Aortic arch
Superior vena cava
Base
Right pulmonary veins
Base of ventricles
Apex of heart
Sinoatrial node
Tricuspid valve
Inferior vena cava
Papillary muscle

Pulmonary artery
Aortic valve
Left pulmonary veins
Atrioventricular node
Mitral valve
Chordae tendinae
Bundle of His

RA
LA
RV
LV

Key:
LA, Left atrium
LV, Left ventricle
RA, Right atrium
RV, Right ventricle

Figure 3.6 Anatomy of the heart: coronal section viewed anteriorly.

valves are located. In addition to the physi-cal support it provides, this skeleton is an important electrical insulator in that it is not capable of transmitting action potentials (see page 42).

On each side of the heart, the atrium is sepa-rated from its corresponding ventricle by an atrioventricular valve formed of double-layered endocardium (the tricuspid and mitral valves). The atrioventricular valves are held in their correct orientation by chordae tendinae: these are fibrous cords attached to the cusps of the valves to prevent inversion of the valves during ventricular contraction. The chordae tendinae originate in papillary muscles that are exten-sions of the ventricular myocardium and aid in their function.

Flow of blood through the heart

The right atrium receives blood from the sys-temic veins (the superior and inferior vena cavae) and transmits blood to the right ven-tricle via the tricuspid valve. The right ven-tricle ejects blood into the pulmonary artery through the pulmonary valve.

After circulating through the lungs, blood returns to the left atrium by the pulmonary veins and then into the left ventricle through the mitral valve. The left ventricle ejects blood to the systemic circulation via the aor-tic valve.

Fetal circulation

Blood flow in the fetus is structurally and physiologically different to that in an adult (**Figure 3.7**). The fetus has three shunts, loca-tions where blood takes a different route from the adult circulation:

- The ductus venosus carries oxygenated blood from the umbilical vein, through the liver to the inferior vena cava.
- The foramen ovale (in the intra-atrial septum) allows direct passage of blood from the right atrium into the left atrium.
- The ductus arteriosus allows blood to flow from the pulmonary artery to the aorta

Blood moves through the cardiac shunts in a right-to-left direction because right-sided pressures are greater than left-sided pressures. This pressure difference is main-tained by two fetal characteristics. First, the lungs of the fetus are collapsed and filled with amniotic fluid, which generates a high pulmonary vascular resistance. Second, the umbilical artery leads to the placenta, which reduces systemic total peripheral resistance.

At birth fetal circulation changes drastically (see page 186).

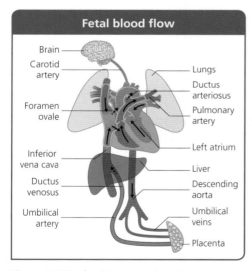

Fetal blood flow

Brain
Carotid artery
Foramen ovale
Inferior vena cava
Ductus venosus
Umbilical artery

Lungs
Ductus arteriosus
Pulmonary artery
Left atrium
Liver
Descending aorta
Umbilical veins
Placenta

Figure 3.7 The fetal circulation has three shunts (labelled in bold) that provide blood with the highest oxygen tension to the brain whilst bypassing the lungs.

Ventricular septal defect (VSD), a hole in the interventricular septum, is the most common isolated congenital cardiac defect. After birth, left-side heart pressures exceeds right-side pressures so blood is shunted from left to right via the defect. Small VSDs cause loud murmurs (from highly turbulent flow) but minimal haemodynamic compromise; large VSDs result in cardiac failure in late infancy.

Electrical conduction through the heart

The sinoatrial node in the right atrium (**Figure 3.6**) is the site at which the heartbeat originates. It is made up of pacemaker cells, specialised myocytes described below.

The pacemaker cells depolarise spontaneously until they initiate an action potential. This then spreads throughout the atrium, causing contraction of atrial muscle which pumps blood into the ventricles. The wave of depolarisation is prevented from spreading from the atria into the ventricles by the presence of the insulating fibrous cardiac skeleton.

There is one gap in the fibrous scaffold; the atrioventricular node in the superior part of the interventricular septum. The presence of the atrioventricular node creates a small delay in transmission of the action potential, which allows complete atrial emptying to take place before ventricular contraction starts. Depolarisation is then rapidly transmitted down the interventricular septum by specialised Purkinje fibres in the bundle of His. Depolarisation of the ventricular myocar-dium thus begins at the apex of the heart and spreads upwards towards the base (adjacent to the atria) (**Figure 3.8**).

Pacemaker cells

Pacemaker cells are cardiac myocytes located in the sinoatrial and atrioventricular nodes. They are said to be electrically unstable because they do not have a stable resting membrane potential (E_m); instead they spontaneously depolarise without an external stimulus (see **Figure 3.9** and caption for events 4, 0 and 3):

4. Pacemaker cells have a relatively high Na^+ permeability (attributed to Na^+ leak channels), which mediates a gradual rise in E_m from the low point following the previous repolarisation: this gradual depolarisation is known as the pre-potential

0. Once the membrane potential reaches about –20 mV, voltage-gated channels become activated as threshold is passed

3. Voltage-gated Ca^{2+} channels and slow voltage-gated Na^+ channels open, with resultant cation influx and an action potential spike.

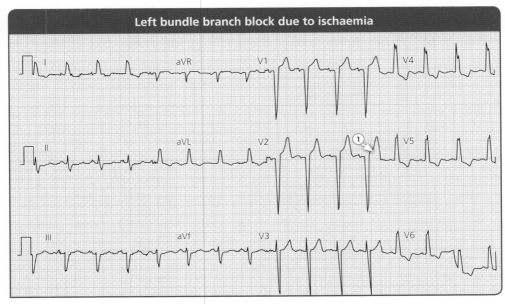

Left bundle branch block due to ischaemia

Figure 3.8 ECG showing left bundle branch block due to ischaemia affecting the left bundle of His. The QRS complex is prolonged ① as the left ventricle depolarises after the right, which makes interpretation of the rest of the ECG difficult.

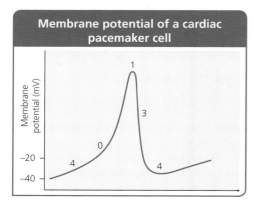

Membrane potential of a cardiac pacemaker cell

Figure 3.9 Changes in the membrane potential of a cardiac pacemaker cell. The pre-potential ④ causes gradual depolarisation until threshold is passed ⓪. Voltage-gated calcium channels mediate depolarisation ①, with potassium exit causing repolarisation ③. The next pre-potential starts immediately after depolarisation ④.

3. Opening of voltage-gated K^+ channels causes K^+ efflux and repolarisation
4. The pre-potential begins immediately after repolarisation ends restarting the cycle

These events follow a standardised numbering, where '2' is not found in pacemaker cells as it represents a plateau phase (as described below).

Normally the activity in the sinoatrial node controls the heart rate because it has the highest intrinsic rate, at 80–100 beats per minute (bpm). If the sinoatrial node fails for any reason, other pacemaker cells in the heart take over. This will result in a lower heart rate of all pacemaker cells. If it is the atrioventricular node that takes over, its cells have an intrinsic rate of around 40–60 bpm. If the atrioventricular node is also damaged then it is possible for ventricular pacemaker myocytes to become the site of action potential initiation. However these have the even lower intrinsic rate of 20–40 bpm. This bradycardia (slow heart rate) will result in low blood pressure, with reduced blood flow to the vital organs.

In rare instances, there is more than one origin of electrical activity; this presents with bigeminy, a sign which can be demonstrated on ECG (**Figure 3.10**).

Electrically stable myocytes

The majority of myocytes forming the atrial and ventricular myocardium do not normally depolarise spontaneously and are referred

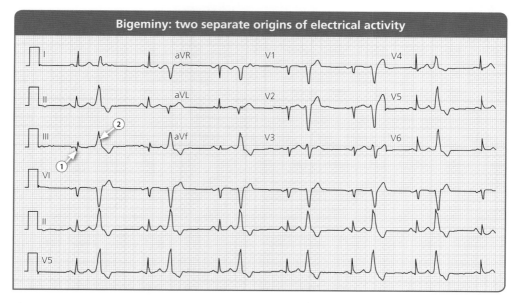

Bigeminy: two separate origins of electrical activity

Figure 3.10 ECG showing bigeminy: two separate origins of electrical activity. Each p–QRS–t ① is followed by an abnormal, prolonged ventricular extrasystole ②. This suggests that, in addition to the sino-atrial node, there is a site of initiation of depolarisation within the ventricular muscle.

to as electrically stable. Like neurones (see page 42) they have a stable resting E_m (4), followed by an action potential if their depolarisation threshold is passed (**Figure 3.11**). At this moment, a variety of voltage-gated channels become activated; the first to open are fast Na^+ channels (1). These open and close very quickly, causing a rapid depolarisation followed by a short fall in membrane potential. Subsequently, voltage-gated slow Na^+ and Ca^{2+} channels open, which are responsible for the plateau phase of the action potential (2). Later, opening of voltage-gated K^+ channels causes repolarisation (3).

Electrically stable myocytes have absolute and relative refractory periods that are, in principle, the same as those in neurones (see page 44), though the long plateau phase in myocytes means their maximal firing rates are substantially lower.

Autonomic innervation of the heart

Innervation by the sympathetic and parasympathetic nervous system influences heart rate and contractility.

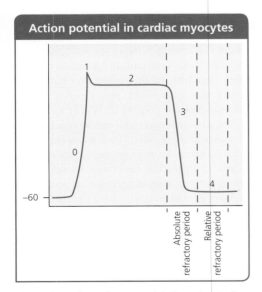

Action potential in cardiac myocytes

1

2

3

0

4

−60

Absolute refractory period

Relative refractory period

Figure 3.11 The action potential of an electrically stable (ventricular) myocyte (4). Depolarisation is caused by Na^+ entry (0) with a short pause (1) before calcium entry maintains the plateau (2). Potassium exit causes repolarisation (3). Refractory periods are illustrated.

Noradrenaline (and circulating adrenaline) bind to β_1-adrenoreceptors on pacemaker cells and ventricular myocardium. By signalling through the cAMP pathway (see page 22), this causes a rise in Na^+ and Ca^{2+} permeability. In pacemaker cells this causes an increase in the pre-potential and action potential gradients, by increasing the rate of cation influx. In ventricular myocytes it increases intracellular Ca^{2+} concentrations, allowing more cross-bridges to form between actin and myosin. The overall effect of sympathetic stimulation on the heart is:

- Higher heart rate, called a chronotropic effect
- Reduced delay at the atrioventricular node before the action potential passes to the ventricles and
- Increased ventricular contractility, called an inotropic effect

Acetylcholine from the vagus nerve (cranial nerve X) binds to muscarinic receptors on pacemaker cells. The effect is a rise in K^+ permeability, which reduces the gradient of the pre-potential and increases the duration and degree of repolarisation. Overall, parasympathetic stimulation slows heart rate at the sinoatrial node, increases delay at the atrioventricular node and increases the refractory period of ventricular myocardium.

Cardiac cycle

The cardiac cycle is the flow of blood through the heart during each beat. **Figure 3.12** illustrates the pressure and volume changes that take place during the cycle and correlates these with of heart sounds and ECG waves. The order of events is the same for right and left sides of the heart; however, the pressures are much higher on the left due to higher systemic vascular resistance.

For ease of explanation, the following section refers to the left of the heart. The same process occurs on the right side. Cross references to the items numbered in Figure 3.12 are given in bold.

Blood enters the atria from the vena cava and pulmonary veins during atrial diastole (the period when atrial muscle is relaxed) because venous pressure is higher than atrial pressure (1).

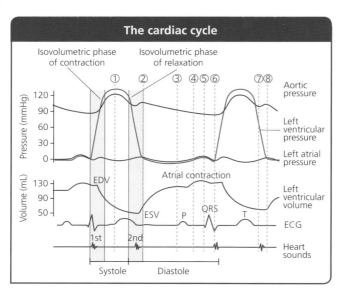

Figure 3.12 The cardiac cycle. EDV, end-diastolic volume; EDS, end-systolic volume.

This begins during ventricular systole (contraction), therefore ventricular pressure is higher than atrial pressure and consequently the atrioventricular valves are closed.

> **Ageing arteries become less elastic and more resistant**; during systole they are less compliant to filling with the increased blood volume. This manifests as **systolic hypertension**. The loss of elastic tissue results in failure of contraction during diastole and therefore normal, or even low, diastolic blood pressure.

Ventricular pressure falls once systole has ended. The inflow of venous blood causes atrial pressure to rise until it exceeds ventricular pressure, causing opening of the atrioventricular valves and allowing the ventricles to begin to fill (2).

The sinoatrial node initiates atrial depolarisation (seen as a P-wave on the ECG), which is immediately followed by atrial contraction (atrial systole) (3). Atrial pressure rises, which is coupled by a step-up in ventricular volume as blood is ejected from the atria into the ventricles (4).

> **Murmurs are caused by turbulent blood flow through the valves** in a normal direction or regurgitant flow through incompetent valves. Soft flow murmurs may be normal, but murmurs usually reflect valvular heart disease.

As described earlier, depolarisation is briefly delayed at the atrioventricular node (seen as the P–R interval) before spreading through the ventricular myocardium (illustrated by the QRS complex). At this point, the maximum ventricular volume has been reached; this is the end-diastolic volume (EDV) (5).

The onset of ventricular systole causes a rise in ventricular pressure. Once it has surpassed atrial pressure the atrioventricular valves close; this is heard as the first heart sound ('lub'). There is then a rapid increase in ventricular pressure during an isovolumetric phase of contraction, so termed because both atrioventricular and aortic valves are closed and therefore left ventricular volume does not change (6).

When ventricular pressure exceeds the aortic pressure, the aortic and pulmonary valves open and blood leaves the ventricles. Towards the end of ventricular systole there is a brief period when aortic pressure is greater than ventricular pressure; however, blood continues to enter the aorta due to the momentum of flow (7). Ventricular myocardium relaxes and begins to repolarise (seen as the T-wave on ECG).

The aortic valve closes (heard as the second heart sound, 'dub') and the isovolumetric phase of relaxation takes place, associated with a rapid fall in ventricular pressure (8). At this point the ventricular volume is at its lowest; this is the end-systolic volume (ESV). Once ventricular pressure falls below that of the atria, the atrioventricular valves open and ventricular filling begins once more.

> **A third heart sound**, in addition to the usual 'lub–dub' first and second sound, is heard if there is rapid ventricular filling and is sometimes normal. **A fourth heart sound** is always pathological and occurs when, during atrial contraction, a jet of blood hits an excessively stiff ventricle. If associated with a tachycardia, a 'gallop rhythm' is audible.

Cardiac output

Cardiac output (CO) is the volume of blood pumped by the heart each minute. It is the product of the volume of blood pumped with each heartbeat, i.e. the stroke volume (SV), and the number of beats per minute, i.e. the heart rate (HR). Stroke volume is the difference in ventricular volume at the beginning and end of contraction, i.e. the difference between end-diastolic and end-systolic volumes. Thus cardiac output is influenced by any process that affects heart rate, end-diastolic volume or end-systolic volume:

$$CO = HR \times SV$$

where

$$SV = EDV - ESV$$

The percentage of ventricular blood pumped out of the heart with each heartbeat is called the ejection fraction and is normally:

$$Ejection\ fraction = SV / EDV$$

The ejection fraction is normally 50–55%.

Sympathetic stimulation increases cardiac output by raising both the heart rate and increasing stroke volume. It does the latter by increasing ventricular contractility, which causes a stronger contraction for any given end-diastolic volume, therefore reducing end-systolic volume. By increasing the stroke volume, sympathetic stimulation increases the ejection fraction. Parasympathetic stimulation reduces cardiac output by slowing the heart rate.

> **Cardiac failure is most often caused by ischaemic heart disease, hypertension or valvular disease.** In cardiac failure, the heart cannot maintain adequate cardiac output at normal atrial pressures. Neural and humoral mechanisms increase end-diastolic volume in order to maintain cardiac output. However, due to progressively increasing end-diastolic volume there is no additional increase in stroke volume and the heart becomes dilated. Inadequate cardiac output leads to poor end-organ perfusion and raised venous pressure manifesting as pulmonary and peripheral oedema (see **Figure 3.14**).

Frank–Starling law of the heart

The Frank–Starling law states that stroke volume increases with increasing end-diastolic volume. This is based upon the length–tension relationship outlined for striated muscle in chapter 2 (see page 57): increasing the pre-contraction length of myocytes facilitates increased cross-bridge formation between filaments and a therefore higher force of contraction.

For the ventricular myocardium, increasing the end-diastolic volume increases the stretch of the ventricular myocytes. At physiological volumes increased length causes increased ventricular force of contraction and a resultant rise in stroke volume (**Figure 3.13**). At very high end-diastolic volume, there is excessive lengthening of ventricular myocytes and thus inadequate overlap for cross-bridge formation. As a result the stroke volume begins to fall, as shown towards the

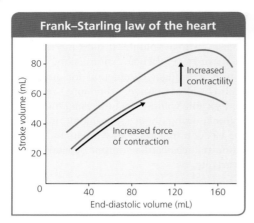

Figure 3.13 The Frank–Starling law of the heart gives a directly proportional relationship between end-diastolic volume and stroke volume until very high end-diastolic volumes are reached. The effect of raised contractility (often referred to as increased sympathetic tone) is demonstrated in the upper curve.

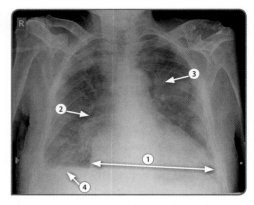

Figure 3.14 Chest X-ray of congestive cardiac failure showing ① cardiomegaly, ② perihilar pulmonary oedema, ③ upper-lobe blood diversion and ④ a right-sided pleural effusion.

right side of the curves in **Figure 3.13**. This is one of the characteristic features of cardiac failure (**Figure 3.14**).

The Frank–Starling effect matches stroke volume to venous return, as well as coupling right and left cardiac outputs. For example, walking causes an increase in venous return from the legs to the right ventricle. The rise in right-side end-diastolic volume is matched by a rise in right-side stroke volume. This passes through the pulmonary circulation as raised left-sided venous return. This raises left-side end-diastolic volume and consequently left-side stroke volume to push more blood into the systemic circulation to compensate for the increased movement of venous blood out of the systemic circulation.

Sympathetic stimulation to increase contractility results in increased stroke volume at any given end-diastolic volume. This is seen as a vertical shift of the Frank–Starling curve (**Figure 3.13**).

Arteries and arterioles

Structure and function

Different arterial and venous vessels have specialisations for their individual functions, however all vessels excluding the microcirculation have the same general structure (**Figure 3.15**):

■ Vessels are lined by the endothelium (specialised epithelium) arranged as a single layer of cells called the tunica intima
■ The endothelium is surrounded by is a muscular layer of very variable thickness, the tunica media

■ The outermost layer surrounding the tunica media is a fibrous sheath, the tunica adventitia.

Between these layers is a variable amount of elastic connective tissue – there is lots in arteries but very little in veins, whereas veins have more collagen.

Arteries convey blood between the heart and capillary beds in the tissues of the body. Arteries and arterioles have smooth muscle in their walls (comprising the tunica media); this allows them to dilate by smooth muscle relaxation and constrict by smooth muscle

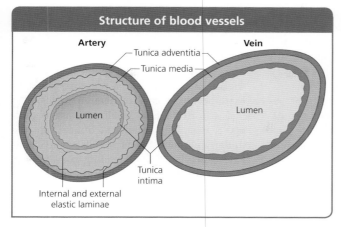

Structure of blood vessels

Artery

Vein

Tunica adventitia

Tunica media

Lumen

Lumen

Tunica intima

Internal and external elastic laminae

Figure 3.15 Veins and arteries both have tunica intima, media and adventitia. However, veins have a wider lumen and arteries have a thicker tunica media with thick internal and external elastic laminae.

Types of artery			
Type	Vessels	Characteristics	Function
Elastic artery	Aorta and its immediate branches	High elastin content in tunica media	Withstand high pressure
		Well-developed internal and external elastic laminae	Transmit systolic and diastolic pressure with minimal energy loss
Muscular artery	Branching arteries leading to capillaries	Thick tunica media	Even out systolic and diastolic pressure
Arteriole	Small vessels	Highly responsive smooth muscle	Regulate total peripheral resistance and flow in capillary beds

Table 3.1 Types of artery and how their structure relates to function

contraction. They decrease in size as distance from the heart increases, and their role changes (**Table 3.1**). Measurement of blood pressure through these vessels illustrates this process (**Figure 3.16**). The large arteries near the heart have a great deal of elastic tissue, which enables them to fulfill their role of transmitting blood pressure from the heart as efficiently as possible, without any change in systolic or diastolic pressure. In progressively smaller vessels there is increasing resistance and progressively less elastic tissue; as a result the difference between systolic and diastolic pressure, i.e. the pulse pressure, narrows. At the level of the arterioles, there is almost no pulse pressure, just one constant blood pressure throughout systole and diastole. The role of the arterioles is to regulate downstream flow to capillaries and upstream blood pressure.

Total peripheral resistance

Total peripheral resistance is the sum of resistance generated by all elements of the systemic circulation. However, the circulations to different organs are effectively acting in parallel, so that a rise in the resistance of blood flow to one organ has relatively little effect on the total peripheral resistance: the main effect of such a rise is to shunt blood away from that organ and towards the others. Conversely, a reduction in the resistance of an organ, for example due to vasodilation in a working muscle, will tend to 'steal' blood from other organs.

As discussed on page 70, resistance is closely related to blood pressure and flow. Where resistance is increased, the pressure (and flow) downstream will decrease but the pressure upstream will increase (see **Figure 3.3**). For example, an increase in vascular resistance in the kidney will increase total peripheral resistance a little and reduce renal blood flow. The increase in total peripheral resistance will increase arterial pressure and consequently blood flow to all other tissues.

Arterioles are the vessels where blood pressure decreases most (**Figure 3.16**). The responsive nature of their vascular smooth muscle means that they are able to regulate their resistance and control blood pressure. They are termed the 'resistance vessels' for this reason. Arterioles regulate total peripheral resistance and arterial blood pressure.

Factors influencing arteriolar tone

There are a number of factors that influence arteriolar tone, which determines vascular resistance:

■ Contraction of the smooth muscle in the vessel wall causes vasoconstriction, i.e. a reduction in vessel diameter and consequently an increase in vascular resistance
■ Conversely, smooth muscle relaxation causes vasodilatation, an increase in vessel diameter which reduces vascular resistance

Endothelial substances

Endothelial cells release a number of factors that regulate arteriolar tone. The most important is nitric oxide (NO), which is released in response to shear stress. This is the force exerted by the movement of blood over the endothelium; it increases with high velocity, pressure or flow. It is important for maintenance of normal blood pressure. In the absence of NO, blood pressure would be extremely high, causing haemorrhages.

Nitric oxide is a small uncharged molecule, which means it can diffuse into the underlying smooth muscle cells where it activates guanylate cyclase leading to a sequence that results in muscle relaxation and vasodilatation (**Figure 3.17**). The endothelium also releases prostaglandins in response to shear stress, these have the same effect as NO.

The endothelium also responds to circulating factors. For example, hormones such as angiotensin II bind receptors on endothelial cells to stimulate release of secondary mediators that influence smooth muscle cells.

Autonomic innervation

The sympathetic nervous system (page 62) is of critical importance in maintaining and regulating arteriolar tone. If NO is the main factor causing vasodilatation, sympathetic noradrenaline is the main mechanism for vasoconstriction. Sympathetic nerves release noradrenaline, which can act at either:

■ α-adrenoreceptors, causing vasoconstriction and a rise in total peripheral resistance or
■ β-adrenoreceptors causing, vasodilation and thus increasing blood flow to the organ

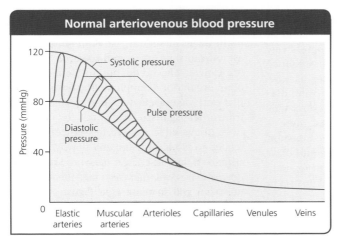

Normal arteriovenous blood pressure

Figure 3.16 The first vessels in the arterial tree, the elastic and muscular arteries, transmit blood pressure with minimal loss. Through the arterioles there is a great fall in blood pressure and the pulse pressure falls until it is eventually lost.

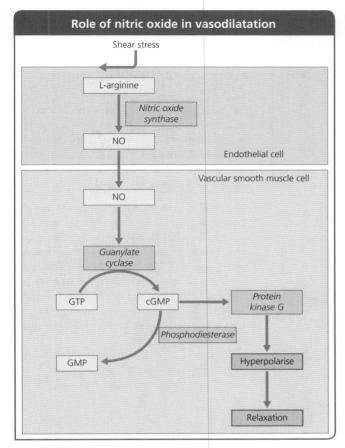

Figure 3.17 Nitric oxide is produced by nitric oxide synthase in endothelial cells in response to shear stress. NO is a small uncharged molecule and diffuses into muscle cells. It increases formation of cGMP by activating guanylate cyclase. Protein kinase G mediates changes that result in hyperpolarisation (which causes inactivation of MLCK and uptake of Ca^{2+} into the sarcoplasmic reticulum) and muscle relaxation, i.e. vasodilatation.

Binding of noradrenaline to α-adrenoreceptors is a key mechanism for control of local tissue blood flow and systemic blood pressure.

> **Vasopressor and inotropic drugs** are used to treat symptomatic low blood pressure and poor cardiac function. In the opposite way to antihypertensive drugs, vasopressor drugs such as noradrenaline promote arteriolar vasoconstriction to increase total peripheral resistance.
>
> Inotropic drugs such as dobutamine activate cardiac β-adrenoreceptors, increasing cardiac output.

Myogenic tone

The myogenic response of the vascular smooth muscle of arterioles is its propensity to contract in response to stretch caused by an increase in blood pressure. Consequently, a rise or fall in blood pressure is coupled to an increase or decrease in resistance, respectively, which limits the change in downstream blood flow. This holds true over a range of pressures, called the autoregulatory range (**Figure 3.18**).

If arterial blood pressure falls below the autoregulatory range the arterioles are already maximally dilated and tissue flow falls with falling mABP. Similarly, if mABP rises higher than the autoregulatory range, downstream flow will increase despite maximum myogenic vasoconstriction.

The arterioles of certain tissues have an especially prominent myogenic response. An example is cerebral arterioles, which reflects the importance of control of cerebral blood flow.

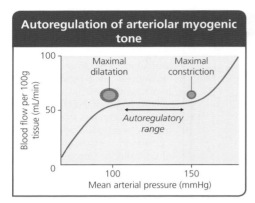

Autoregulation of arteriolar myogenic tone

Figure 3.18 Within the autoregulatory range a rise in pressure in the arterioles perfusing a tissue will cause reflex constriction, which increases resistance and maintains constant blood flow through the tissue.

> **Severe hypertension which exceeds the autoregulatory range of the cerebral arterioles may result in an intracerebral haemorrhage,** a bleed that occurs deep inside the brain and represents a form of stroke. Such hypertension can be caused, for example, by pre-eclampsia in pregnancy or by renal artery disease.

Metabolic hyperaemia

The matching of blood flow to the metabolic activity of a tissue is termed metabolic hyperaemia. The mechanistic details vary between organs, but the premise is the same: increased metabolic activity creates vasoactive factors that act on local arterioles to cause vasodilatation and an increase in flow into tissues. Examples of vasoactive factors include:

- low pH due to accumulation of CO_2 or lactic acid
- high adenosine released from contracting cardiac myocytes
- high K^+ due to release from muscles or nerves

The local, paracrine, action of the vasoactive mediators means that blood flow is directed to specifically to areas of activity and away from inactive tissues.

Other factors

Two important vasoconstrictors are antidiuretic hormone (ADH, also called vasopressin) and angiotensin-II. Both of these have major roles in osmoregulation and volume regulation (see page 152). Angiotensin-II and ADH are released in response to a fall in effective circulating volume (or blood pressure) and cause systemic vasoconstriction to increase total peripheral resistance, raising mean arterial blood pressure.

Serotonin, a potent vasoconstrictor which helps to reduce bleeding, is released when platelets become activated following tissue damage.

> **Anti-hypertensive drugs exploit** factors influencing myogenic tone in arteriolar smooth muscle. Calcium channel blockers (e.g. amlodipine) prevent Ca^{2+} entry needed for vascular smooth muscle contraction. α-Adrenoreceptor antagonists (e.g. doxazosin) are highly potent anti-hypertensives.

Microcirculation

The microcirculation consists of the smallest blood vessels, the capillaries, and the vessels that drain into and out of them. Capillaries arise from arterioles and form a capillary bed (a series of interconnecting channels through a tissue).

Structure and function

Movement of fluid and the exchange of substances between the blood plasma and the interstitial (intercellular) fluid occurs in the microcirculation. The smallest vessels in

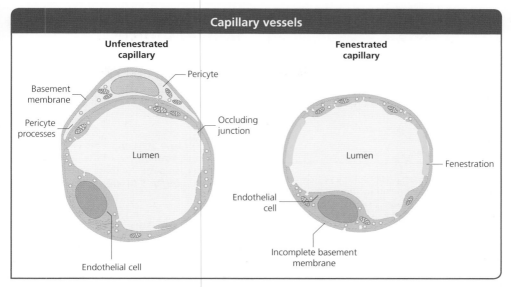

Figure 3.19 Unfenestrated capillaries have occluding junctions between endothelial cells and are associated with supporting pericytes that sit within the basement membrane. Fenestrations are made of double plasma membrane.

the circulatory system are capillaries (**Figure 3.19**), which consist of a single layer of endothelial cells supported by a basement membrane and occasional pericytes. The latter are supporting cells that can cause capillary contraction and increase the barrier between capillaries and tissues. They are only found on non-fenestrated capillaries. The endothelial cells are flattened and mostly very thin and they are joined by occluding junctions. This makes it relatively simple for molecules to diffuse through or between cells. In addition, there is extensive vesicular trafficking, which helps to move material across the endothelium in a process called transcytosis.

There are two types of capillary: unfenestrated (continuous) and fenestrated (**Figure 3.19**).

Fenestrated capillaries

In areas where a particularly high permeability to water and/or solute is required, fenestrated capillaries are found. Fenestrations are tunnels that pass completely though the endothelial cell and are lined with double plasma membrane that is continuous with the cell membrane. Fenestrations are closed by a thin diaphragm. In addition fenestrated vessels have relatively leaky occluding junctions and an incomplete basement membrane.

Fenestrated capillaries are found in the kidney, intestine, liver and spleen, as well as some exocrine glands and the choroid plexus. A specialised form – sinusoidal or discontinuous capillaries – is found in the liver and spleen. These have larger fenestrations and the gaps between cells are much wider than other fenestrated capillaries.

Flow through capillary beds

Due to their large total cross-sectional area the blood velocity in capillaries is very low and they are only just large enough to admit one erythrocyte (red blood cell) at a time.

Arteriolar vasoconstriction causes a reduction in hydrostatic pressure downstream and at the arteriole's opening into the capillary bed. This is combined with contraction of precapillary sphincters to cause an erythrocyte to impact at the capillary opening such that flow through that capillary ceases (**Figure 3.20**). In this way capillary beds are described as 'open' or 'closed'; at any one time many capillary beds are closed. Blood flow to the tissue

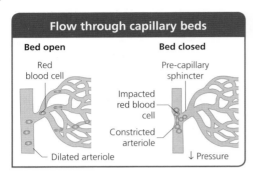

Flow through capillary beds

Bed open	Bed closed
Red blood cell	Pre-capillary sphincter
	Impacted red blood cell
	Constricted arteriole
Dilated arteriole	↓ Pressure

Figure 3.20 Vasoconstriction of the pre-capillary arteriole, coupled with contraction of pre-capillary sphincter, causes a fall in pressure at the opening of the capillary bed. A red blood cell impacts at the opening and closes the capillary bed.

increases, in response to the production of local vasodilators, by opening of more capillaries. If all capillaries were perfused at once then blood pressure would fall dramatically, as happens in septic shock.

Diffusion of solutes

Substances in solution, for example O_2, CO_2, glucose and lipids, move into tissues by diffusion. Fick's law describes the factors associated with the rate of diffusion:

$$\text{Rate of diffusion} \propto \frac{\text{concentration gradient} \times \text{surface area} \times \text{permeability}}{\text{thickness}}$$

The concentration gradient is influenced by the metabolic activity of the tissue. A more active tissue uses glucose and O_2 and produces CO_2 at a higher rate, increasing the gradient for diffusion.

The surface area available for diffusion is influenced by the number of capillary beds open. Arteriolar vasodilatation and opening of capillaries increases the available surface area and rate of diffusion.

The thickness and permeability of a given capillary remains constant. Fenestrated capillaries have a higher diffusion rate than continuous ones for this reason.

Movement of fluid: Starling's forces

Movement of fluid across the capillary wall is determined by the balance of hydrostatic and osmotic forces. These are termed Starling forces.

> Don't confuse Starling forces with the Frank–Starling law of the heart discussed on page 79: these are the same Starling but different principles.

Hydrostatic pressure
The hydrostatic pressure is what we normally think of as the blood pressure. Because the fluid is being pumped, it is at a higher pressure than the surrounding tissue. Hydrostatic pressures are indicated by P.

> **Oedema,** swelling due to accumulation of fluid in the soft tissues, occurs as a result of a shift in the balance of Starling's forces. For example, patients with right-sided cardiac failure have raised venous pressure, which reduces fluid reabsorption at the venous end of capillaries therefore these patients develop ankle oedema.

Osmotic pressure
Osmotic pressure is generated by a concentration gradient: if there is a higher solute concentration in one solution than another, water will be 'drawn' towards the concentrated solution. Alternatively, you can think of the water concentration being lower in one solution, and water flowing down its concentration gradient.

Many solutes move fairly freely across the capillary wall and will exert little osmotic pressure because they fully equilibrate.

Oncotic pressure
Oncotic pressure is the osmotic pressure exerted by solutes that are unable to cross

the capillary wall and so are trapped inside the capillary. The primary contributors to oncotic pressure are plasma proteins. Thus oncotic pressure is much higher inside the capillary than outside it, providing a force that counterbalances the hydrostatic pressure. Oncotic pressures are indicated by Π (see below).

Relationship between hydrostatic and oncotic pressure

In the microcirculation, there is a hydrostatic pressure for the capillary (P_{cap}) and tissue space (P_{TS}), and an oncotic pressure for each of them (Π_{cap} and Π_{TS}, respectively). P_{TS} is usually very low; also there should be virtually no plasma protein in the tissue space, so Π_{TS} should be almost zero. Consequently, under physiological conditions, fluid movement across the capillary wall is primarily dependent on the balance of P_{cap} and Π_{cap}. Fluid movement can be summarised as:

$$\frac{\text{Tissue fluid}}{\text{formation}} \propto (P_{cap} + \Pi_{TS}) - (\Pi_{cap} + P_{TS})$$

The effect of this along the length of an arteriole is shown in **Figure 3.21**. At the arterial end of the capillary P_{cap} is greater that Π_{cap}, so fluid moves out into the tissue space.

However, resistance along the length of the capillary causes a fall in P_{cap}, so that by the venous end Π_{cap} is greater that P_{cap} and fluid is reabsorbed from the tissue space. As a consequence, there is a constant turnover of interstitial fluid but, under normal circumstances, little or no net fluid accumulation.

The movement of fluid out of the arterial end of the capillary and into the tissue concentrates plasma proteins, and causes a rise in Π_{cap}. In most capillaries this is a small rise which is unlikely to play the main role in fluid reabsorption. However, as discussed on page 137, when a large volume is filtered at the glomerular capillaries the changes in oncotic pressure are more marked.

Arteriolar vasodilatation increases P_{cap} and therefore shifts the balance of Starling's forces for the entire length of the capillary towards tissue fluid formation.

> **Cellulitis** causes oedema by a completely different mechanism: increased capillary permeability, promotes leakage of proteins out of the capillary, which reduces capillary oncotic pressure. As a result less fluid is reabsorbed at the venous end of capillaries, resulting in a build up of tissue fluid.

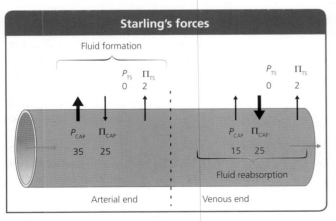

Figure 3.21 Starling's forces along the length of a capillary. Tissue fluid is formed at the arterial end and reabsorbed at the venous end as hydrostatic pressure falls.

Starling's forces

Fluid formation

| P_{TS} | Π_{TS} |
| 0 | 2 |

| P_{TS} | Π_{TS} |
| 0 | 2 |

| P_{CAP} | Π_{CAP} |
| 35 | 25 |

| P_{CAP} | Π_{CAP} |
| 15 | 25 |

Fluid reabsorption

Arterial end   Venous end

Lymphatic vessels

Capillaries reabsorb most but not all of the fluid formed in tissues. Approximately 4 litres/day passes into the lymphatic system, a series of low-pressure vessels with valves (similar to the structure of veins) that transport fluid, lipids and immune cells back into the circulation via the thoracic ducts (large lymphatic ducts that empty into subclavian veins).

> **Lymphatic vessels and lymph nodes are a common site for early metastasis in cancer.** As part of surgical resection, lymphatic vessels draining the tumour bed may be removed. When axillary lymph nodes are removed during breast cancer surgery, lymphoedema, a build-up of tissue fluid with swelling of the affected limb, may occur post-operatively.

Small lymphatic capillaries are found in every tissue. These are small vessels lined by a single layer of endothelium. This has pores through which fluid drains from the tissue space into the capillaries. The fluid is then known as lymph, and will only pass in one direction: back towards the heart. From the lymphatic capillaries the excess tissue fluid drains into progressively larger lymphatic vessels that ultimately re-join the circulation (**Figure 3.22**).

The lymphatic system has a vital immune role. It facilitates movement of white blood cells from the tissues into lymph nodes and the spleen. Additionally, the porous nature of lymphatic capillaries allows them to assist in uptake of proteins and tissue debris for immune activation.

Lymphatic vessels (lacteals) are also necessary for absorption of lipids from the gut, as discussed in Chapter 7.

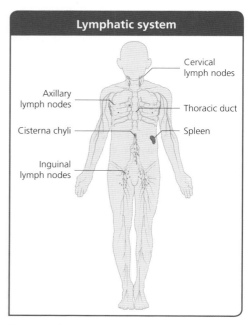

Figure 3.22. The major groups of lymph nodes, lymphatic channels and spleen are illustrated. The cisterna chyli is an enlarged lymphatic channel underneath the diaphragm. The spleen is part of the lymphatic system; immune cells reach it from the blood.

Veins

Structure and function

Veins carry blood from the peripheries back to the heart. They have a larger diameter than arteries and consequently contain more of the total blood volume. Venous pressure is much lower than arterial pressure, so there are additional mechanisms in place to maintain flow back towards the heart. Many veins contain valves, which are formed of folds of tunica intima and prevent retrograde flow. The valves act in conjunction with the other mechanisms described below.

The walls of veins contain less smooth muscle than arteries, minimal elastin and much more collagenous tissue. Veins are highly compliant; however at high volumes their collagen becomes taught and their compliance falls. Contraction of venous smooth muscle (venoconstriction) reduces their compliance and increases their hydrostatic pressure.

> **Varicose veins are dilated, tortuous vessels in the lower limbs** characterised by incompetent valves and inefficient flow. When valves cease to function normally, blood pools in the leg veins and the skeletal muscle pump is unable to effectively promote flow back to the heart. Persistently pooled blood gives rise to the features of chronic venous stasis: eczema, oedema and ulcers.

Flow through veins

A number of mechanisms influence flow of blood through the veins, and hence influence venous pressure:

- **Skeletal muscle pump**: contraction of skeletal muscles causes compression of adjacent veins and forces the blood to flow back towards the heart, with retrograde flow prevented by valves (**Figure 3.23**)
- **Respiratory pump**: during inspiration there is negative pressure generated inside the thorax due to the diaphragm flattening and descending, with increased intra-abdominal pressure; these help to draw blood back from the abdomen into the thoracic veins and then into the heart
- **Venoconstriction**: contraction of smooth muscle raises venous hydrostatic pressure and helps maintain flow
- **Posture**: flow in veins is greatly affected by gravity due to the weight of a standing column of blood. During standing, blood

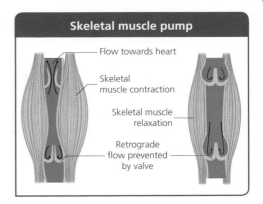

Skeletal muscle pump

Flow towards heart

Skeletal muscle contraction

Skeletal muscle relaxation

Retrograde flow prevented by valve

Figure 3.23 Contraction of skeletal muscle causes compression of adjacent veins. In the presence of valves, retrograde flow is prevented and blood moves towards the heart.

pools in the veins of the legs and there is heavy reliance upon the skeletal muscle pump for return flow to the heart

Central venous pressure

Central venous pressure is the pressure in the systemic veins closest to the heart, i.e. the superior and inferior vena cavae. It is an important determinant of cardiac output, being the main factor that controls end-diastolic volume and, according to the Frank–Starling law, stroke volume (see page 79).

All of the components previously described as influencing venous pressure make a contribution to CVP. Additionally, blood volume is key: veins contain over 60% of the blood volume and yet, because their walls are inelastic and highly compliant, at low volume venous hydrostatic pressure is low, e.g. 5 mmHg (in contrast to arterial pressure of 90 mmHg).

Coronary circulation

Structure

The tissues of the heart receive their blood supply from the coronary arteries. These are the first branches of the ascending aorta. They arise immediately superior to the aortic

valve, from the aortic sinuses. These sinuses are bulges in the aortic wall that help encourage flow into the arteries when the aortic valve is closed, i.e. during diastole.

The heart is supplied by the right and left coronary arteries (**Table 3.2**). The left coronary

Cardiac blood supply	
	Supplying vessel
Right ventricle	Right coronary artery
Anterior interventricular septum	Anterior interventricular artery (from left coronary artery)
Lateral left ventricle	Left circumflex artery (from left coronary artery)
Posterior interventricular septum	Right coronary artery

Table 3.2 Blood supply to the ventricular muscle

artery divides into the left circumflex and anterior interventricular artery, which anastomoses with the posterior interventricular artery.

> Knowledge of the areas of myocardium supplied by each coronary vessel is important for interpreting ECGs and predicting the affected vessel. The atria are supplied by small branches of the coronary arteries, but atrial ischaemia has less impact on cardiac output than does ventricular ischaemia, so it is more important to learn ventricular supply in detail.

The coronary vessels give rise to smaller branching arteries and arterioles that perforate the myocardium to supply the cardiac tissue.

Coronary flow during the cardiac cycle

As the coronary branches run through the myocardium they are subject to the transmural pressure generated by systole. The left ventricular pressure rises to approximately 120 mmHg during systole, and the innermost (subendocardial) myocardium is subject to this pressure. This exceeds the systolic pressure in the artery, so the subendocardial myocardium is not perfused during systole because the arterioles are completely occluded.

The outermost (subepicardial) myocardium immediately beneath the epicardium is subject to a lower transmural pressure, so some perfusion occurs during systole.

Left coronary artery flow

A plot of left coronary artery flow during the cardiac cycle shows that most flow occurs during diastole (**Figure 3.24**). Left ventricular myocardial blood flow is lowest during the isovolumetric phases of systole because left ventricular pressure is high but coronary flow is low. Flow increases during systole as coronary artery pressure rises, but is minimal compared to the blood delivered during diastole.

Right coronary artery flow

Because the tension in the wall of the right ventricle is much lower than in the left, perfusion of the right ventricle is more equally divided between systole and diastole.

Metabolic hyperaemia (functional hyperaemia)

Hyperaemia is an increase in blood flow. Metabolic hyperaemia is an increase that occurs in normal circumstances (reactive hyperaemia occurs after a pathological reduction in flow).

The myocardium has a very high energy demand. It is only able to perform aerobic, not anaerobic, metabolism and normal activity extracts almost all the oxygen supplied by the coronary circulation. Therefore an increase in cardiac work must be coupled with an increase

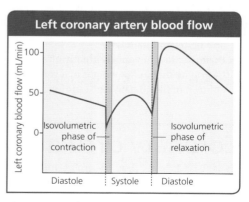

Figure 3.24 Left coronary artery blood flow through the cardiac cycle. Almost all flow is delivered during diastole, with the lowest flow occurring during the isovolumetric phases.

in coronary blood flow to provide the necessary increase in oxygen supply. Cardiac work increases with rises in HR, SV or TPR.

$$\text{Cardiac work} \propto \text{HR} \times \text{SV} \times \text{TPR}$$

However, a rise in cardiac work is potentially associated with a reduction in coronary blood flow. This is because as the heart rate rises diastole shortens more than systole, which limits the time for coronary flow. Furthermore, an increase in stroke volume or total peripheral resistance is associated with a rise in ventricular pressure, further compromising the coronary flow.

The myocardium uses metabolic hyperaemia to increase its blood supply when needed. Hypoxia stimulates upregulation of 5' nucleotidase (5'NT), which catalyses formation of adenosine from 5' AMP (**Figure 3.25**). Adenosine causes vasodilatation of coronary arterioles, increasing flow to match demand.

> **Angina is a manifestation of sublethal cardiac ischaemia usually** caused by build-up of fatty plaques in the coronary vessels (coronary atherosclerosis). When cardiac work increases on exertion, despite maximum dilatation from adenosine release, limited blood flow results in myocardial ischaemic, causing chest pain. Anti-angina drugs causing NO release provide initial symptomatic relief through vasodilation increasing perfusion (see **Figure 3.17**) and venodilation reducing cardiac work.

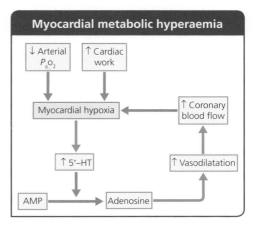

Figure 3.25 Myocardial metabolic hyperaemia is mediated by hypoxia-induced upregulation of 5' nucleotidase (5' NT), which increases production of the vasodilator adenosine.

Blood pressure

Factors that influence arterial blood pressure

This is usually described by giving both the maximal and the minimal pressures reached during the cardiac cycle:

- systolic blood pressure (SBP) is the maximum pressure reached in the aorta during systole

- diastolic blood pressure (DBP) is the minimum pressure in the aorta; it occurs at the end of diastole, just before the aortic valve opens for the next cycle (**Figure 3.26**).

When the left ventricle contracts, up to 60% of the force of each stroke volume is directed against the walls of the elastic arteries and stretches them. As stretching of the aorta is the main determinant of SBP (see below),

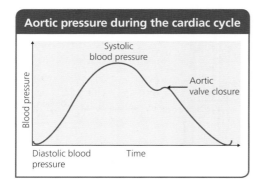

Aortic pressure during the cardiac cycle

Systolic blood pressure

Aortic valve closure

Blood pressure

Diastolic blood pressure

Time

Figure 3.26 . The minimum pressure, at the opening of the aortic valve, is diastolic pressure. The maximum pressure reached is systolic pressure. Valve closure causes a small increase in pressure during diastole.

stroke volume is the most important cardiac factor determining SBP.

In contrast, diastolic blood pressure is influenced by two factors: heart rate and total peripheral resistance:

- A rise in heart rate shortens diastole; this reduces the time for blood to flow out of the aorta and for aortic pressure to fall, therefore the aortic pressure (i.e. DBP) is higher when the aortic valve opens for the next cycle.
- Increasing total peripheral resistance slows the rate of outflow from the aorta, therefore raising DBP

Mean arterial blood pressure (mABP)

mABP is closer to diastolic blood pressure because around two-thirds of the cardiac cycle is diastole. For this reason, it is calculated as:

$$mABP = DBP + (SBP/3)$$

Baroreflex

Mean arterial blood pressure is tightly controlled by the baroreflex to ensure normal body function. It operates as a classic homeostatic feedback loop (see page 29).

Mechanoreceptors

Systemic arterial blood pressure is measured by mechanoreceptors in the wall of the carotid sinus, a dilated area at the bifurcation of the common carotid artery, and the aortic arch. These respond to both the absolute blood pressure and to the rate of change of pressure.

The mechanoreceptors are activated by stretch in the vessel walls, i.e. by an increase in blood pressure. This stimulates increased activity in their afferent nerves: cranial nerves XI (glossopharyngeal) for the carotid sinus and X (vagus) for the aortic arch.

Neural integration and output

The afferents pass to the nucleus tractus solitarius in the medulla oblongata. This nucleus provides an excitatory output to the nucleus ambiguus, the main nucleus for the vagus and an inhibitory output to the sympathetic nuclei. The effect is to

- increase parasympathetic stimulation of the heart, reducing heart rate (reduction below 60 bpm is defined as bradycardia), and
- reduce sympathetic activity in the circulatory system, resulting in vasodilation and a drop in total peripheral resistance

In addition, the nucleus tractus solitarius communicates with the paraventricular and supra-optic nuclei, which release antidiuretic hormone (ADH). In the presence of increased activity in the nucleus tractus solitarius, ADH secretion falls and this causes a drop in circulating volume as described on pages 000.

Response to a fall in blood pressure

A fall in arterial blood pressure is detected by carotid and aortic mechanoreceptors, which reduce the frequency of their action potentials in response to reduced stimulation.

In addition, low-pressure baroreceptors in the atria and pulmonary circulation play a role if the drop in blood pressure is due to hypovolaemia. The reduction in activity of the nucleus tractus solitarius results in a number of outputs that act to raised blood pressure:

- A fall in the vagal output to the heart, raising heart rate
- A reduction in the inhibition of sympathetic output: consequently, total peripheral resistance increases due to systemic vasoconstriction (particularly in the skin, gut, kidney and skeletal muscle), stroke volume increases due raised ventricular contractility and heart rate rises
- An increase in ADH synthesis from the hypothalamus and its subsequent release from the posterior pituitary gland, which causes systemic vasoconstriction and water reabsorption, which help to counter hypotension
- Sympathetic signalling to the kidney, which stimulates the renin–angiotensin–aldosterone system (RAAS), which acts to raise blood volume and vasoconstricts using Ang-II (the RAAS is discussed in detail in Chapter 5)

These mechanisms together increase stroke volume, heart rate and total peripheral resistance – the determinants of blood pressure.

> **Vasovagal syncope (fainting) occurs in response to some strong emotional stimuli, or forceful ventricular contraction on low end-diastolic volume.** This is a neuro-cardiovascular reflex that causes an abrupt increase in parasympathetic activity and reduction in sympathetic activity, decreasing blood pressure below the brain's autoregulatory range. This precipitates transient loss of consciousness (syncope); the patient recovers rapidly when heart rate increases and blood flow to the brain is restored.

Blood cells and the immune system

Composition of blood

Blood volume in a healthy adult is approximately 5 litres (80 mL/kg), of which roughly half is cells and half is fluid.

The cellular components

This consists of:

- red blood cells (also called RBCs, red cells and erythrocytes)
- white blood cells (also called WBCs, white cells and leukocytes) and
- platelets

The fraction of the blood composed of RBCs is called the haematocrit. This is almost the same as the cellular fraction, because WBCs and platelets together comprise less than 1% of the cellular fraction.

All blood cells are formed in the bone marrow from haematopoietic stem cells in a process termed haematopoiesis or haemopoiesis (**Figure 3.27**). These stem cells first differentiate into either myeloid or lymphoid progenitors (stem cells), which then continue to differentiate to produce the specialised cells discussed in this chapter.

The liquid component

Plasma is the fluid in which the blood cells are suspended. It is formed of:

- Water
- Solutes such as glucose, Na^+, Cl^-
- Lipids and other insoluble particles, and
- Plasma proteins such as albumin
- Clotting factors (substances that promote clotting – see page 96)

If blood is allowed to clot, the fluid that remains is called serum. This has a composition very similar to plasma but lacks clotting factors.

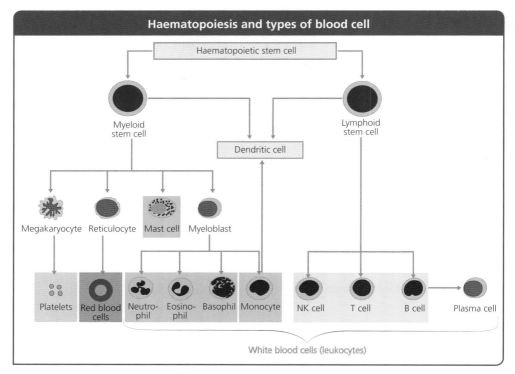

Figure 3.27 Differentiation of haematopoietic stem cells.

Red blood cells

RBCs facilitate gas transport around the body. Gas transport is discussed in Chapter 4 (page 115).

Structure and function

RBCs originate from common myeloid stem cells, which differentiate into erythroid progenitor cells, which mature as erythroblasts then normocytes into fully differentiated erythrocytes (RBCs). This process is accelerated by erythropoietin (EPO), a peptide hormone released from renal tubular cells in response to hypoxia. During maturation RBCs lose their nuclei and mitochondria and take up a characteristic biconcave, discoid shape. This gives them a large surface area for gas exchange and also makes them flexible, allowing them to pass through capillaries.

RBCs contain a high concentration of haemoglobin (see page 120): each RBC carries around one billion oxygen molecules. They also contain carbonic anhydrase, which is crucial for CO_2 carriage by converting it to bicarbonate (see page 122).

Red cells have a lifespan in the circulation of about 120 days.

Blood groups

On their surface, RBCs express antigens, molecules against which an immune response can be mounted; it is these that define the blood groups. Infusion of cells carrying unmatched antigens leads to a transfusion reaction, as the immune system recognises the blood as foreign and attacks it. Clinically the most significant blood group system is the ABO system (**Table 3.3**). A patient produces antibodies against antigens that she doesn't express. Thus a person with type O blood is a universal donor: donated type O blood will not normally provoke a response in anyone because it lacks both antigen A and antigen B. In contrast, a person with type AB blood produces neither type of antibody and is therefore a universal recipient.

ABO blood groups			
Blood group	Antigens present on RBC	Antibodies present in serum	Blood that can be received safely
O (universal donor)	Nil	Anti-A, and anti-B	Any (O, A, B, or AB)
A	A-antigen	Anti-B	A or O
B	B-antigen	Anti-A	B or O
AB (universal recipient)	A-antigen, and B-antigen	Nil	A, B, AB, or O

Table 3.3 The ABO blood group system

There are more than 40 other red cell antigens that can cause reactions but they do so more rarely than AB antigens. One notable example is the Rhesus antigen, which is the next most common cause of blood-group reactions. Normally this does not provoke a reaction the first time it is given, but a Rhesus-negative patient who is given Rhesus-positive blood will develop an immune response and thus react strongly against a subsequent Rhesus-positive transfusion.

> A Rhesus-negative woman carrying a Rhesus-positive baby may produce anti-Rhesus antibodies if their blood mixes during delivery. In subsequent pregnancies with Rhesus-positive babies, rapid anti-Rhesus response produces antibodies which cross the placenta into the fetus causing haemolysis, leading to jaundice and, if untreated, brain damage and potentially death of the fetus.

Platelets and haemostasis

Haemostasis is the process of stopping blood loss from damaged vessels. It is achieved by:

- Aggregation of platelets (see **Figure 3.27**), which form a mass that acts as a physical barrier to blood loss, and
- Coagulation, i.e. clotting, of blood via activation of the coagulation cascade

Haemostasis occurs in both arterial and venous vessels:

- **Thrombosis** generally refers to events that stop arterial bleeding in a high-pressure,

high-flow setting; this is usually initiated by platelet aggregation
- **Coagulation** is cessation of venous bleeding in a low-pressure, low-flow setting, which is predominantly dependent on clotting factors.

Thrombosis and coagulation both ultimately result in the formation of a thrombus. A thrombus is a solid piece of material in a vessel, arterial or venous. It is formed of platelets, dead cells and insoluble fibrin, a protein that cross links to make a mesh that partially or completely occludes blood vessels.

> If part of a thrombus breaks away and travels in the blood stream it is called a **thromboembolus,** an embolus being a solid piece of material traveling in the circulation. The most common type is a venous thromboembolism, where part of a clot from a deep vein in the pelvis breaks off and travels to the lungs, where it causes infarction of lung tissue.

Platelet structure and function

Platelets are anuclear fragments of cells that bud-off megakaryocytes (large, multinucleate, myeloid-derived cells; see **Figure 3.27**) in the bone marrow. Platelets are continuously produced in the bone marrow; they persist in the blood for only about 10–12 days. Their primary function is haemostasis, but they are also involved in pathological inflammation.

Platelets contain three types of granules:

- α-granules contain a range of clotting factors

- Dense granules contain ATP, ADP, serotonin (a potent vasoconstrictor), and Ca^{2+}
- Glycogen granules

A glycoprotein (GpIb) is constitutively expressed on the surface of platelets (see below).

Platelet aggregation and thrombosis

Platelet aggregation is initiated by damage to the endothelium, which exposes the underlying extracellular matrix. A constitutively produced circulating protein, von Willebrand factor (vWF) binds to the collagen of the extracellular matrix, which then forms a bond with the constitutively expressed GpIb on the surface of platelets (**Figure 3.28**). When vWF binds to GpIb they are activated; this results in translocation of glycoprotein IIb/IIIa (GpIIb/IIIa) to the platelet surface (GpIIb/IIIa is a complex formed from glycoproteins IIb and IIIa). Platelets then make strong bonds with each other between GpIIb/IIIa and vWF, which binds platelets together. This process continues, with an expanding aggregate of platelets.

Coagulation of clotting factors (see below) helps bind the platelets together and in combination 'plug' or seal over the damaged area, achieving haemostasis. The processes of platelet activation and coagulation occur simultaneously.

Platelet activation

There are several factors that activate platelets by binding to them and promoting aggregation:

- Adenosine diphosphate (ADP)
- Thrombin, an enzyme activated by the coagulation system (see below)
- Calcium
- Thromboxane A_2, a lipid signalling molecule

Upon activation the platelets degranulate, i.e. release the contents of their granules. These promote platelet aggregation and activation of the coagulation cascade and augment certain inflammatory responses.

Coagulation system

The coagulation system is a group of soluble clotting factors in circulation that, when activated, trigger a cascade of reactions that ultimately results in the formation of a mesh of insoluble fibrin, i.e. a clot to seal damaged vessels (**Figure 3.29**). Each of the clotting factors is a pro-enzyme, i.e. a precursor molecule that becomes an active enzyme when part of the molecule is cleaved. In the cascade, active enzymes are indicated by 'a', e.g. factor Xa (FXa) is the active form of factor X (FX).

All the clotting factors have a short half-life and are synthesised in the liver. Several (FII, FVII, FIX, and FX) require vitamin K for their production. The reactions of the coagulation system often take place on the surface of platelets and require Ca^{2+} as a co-factor.

The coagulation system is divided into 'extrinsic' and 'intrinsic' pathways, depending on the method of initiation, as described below.

The extrinsic pathway

This is triggered by endothelial damage, which exposes underlying tissue factor (TF).

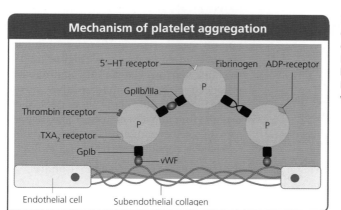

Figure 3.28 Platelets constitutively express GpIb on their surface, but once activated they express GpIIb/IIIa, which mediates strong bonds between them. Gp, glycoprotein; P, platelet; TXA$_2$, thromboxane; vWF, von Willebrand factor.

Mechanism of platelet aggregation

5'–HT receptor
Fibrinogen   ADP-receptor
GpIIb/IIIa
Thrombin receptor
TXA$_2$ receptor
GpIb
vWF
Endothelial cell
Subendothelial collagen

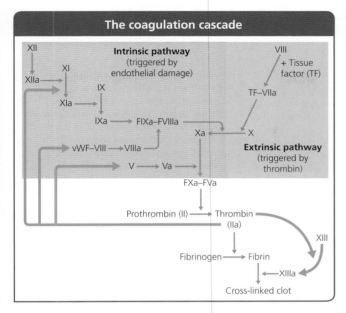

Figure 3.29 Activation of the coagulation of clotting cascade occurs via the extrinsic or intrinsic pathways, but both converge on generation of thrombin, which forms an insoluble fibrin mesh.

Factor VII (FVII) binds to tissue factor, activating factor VII to FVIIa-TF; this complex is then able to activate FX, which associates with its co-factor, FV, to form FXa-FVa (a small amount of active FV is present spontaneously). FXa-FVa converts prothrombin (FII) into thrombin (FIIa), which cleaves soluble, circulating fibrinogen (a soluble precursor of fibrin) into insoluble fibrin.

The small amount of thrombin generated by the extrinsic pathway is insufficient to result in formation of a full fibrin clot. Instead, it triggers the intrinsic pathway to do this (see below). The thrombin initially produced by the extrinsic pathway has four main actions:

- Activation of FV
- Activation of FVIII (by cleavage from circulating FVII–vWF complexes)
- Activation of FXI
- Activation of platelets

The extrinsic pathway is rapidly terminated by the extrinsic pathway inhibitor (EPI) that blocks activation of FX by FVIIa-TF.

The intrinsic pathway

This is triggered by thrombin generated by the extrinsic pathway or from platelet degranulation. FIXa–FVIIIa complexes activate FX, which is able to generate large amounts of thrombin and therefore a fibrin mesh or clot is formed.

Thrombolysis (fibrinolysis)

Thrombolysis is the process of cleaving insoluble fibrin into soluble degradation products, to remove clots (**Figure 3.30**). This cleavage is mediated by plasmin, which circulates as inactive plasminogen and is activated by tissue plasminogen activator (tPA). The source of tPA is intact (undamaged) endothelial cells, which release it in response to the presence of thrombin.

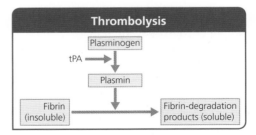

Figure 3.30 Mechanism of thrombolysis: plasmin breaks down insoluble fibrin into soluble degradation products. tPA, tissue plasminogen activator.

This limits thrombus enlargement and also helps the thrombus to be broken down once the causative damage has been repaired.

> **Thrombolysis is used therapeutically in the treatment of ischaemic stroke and myocardial infarction,** by administration of synthetic ('recombinant') tPA to reopen blocked vessels. It carries the risk of worsening bleeding if thrombus is covering a vascular defect. A CT of the head is done before giving tPA to check for appearances suggestive of haemorrhagic stroke.

Anti-coagulation systems

The body has several systems to prevent unnecessary activation of the coagulation cascade:

- **The antithrombins** (e.g. antithrombin III) inhibit thrombin and other active clotting factors, blocking progression of the cascade.
- **The anticoagulant heparin** works by activating antithrombin III, making it rapidly effective.
- **The protein C system** is an anti-coagulant complex of proteins (**Figure 3.31**). In response to the presence of thrombin, thrombomodulin is expressed on the surface of intact endothelial cells. Circulating protein C and its cofactor

protein S bind to thrombomodulin and break down FVa and FVIIIa.

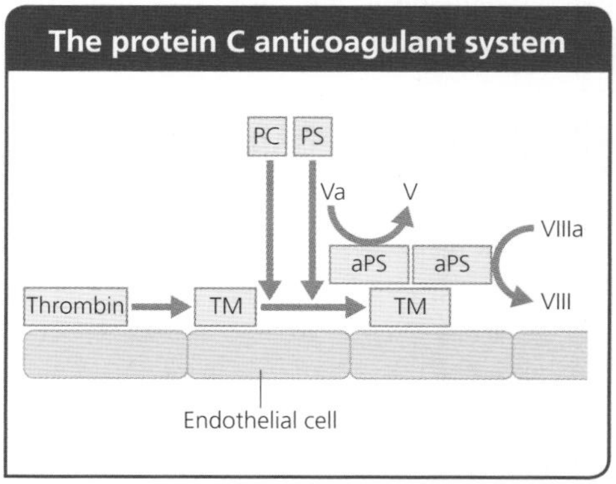

> The anticoagulant drug warfarin antagonises the effects of vitamin K, preventing the formation of clotting factors. The onset of warfarin coagulation is much slower (2–3 days) than heparin anticoagulation (<12 hours). Over-anticoagulation has serious clinical consequences due to spontaneous bleeding (e.g. **Figure 3.32**).

> Qualitative or quantitative defects in platelets or clotting factors result in increased tendency to bleed (haemophilia) or propensity to clotting (thrombophilia). Hereditary examples include haemophilia A (due to FVIIIa deficiency) and increased venous thromboembolism in protein C deficiency (due to excess active FVa and FVIIIa).

White blood cells and the immune response

White blood cells, also called leukocytes, are derived from both the myeloid and lymphoid

The protein C anticoagulant system

Figure 3.31 When protein C (PC) and S (PS) bind to thrombomodulin (TM) on intact endothelial cells, they inactivate active FVa and FVIIIa.

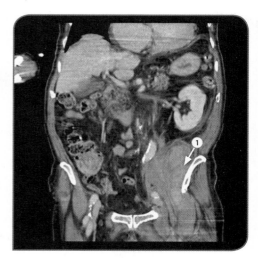

Figure 3.32 CT of the abdomen showing an enormous haematoma ① in psoas major muscle. This man was over-anticoagulated with warfarin and spontaneously bled into the muscle.

lineages. They play various roles in the body's immune responses:

- **The innate immune response**: derivatives of myeloid stem cells are generally involved in the innate immune response, which provides non-specific defence against infection (sometimes called natural immunity)
- **The adaptive immune response**: derivatives of lymphoid stem cells (lymphocytes) co-ordinate the adaptive immune response, which develops in response to an infection and provides defence specific to that pathogen (sometimes called acquired immunity)

Complement system

Complement molecules are soluble pro-enzymes involved in the response to foreign or 'non-self' molecules. The complement system is a cascade of reactions that produces a number of different complement molecules that have roles in both the innate and adaptive immune responses. The complement cascade is activated in three ways (see **Figure 3.33**):

- it is initiated by generic pathogenic bacterial markers, as part of the innate immune response: the **alternative pathway**
- it is initiated by immunoglobulin from the adaptive response: the **classical pathway**
- it is initiated by mannose (a bacterial pathogenic molecule): the **mannose-binding lectin pathway**

Activation triggers a series of cleavage reactions (**Figure 3.33**) The result is formation of proteins, some of which are enzymes, that help to attract neutrophils, activate mast cells, and kill bacteria (**Table 3.4**).

Macrophages

These are myeloid cells that circulate in the blood as monocytes but become macrophages when resident in tissue. They are phagocytic cells that engulf and destroy foreign cells, such as bacteria, as well as fragments of the body's own cells.

> **Macrophages are implicated in a wide range of conditions, including rheumatoid arthritis, malignancy and atherosclerosis. They drive an inflammatory response that promotes damage to cartilage in rheumatoid arthritis. They secrete pro-growth cytokines in cancer. And they take up fat and damage artery walls in atherosclerosis.**

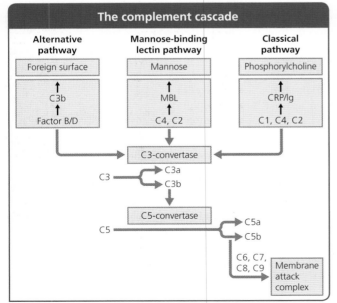

The complement cascade

Alternative pathway	Mannose-binding lectin pathway	Classical pathway
Foreign surface	Mannose	Phosphorylcholine
↑ C3b ↑ Factor B/D	↑ MBL ↑ C4, C2	↑ CRP/Ig ↑ C1, C4, C2

C3-convertase

C3 → C3a / C3b

C5-convertase

C5 → C5a / C5b

C6, C7, C8, C9 → Membrane attack complex

Figure 3.33 In the complement cascade, a series of proteins undergo successive cleavage to generate several protein complexes (complement molecules) that have antibacterial functions.

Functions of complement		
Function	Description	Mechanism
Opsonisation	Increases the ability of phagocytic cells to engulf bacterial pathogens	C3b binds to 'foreign' surfaces, which activates complement receptors (CR1) on phagocytes
Neutrophil chemotaxis	Attracts neutrophils to site of bacterial entry	Neutrophils migrate along a concentration gradient of C5a
Mast cell degranulation	Releases inflammatory mediators from mast cells (see page 101)	C5a binds to receptors on mast cells
Membrane attack complex (MAC)	MAC inserts into bacterial membranes causing their lysis	C5b and C6-9 form a complex that directly damages or kills bacteria

Table 3.4 Functions of complement

Role in innate immunity

Macrophages become activated when they recognised foreign molecules – antigens – on bacteria. They then secrete a number of cytokines that augment (enhance) the innate immune response. Amongst their other effects (**Table 3.5**), cytokines attract neutrophils to the site of infection. In most bacterial infections the majority of the killing of pathogens is mediated by neutrophils (see below), though macrophages are able to phagocytose and kill bacteria themselves. Any cell that can phagocytose is a phagocyte; this term encompasses macrophages, antigen-presenting cells (dendritic cells) and neutrophils.

Role in antigen processing

Macrophages process antigens from bacterial material they have phagocytosed. They then 'present' the processed antigens to CD4$^+$ T cells (described later), to mediate an adaptive immune response against bacteria. This process is needed to produce high-affinity antibody, i.e. antibody directed against specific bacterial pathogens.

The reticuloendothelial system and red cell destruction

Monocytes and macrophages are the principal cells of the mononuclear phagocyte system, also called the reticuloendothelial system. As well as circulating in the blood, they are resident in many tissues. In the spleen, liver and bone marrow they play a role in phagocytosis and destruction of effete

Acute-phase cytokines	
Cytokine	Function
IL-1	Pyrogen that acts on the hypothalamus to induce fever
IL-6	Acts on the liver to increase synthesis of acute phase proteins (C-reactive protein, MBL and ferritin)
IL-8	Chemotactic factor for neutrophils
TNF-α	Increases leukocyte adhesion to endothelium, raises capillary permeability, chemoattractant for macrophages

Table 3.5 Cytokines released by activated macrophages

(worn out) red blood cells and the recycling of haemoglobin.

Granulocytes

The term granulocyte encompasses

- Neutrophils
- Mast cells
- Basophils
- Eosinophils

These are myeloid-derived cells containing abundant granules (vacuoles containing substances such as enzymes). Each type of granulocyte has specialised functions. They are often called polymorphs, because they have multilobed nuclei.

Neutrophils

These comprise two-thirds of the body's white blood cells. They are the main bacteria-killing cells of the immune system. They have a lifespan of less than a day, so their numbers fall rapidly if their production ceases, for example as a result of bone marrow failure during chemotherapy.

Large numbers of neutrophils are stored in the bone marrow and released into the circulation when bacterial infection is identified. Macrophages complement and mast cells help co-ordinate the 'recruitment' (attraction) of neutrophils to the site of infection.

Neutrophils phagocytose bacteria. Once bacteria have been endocytosed, the phagocytes utilise several killing mechanisms, including:

- generation of superoxide radicals,
- formation of toxic nitric oxide compounds
- release of proteolytic enzymes from lysosomes

This takes place in bacteria-containing phagolysosomes (formed from fusion of phagosomes and lysosomes). Once a neutrophil has become filled with dead bacteria it dies and may be phagocytosed itself by a macrophage. The pus associated with infected wounds is made up largely of dead neutrophils and cellular debris from other dying cells.

Mast cells and basophils

Mast cells and basophils are closely related inflammatory cells. They both have granules that contain key inflammatory mediators: histamine, serotonin, and tryptase. In addition to degranulation (release of granules), upon activation mast cells synthesise:

- Prostanoids (mediators of inflammatory and other reactions, including vasoconstriction)
- Eosinophil chemotactic factor and
- Tumour necrosis factor-α (TNF-α)

Mast cell activation (by C3a) is a physiological response to infection, helping with the clearance of bacteria and worms. However mast cells have probably been most studied for their role in hypersensitivity, particularly type I hypersensitivity or allergic reactions. In this situation, mast cells are activated by IgE that has bound an allergen, i.e. a non-pathogenic antigen that evokes an allergic response (e.g. pollen).

Eosinophils

Granulocytes are primarily concerned with defence against fungal and parasitic infection, through interaction with mast cells and IgE. Their numbers remain low in the circulation unless such infection is present, in which case their numbers increase, as they do in chronic allergy as well.

Lymphocytes

Lymphocytes comprise B cells, T cells (also called T lymphocytes) and natural killer (NK) cells. They are mononuclear cells that, with the exception of NK cells, mediate the adaptive immune response. In addition, some subsets of all three types act as memory cells that provide a rapid, effective response on re-exposure to an antigen that has been encountered previously.

Each T-cell and each B-cell expresses a single randomly generated surface receptor that is specific to one molecular sequence (epitope) on an antigen. With several million different T-cells and B-cells, they are together able to respond to almost any molecular sequence. Therefore the body is capable of mounting a response to almost any pathogen despite each lymphocyte only responding to one antigen.

B cells

B cells produce immunoglobulins (antibodies), molecules that bind to antigens of any structure, for example protein, carbohydrate, nucleic acid or lipid (**Figure 3.34**). Each B cell will only ever produce immunoglobulin specific to one antigen:

1. Newly formed B cells are termed naive B cells; they have membrane-bound immunoglobulin, which functions as their surface receptor
2. After a naive B cell binds antigen, it interacts with a T cell specific to the same antigen (a Th2 CD4$^+$ cell – see below)
3. This activates the B cell, enabling it to:
   a Transform into a plasma cell that secretes the immunoglobulin as free antibodies or
   b Become a memory cell, which stays in the lymph nodes, spleen or bone

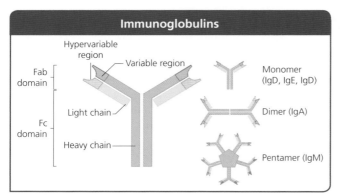

Figure 3.34 The hypervariable part of the antigen binding site is show in red in a generalised immunoglobulin. Depending on the antibody subtype, several immunoglobulins may combine to form functional units as dimers or pentamers.

marrow, waiting to be exposed to the same antigen again

B cells can also switch production from one to another of the five different types of immunoglobulin (**Figure 3.34**):

- IgG is the most abundant and highly specific to a single antigen
- IgA is important in the gut and respiratory tract, to prevent pathogen entry
- IgM activates complement,
- IgE is involved in allergy, activating mast cells, and
- IgD is of unknown function.

T cells

T lymphocytes have a range of roles in the immune system:

- CD4+ T cells contribute to the production of antibodies by B cells
- CD8+ T cells are cytotoxic, i.e. they recognise abnormal cells and destroy them
- Other T cells act as memory cells or suppress activity of the immune system

CD (cluster of differentiation) proteins are surface markers of immune cells. CD4 and CD8 are found on the surface of T ells. CD4 and CD8 are present in a complex with T-cell receptors on the T-cell membrane. CD4 and CD8 allow T-cell receptors to interact with large molecules called major histocompatibility complexes (MHCs, see below) in order to bind antigen. CD4+ and CD8+ T cells have different functions in the immune system, as described below.

Antigen presentation and major histocompatibility complexes

Unlike the receptors on B cells, those on T cells are unable to bind free antigen. Instead, the T-cell receptors (TCRs) recognise fragments of protein antigens when these are bound to major histocompatibility complexes (MHCs, also called human leukocyte antigens, HLAs) on 'antigen-presenting' cells. TCRs can only bind peptide antigens.

The formation of peptide fragments from antigens by the cell and the loading of these peptides onto MHC molecules on the cell's surface are called antigen presentation (**Figure 3.35**). There are two broad groups of MHC molecule involved in the adaptive immune system, class I and class II.

Antigen presentation by MHC class I (Figure 3.35a)
Endogenous proteins from almost every cell in the body are broken down, loaded onto MHC class I, and presented on cell surfaces. If a cell is infected by a virus or contains other abnormal proteins, pathogenic peptides are presented on its surface in this manner. CD8+ 'cytotoxic' T-cells bind to the antigen–MHC class I complex, and this leads to the destruction of the cell containing the virus.

Antigen presentation by MHC class II (Figure 3.35b)
In contrast, only a few cells express MHC class II: macrophages, B cells, and Langerhans' cells. These 'professional' antigen-presenting cells endocytose exogenous (extracellular) antigen and present it, together with MHC class II, to CD4+ 'helper'

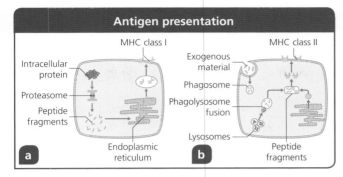

Figure 3.35 The mechanism for (a) endogenous and (b) exogenous antigen presentation, in which peptides are loaded into MHC class I and class II, respectively.

T cells (see below). The T cells then secrete cytokines which enhance the activity of the presenting cell. Cytokines also diffuse locally, attracting other cells of the immune system, such as macrophages.

Helper T cells

There are two main forms of helper T cells, which have slightly different actions (**Table 3.6**).

Th1 CD4⁺ T cells Th1 helper T cells are primarily involved in augmenting macrophage clearance of bacteria. After macrophages have engulfed bacteria, they present fragments complexed with MHC class II molecules to CD4⁺ T cells. If the CD4⁺ T cell's TCR is specific to that epitope then the Th1 cell provides stimulatory signals to the macrophage to cause macrophage activation.

Th2 CD4⁺ T cells Th2 cells are needed in the production of high-affinity antibody. As described above, naive B cells present antigen to Th2 CD4⁺ T cells. The Th2 CD4⁺ T cells signal the B cells to convert into plasma cells and to start producing specific antibodies.

NK cells

Among lymphocytes, NK cells are unique in that they that do not have antigen-specific receptors. Therefore, rather than being a component of the adaptive immune system, responding to specific antigens, they are part of the innate immune response. The targets of NK cells are often virally infected cells, but NK cells are also thought to target cancer cells. NK cells interact with and induce apoptosis in the target cell, i.e. induced or programmed, controlled cell death that takes place in an energy-dependant manner. They do this using the same mechanisms as cytotoxic T cells.

CD4⁺ T-cell responses		
	Th1 response	Th2 response
Pathogen targeted	Intracellular bacteria	Extracellular pathogens
Immune method	Macrophage-mediated bacterial killing	Antibody production
Cells involved	Th1 CD4⁺ T cells and macrophages	Th2 CD4⁺ T cells and B cells
Cytokines	IL-3, IL-12, TNF-α, and IFN-γ	IL-4, IL-5, IL-10, and IL-13

IL, interleukin; TNF, tumour necrosis factor.

Table 3.6. A summary of T helper cell (CD4⁺) responses

Whether an NK cell is activated by a target cell depends on a number of factors:

An 82-year-old man presents to his GP with fatigue and easy bruising. Blood tests demonstrate severe anaemia (Hb 58 g/L), thrombocytopenia (platelets 12 x 10⁹/mL) and hugely raised white cell count (white cells 154 x 10⁹/mL).

Leukaemias are malignancies in white blood cells or their progenitors, grouped into acute and chronic, based upon their rate of progression. Acute leukaemia results from malignancy in early progenitor cells with a high rate of division and multiplication; chronic leukaemia arises in a relatively highly differentiated white cell that has suffered a pathological failure to undergo apoptosis (cell death). Abnormal cells displace normal cells from the bone marrow, causing bone marrow failure with anaemia, bleeding (from low platelets) and severe infections.

- Absence of MHC class I on the surface of the target cell: many viruses cause downregulation of MHC class I and this is detected by NK cells
- Presence of IgG bound to the target cell's surface
- Presence of molecular 'stress signals' on the target cell's surface

Interferons

Every cell in the body is able to mount its own antiviral response using interferons (IFN), which have autocrine (within the same cell) and paracrine (on nearby, neighbouring cells) actions as they:

- Activate endonuclease, which breaks down the RNA necessary for viral protein synthesis
- Increase MHC class I expression so that presence of viral proteins is increased
- Activate NK cells to kill virally infected cells

Answers to starter questions

1. The intrinsic rhythm of the heart is generated by pacemaker cells in the sinoatrial or atrioventricular nodes. These cells depolarise spontaneously because of their high sodium permeability. This results in regular depolarisations that spread through the myocardium causing contraction.

2. Blood pressure is tightly controlled to maintain a sufficient supply of blood to the tissues. If pressure is consistently too high, this can cause severe complications, such as stroke, chronic kidney disease and coronary heart disease.

3. As the heart contracts it generates a transmural pressure gradient between the ventricular chamber and the epicardial surface. Cardiac cells immediately underneath the ventricle are subject to ventricular pressures: up to 120 mmHg during systole. This is much greater than the pressure in the left coronary vessels during systole, so almost all blood flow to the heart is delivered in diastole. When cardiac work increases (rise in heart rate or contractility) the flow provided during diastole is further reduced because the duration of diastole decreases and the transmural gradient increases.

4. Metabolic hyperaemia is the process of regulating blood flow according to tissue activity. When metabolic activity increases in a tissue it releases a factor that acts as a vasodilator on local arterioles, raising blood flow in the area. For example, K^+ is released during the action potentials of skeletal muscle, causing vasodilatation that increases blood flow to the muscles.

5. Fainting (syncope) occurs when tissue blood flow to the brain falls below the level required for normal cognitive function. Flow is autoregulated by the myogenic tone of cerebral arterioles. A drop in heart rate or systemic vasodilatation can cause cerebral blood pressure to fall, causing syncope because there is not enough perfused brain to maintain consciousness.

Chapter 4
Respiratory system

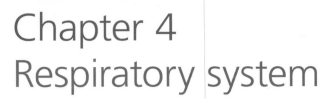
Starter questions

Answers to the following questions are on page 130.

1. What prevents our lungs from collapsing?
2. How is more oxygen delivered to the most active tissues?
3. Why is carbon monoxide inhalation dangerous?
4. What controls the duration of each breath?
5. Why do lung diseases cause heart failure?

Introduction

Respiration is broadly defined as the physical and chemical processes by which the body:

- obtains the oxygen required for energy-producing reactions in cells
- removes the carbon dioxide formed as a waste product of these reactions

Respiration involves:

- ventilation (or breathing) to produce movements of the chest to inflate and deflate the lungs and thereby inhale and exhale air

- passive diffusion of gases between air-filled spaces of the lungs and the adjacent blood vessels

Blood gases are maintained at optimal pressures (sometimes called tensions) by neural control of the rate and depth of breathing. This control is provided by the integration of multiple reflexes.

If breathing ceases, cardiac arrest and hypoxic brain damage ensue within minutes as a result of oxygen starvation.

Case 3 Laboured breathing in a premature baby

Presentation

Jenna Rose, aged 32 years, is 28 weeks pregnant. Until now, her pregnancy has been uneventful; however, she has suddenly entered labour. Evidence of fetal distress leads to an urgent forceps-assisted delivery.

However, at birth, the baby is bluish and grunting. His breathing is laboured, he has no cry or cough and his chest is indrawn along the costal margin (subcostal recession).

Analysis

These signs indicate severe respiratory distress, requiring assisted ventilation with a facemask for positive-pressure ventilation. There are several potential causes, however, in premature neonates, particularly those born before 30 weeks, the most probable cause is lung surfactant deficiency.

Production of surfactant begins at 24 weeks' gestation, but reserves normally accumulate slowly. If there is enough time before delivery, two doses of corticosteroids are given to the mother, 12–24 h apart, to stimulate surfactant production.

Surfactant deficiency greatly increases respiratory effort and makes it extremely difficult for the baby to take its initial breaths. Before the first breath, the lungs are filled with (amniotic) fluid, which must be forced out of the alveoli by air pressure on inflation. Positive pressure ventilation is required to facilitate this process if the neonate is unable to generate the necessary respiratory effort on its own.

Further case

2 weeks later, the baby requires intubation and respiratory support with high ventilation pressures in the neonatal unit.

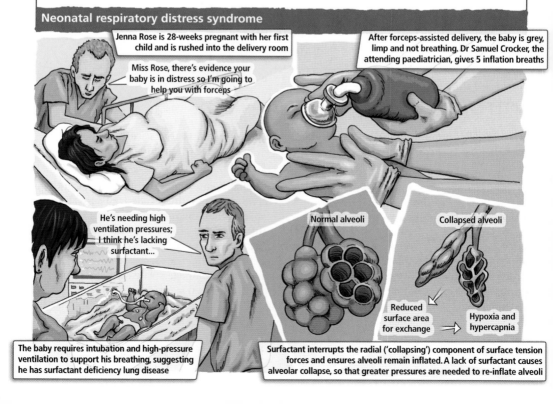

Neonatal respiratory distress syndrome

Jenna Rose is 28-weeks pregnant with her first child and is rushed into the delivery room

Miss Rose, there's evidence your baby is in distress so I'm going to help you with forceps

After forceps-assisted delivery, the baby is grey, limp and not breathing. Dr Samuel Crocker, the attending paediatrician, gives 5 inflation breaths

He's needing high ventilation pressures; I think he's lacking surfactant...

Normal alveoli

Collapsed alveoli

Reduced surface area for exchange

Hypoxia and hypercapnia

The baby requires intubation and high-pressure ventilation to support his breathing, suggesting he has surfactant deficiency lung disease

Surfactant interrupts the radial ('collapsing') component of surface tension forces and ensures alveoli remain inflated. A lack of surfactant causes alveolar collapse, so that greater pressures are needed to re-inflate alveoli

Case 3 *continued*

A chest X-ray show patchy areas of consolidation. A sudden deterioration in his condition is determined to be the result of a pneumothorax (air in the pleural space). However, after insertion of a chest drain he recovers and is discharged from hospital.

Further analysis

Surfactant reduces surface tension in the lung. Without it, the lung is poorly compliant so that large forces are required for inflation; alveoli remain collapsed, and small alveoli empty into larger ones. A huge amount of effort is needed to breathe due to the reduced ability to expand, and mechanical ventilation is required if there are signs of acute respiratory distress.

When many alveoli remain collapsed, as indicated by the patchy consolidation on X-ray, the surface area available for diffusion is reduced. A consequence of using high ventilation pressures is an increased risk of pneumothorax, which can be difficult to manage. Neonates with chronic lung disease may require supplemental oxygen for months, but most have normal long-term respiratory function.

Properties of gases

A gas consists of individual molecules existing separately in space and able to move independently of each other. A gas-filled space may contain a single element, for example pure oxygen, or a single compound. Alternatively, it may contain a mixture of elements or compounds; an example is the earth's atmosphere, which comprises 74% nitrogen, 21% oxygen and a small amount of water, carbon dioxide and other substances.

Understanding lung physiology requires discussion of the physical characteristics of gases, which are most easily explained by considering their behaviour in a container, i.e. in an enclosed space or system.

Partial pressure

The pressure exerted by a gas is the force its molecules generate against the walls of the container, as a result of their random movement. Such pressure is exerted by all gases in a container, for example each of the gases within the alveoli. The pressure attributable to a particular gas, irrespective of whether it is the only gas in the system or one of a mixture of gases, is termed its partial pressure.

The partial pressure of a gas drives its diffusion through and between spaces, in a similar way to the concentration of a substance providing the impetus for its diffusion through a liquid and between compartments.

Dalton's law

This law describes the principle that the total pressure in a system (P_{total}) equals the sum of the partial pressures (P_1, P_2, P_3, etc.) for each of its constituent gases:

$$P_{total} = P_1 + P_2 + P_3 + ... P_n$$

Boyle's law

Boyle's law describes the relationship between the pressure of a gas and the volume (V) it occupies:

$$PV = \text{a constant, } k$$

Therefore,

$$P \propto \frac{1}{V}$$

For one gas and the volume (V_1) it occupies in a mixture of gases, the equation can be rearranged in a series of steps in a way that has multiple applications in the respiratory system:

$$\frac{P_1}{P_{total}} = \frac{V_1}{V_{total}}$$

In this form, Boyle's law explains that the partial pressure of a gas in a system is proportional to the fractional volume that it occupies in the whole system. Rearrangement of this equation shows that the partial pressure of each gas reflects its relative or fractional concentration in the system:

$$P_1 = P_{total} \times \left(\frac{V_1}{V_{total}}\right)$$

In other words,

$$P_1 = P_{total} \times \text{fractional concentration of gas}_1 \text{ in mixture}$$

As an example, the P_{total} of air (at sea level) is 100 kPa, and oxygen comprises 21% of air by volume, so Po_2 at sea level is 21 kPa.

Flow dynamics

Many of the principles of movement of fluid through tubes apply equally to the movement of gases (see page 70). The relationship between flow, velocity and total cross-sectional area is particularly significant:

$$\text{flow} = \text{velocity} \times \text{total cross-sectional area}$$

As the airways divide from the trachea to the alveoli, their total cross-sectional area greatly increases. Therefore, to maintain uniform flow throughout the lung, the velocity of gas

flow must be extremely low in the smallest airways (**Figure 4.1**).

At high altitudes, oxygen comprises 21% of inspired air, as it does at sea level, but the atmospheric pressure is much lower. Applying Boyle's law, if atmospheric pressure is reduced to 50 kPa instead of the 100 kPa at low altitudes, the Po_2 is 10 kPa instead of 21 kPa. At 10 kPa, less oxygen dissolves in the blood. Therefore, an artificial oxygen supply is required to exercise at high altitudes, unless there has been a period of acclimatisation to increase oxygen carriage.

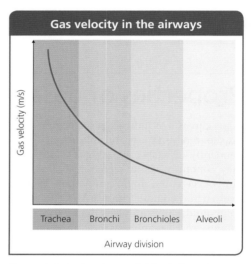

Gas velocity in the airways

Figure 4.1 As the airways divide, their total cross-sectional area increases. Constant flow of air results in an exponential reduction in gas velocity from the trachea to the alveoli.

Lungs, pleurae and muscles of respiration

The respiratory system comprises the tubes leading from the mouth and nose to the lungs, the lungs themselves, and the structures in the chest that move air into and out of the lungs.

This section focuses on the lungs, pleurae and muscles of respiration, because of their key roles in ventilation.

The lungs

These soft, flexible organs are in the thorax. They are bounded by the chest wall, which comprises a bony skeleton and the muscles of respiration.

If the lungs were simply two air-filled sacs, their internal surface area would be insufficient

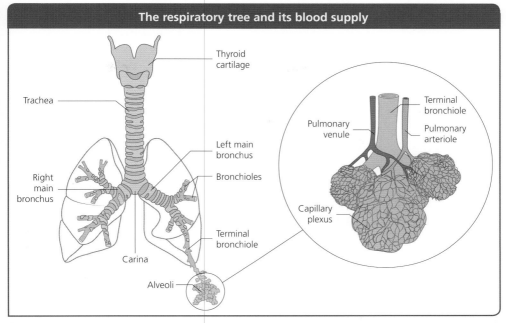

The respiratory tree and its blood supply

Thyroid cartilage

Trachea

Left main bronchus

Bronchioles

Right main bronchus

Terminal bronchiole

Carina

Alveoli

Terminal bronchiole

Pulmonary venule

Pulmonary arteriole

Capillary plexus

Figure 4.2 The trachea separates into two bronchi, which divide into successively smaller bronchioles with about 25 orders of branching from the trachea to the terminal bronchioles. About 500 million alveoli arise from the terminal bronchioles to provide an area of 75 m² for gaseous exchange between the alveolar cavities and the dense network of capillary vessels in the alveolar walls.

for the amount of gaseous exchange necessary to meet the demands of cellular respiration. Therefore multiple branching of the airways creates the huge surface area required for adequate gaseous exchange (**Figure 4.2**).

The pleurae

The lungs and the inner face of the chest wall are covered by pleurae, thin layers of epithelial cells and connective tissue.

- The visceral pleura covers the lungs
- The parietal pleura lines the chest wall

The two pleural sacs are in continuity with each other at the lung hilum, such that there is a potential cavity between them (the pleural space; **Figure 4.3**), similar to that between the layers of the pericardium (see page 73).

The pleural space contains a small amount of fluid, which:

- lubricates the two pleural layers so that they can move freely over each other during breathing

- holds the parietal and visceral pleurae together, by acting as a vacuum seal

In this way, the pleural space keeps the lungs expanded against the chest wall.

Muscles of respiration

These are the intercostal muscles and the diaphragm. The diaphragm is a sheet of musculofibrous tissue that separates the thoracic and abdominal cavities.

Accessory muscles of respiration

Attached to the ribcage are the accessory muscles of respiration, which aid the intercostal muscles and diaphragm in the effort of breathing. The accessory muscles are:

- In the neck: sternocleidomastoid, trapezius and the scalene muscles
- In the thorax: serratus anterior and the pectoral muscles
- In the abdomen: rectus abdominis and the oblique muscles

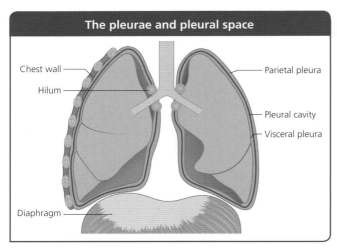

The pleurae and pleural space

Chest wall

Hilum

Parietal pleura

Pleural cavity

Visceral pleura

Diaphragm

Figure 4.3 The parietal pleura (lining the chest wall) and the visceral pleura (lining the lung) are in continuity with each other at the lung hilum. This arrangement creates a potential cavity, the pleural space. Formation of radiographically opaque plaques on the pleurae is strongly associated with asbestosis (see **Figure 4.5**).

Ventilation

Ventilation, or breathing, is the mechanical movements responsible for inspiration and expiration, which enable the exchange of gases in the lungs.

Various factors affect ventilation:

- lung volumes and capacities
- pleural pressure
- compliance and elasticity
- surface tension and pulmonary surfactant
- resistance

Lung volumes and capacities

The four lung volumes and three capacities (each of which consists of two or more lung volumes) are shown in **Figure 4.4**.

- Tidal volume (V_T) is the volume of air that moves into or out of the lungs with each breath at rest; it is usually about 500 mL
- Inspiratory reserve volume (IRV) is the additional volume taken into the lungs with effort after inspiration of V_T

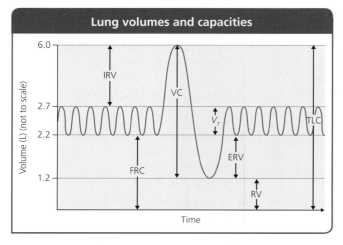

Lung volumes and capacities

Volume (L) (not to scale)

6.0

2.7

2.2

1.2

IRV

VC

V_T

TLC

FRC

ERV

RV

Time

Figure 4.4 Lung volumes and capacities. ERV, expiratory reserve volume; FRC, functional residual capacity; IRV, inspiratory reserve volume; RV, residual volume; TLC, total lung capacity; VC, vital capacity; V_T, tidal volume.

- Expiratory reserve volume (ERV) is the additional volume expelled from the lungs with effort after expiration of V_T
- Residual volume (RV) is the volume of air that remains in the lungs after exhalation of the ERV (the lungs cannot normally collapse completely)
- Functional residual capacity (FRC) is the volume (about 2.7 L) left in the lung after expiration of V_T; it is ERV and RV combined
- Vital capacity (VC) is the total volume of air that can be moved in or out of the lungs with effort; it is the sum of IRV, V_T and ERV
- Total lung capacity is the maximum volume contained by the lungs and therefore the sum of all four volumes

> In restrictive lung diseases such as pulmonary fibrosis, lung volumes (particularly RV and FRC) are reduced. Resulting inadequate ventilation and oxygenation can result in respiratory failure.

Minute ventilation

The volume of air entering or leaving the lungs in a given time period depends on the respiratory rate as well as the volume of air moved into or out of the lungs with each breath. For example, the volume of air breathed in a minute (the minute ventilation) is calculated as follows:

$$\text{minute ventilation } (V) = V_T \times \text{frequency } (f)$$

Dead space

This is the volume of air in the airways that is unavailable for gaseous exchange. It has two components:

- **anatomical dead space** (typically 150 mL) is the total volume in the conducting zone, where no gaseous exchange occurs, i.e. the conducting bronchioles and above
- **alveolar dead space** is the volume in the respiratory zone (i.e. the respiratory bronchioles and below) where gaseous exchange is not occurring. It is zero in healthy people and increases, for example, if alveoli fill with fluid (e.g. pneumonia) or rupture (e.g. emphysema)

Pleural pressure

Between the visceral pleura over each lung and the parietal pleura over the chest wall is the fluid-containing pleural space (**Figure 4.6**). The two layers of pleura are pulled apart by the propensity of the chest wall to expand and the lung to recoil. Thus these opposing forces generate a negative pressure (relative to atmospheric pressure) in the pleural space between them.

Compliance and elasticity

Pulmonary compliance affects ventilation, because patients whose lungs have poor compliance must use greater effort to inhale a normal volume of air.

The compliance of a structure is the volume it achieves when subjected to a given distending pressure:

$$\text{compliance} = \text{change in volume/change in pressure}$$

Therefore a highly compliant structure requires only a small pressure to produce a large increase in volume.

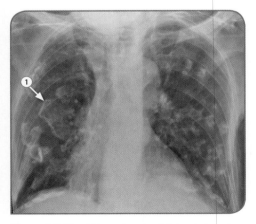

Figure 4.5 Chest X-ray showing bilateral pleural plaques ①. These are calcified areas of pleura that occur in response to asbestos exposure. The plaques themselves are not harmful or malignant but can have a shocking appearance on X-ray.

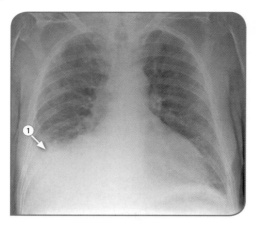

Figure 4.6 Chest X-ray showing a right-sided pleural effusion ①. This collection of fluid in the pleural space was due to an underlying infection that had stimulated production of reaction fluid by the pleura.

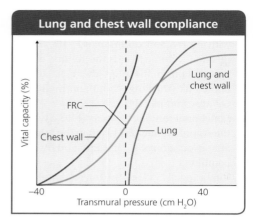

Figure 4.7 Compliance curve for lung, chest wall and both structures together, showing changes in volume with changes in distending pressure. FRC, functional residual capacity.

Elasticity is the inverse of compliance:

elasticity = 1/compliance = change in pressure/change in volume

A highly elastic structure has a propensity to maintain its volume. When subjected to a force that increases its volume, it stores potential energy. This energy returns the structure to its original volume when the distending pressure is removed.

The content and arrangement of connective tissues (e.g. elastin, collagen and glycosaminoglycans) in a structure determine its compliance and elasticity. The elasticity of the lung and visceral pleura confer a tendency for the lung to collapse, whereas chest wall elasticity confers a tendency to expand. However, the lung and visceral pleura are held to the chest wall and parietal pleura by the fluid in the pleural space, and negative pleural pressure ensures that the lung and chest wall act as a single structure.

Static compliance (i.e. compliance in the absence of airflow) of the lungs and chest wall is shown in **Figure 4.7**. Compliance is greatest at about FRC, i.e. after a normal expiration, when there is zero distending pressure. Therefore minimum force is required to inflate the lungs by the usual amount, V_T, and expiration is passive, thereby minimising the effort required for quiet breathing. Substantially more force is required for forced inspiration or expiration.

Respiratory muscles use energy to expand the ribcage (**Figure 4.8**). The resulting movement of the parietal pleura away from the visceral pleura (and lung) further reduces the negative pleural pressure that connects the lungs and chest wall. As the whole lung expands, a distending pressure is exerted throughout the lung that opens each airway to increase the volume of the lungs and airways.

A rearrangement of Boyle's law describes how these changes produce ventilation:

$$V_1 \times P_1 = V_2 \times P_2$$

As alveolar volume increases from V_1 to V_2, there is a proportional decrease in intrathoracic pressure from P_1 to P_2 to maintain equilibrium. Consequently, airway pressure decreases to below atmospheric pressure, causing gases from outside the body to move into the alveoli.

This process is reversed in expiration. Passive recoil of the chest wall and lung towards their positions at resting volume occur at FRC, i.e. at the end of a normal breath. Pleural pressure increases and causes gases to move from the alveoli to outside the body. The increase in alveolar pressure also generates a pressure on the lung's airways, which can cause their

Mechanism of ventilation

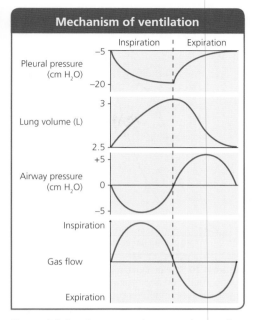

Figure 4.8 Respiratory muscles cause chest wall movement that reduces pleural pressure and thereby causes the lung to inflate. Airway pressure decreases to below atmospheric pressure, causing air to be inhaled.

collapse and the trapping of air in the lung. This is seen in patients with disease that increases small airway resistance, such as chronic obstructive pulmonary disease (COPD).

Surface tension and pulmonary surfactant

Pulmonary compliance also depends on the surface tension of the mucoid lining of the alveoli. Pulmonary surfactant decreases this surface tension, thereby increasing pulmonary compliance and reducing the effort needed to expand the lungs.

Surface tension

Much of the elastic recoil of the lung is the result of surface tension effects at air–water interfaces; a lung filled with fluid is much more compliant. These surface tension effects arise because all alveoli are covered in a thin layer of fluid. The van der Waals forces between adjacent water molecules in this fluid exert radial and circumferential forces that favour alveolar collapse (**Figure 4.9**). Therefore, for alveoli to remain at constant volume, these forces must be countered by an equal, opposing force from their internal gas pressure.

The internal pressure (P) required to keep a fluid-lined sphere such as an alveolus inflated is calculated by Laplace's law:

$$P = 2T / r$$

In this equation, T is wall tension, the pulling force exerted on the alveolar wall, and r is the radius. Surfactant maintains a nearly constant T.

Accordingly, small alveoli (with a small r) require a higher internal pressure to remain inflated. Theoretically, this implies that the high pressure in small alveoli would equalise by transfer to low pressure larger alveoli. However, this is inhibited by surfactant.

Surfactant

Surfactant is a phospholipid that is amphiphilic, i.e. both hydrophilic and hydrophobic,

Forces of alveolar surface tension

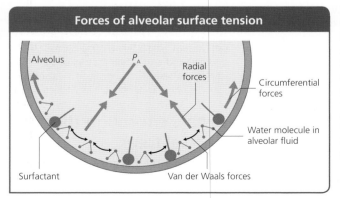

Figure 4.9 The van der Waals forces between water molecules in the fluid lining the alveoli cause circumferential and radial (collapsing) forces. These forces are equally opposed by alveolar air pressure (P_A). The dual hydrophilic–hydrophobic nature of surfactant enables it to decrease the attraction between water molecules in the alveoli, thereby greatly reducing surface tension.

secreted by type 2 pneumocytes of the alveolar epithelium. The large surfactant molecules come between the water molecules in the fluid lining the inner alveolar surface, with their hydrophobic lipid tails projecting into the gases in the alveolus (**Figure 4.9**). The effect is to interrupt van der Waals forces between the water molecules and thereby reduce surface tension.

The action of surfactant has three consequences.

■ Lung compliance is increased, reducing the effort required for breathing
■ The internal pressure required to maintain alveolar inflation is reduced; surfactant has a greater effect in smaller alveoli, so it helps to prevent small alveoli emptying into large ones
■ Increased compliance means smaller forces are required for airway movement, minimising the amount of fluid drawn into the alveoli that inhibits gaseous exchange

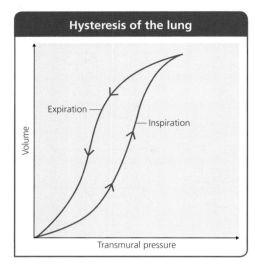

Figure 4.10 The dynamic resistance of the lung during inspiration and expiration is not linear or equal, because of differences in resistance to the movement of gases through the large airways.

Resistance

The movement of air during ventilation is inherited by airway resistance – the forces of friction and stiffness opposing air flow. It is calculated as the ratio of pressure to the rate of flow (see page 107). The respiratory muscles expend energy to move the chest wall to expand the lungs, thereby enabling the intake of air. A small amount of resistance is generated by the stiffness of tissues of the lung and chest wall. However, 80–90% of resistance is dynamic resistance; the effect of friction on inhibiting air flow.

When dynamic resistance is plotted on the compliance curve, it is apparent that airway resistance during inspiration and expiration are unequal. This is an example of hysteresis – when a physical property varies due to delayed effects – and is due to changes in compliance during the ventilatory cycle (**Figure 4.10**).

■ **In early inspiration**, resistance is high while alveoli are recruited as they have low compliance due to surface tension
■ **In early expiration**, alveoli have low compliance because of resistance to flow through the bronchial tree

> **A 10-year-old boy presents to the emergency department with breathlessness and a cough.** He complains of a feeling of tightness in his chest. His parents say that he has been waking up coughing at night for the past few weeks. A wheeze throughout his chest is audible on auscultation.
>
> Asthma is a common obstructive airway disease. It is characterised by fully reversible airway obstruction (unlike chronic obstructive pulmonary disease, in which the obstruction is irreversible). Acute asthma attacks usually have a trigger, such as intercurrent viral illness or exposure to an allergen; untreated patients may have milder symptoms between attacks. Treatment includes avoidance of precipitating factors, and administration of bronchodilators (e.g. salbutamol, a β_2-adrenergic receptor agonist) and anti-inflammatory drugs (corticosteroids).

Resistance through the bronchial tree

Resistance to airflow is greatest in the upper respiratory tract (the larynx and pharynx) and large airways. These parts of the respiratory tract, in accordance with Poiseuille's law (see page 71), have the smallest total radius and therefore highest resistance to air flow. The radius of the thorax, for example, is smaller than the sum of all the radii of the bronchioles.

Furthermore, large airways are more likely to have turbulent flow. The probability of turbulence occurring is described by the Reynolds number (see page 71). Turbulent flow is more likely in airways with larger lumens, higher flow velocity and increased branching. Turbulent flow is less energy-efficient because of its chaotic, irregular nature, therefore it increases resistance.

Bronchodilation and bronchoconstriction

Bronchioles, as small airways, have only a small contribution to the total resistance in the respiratory system. However, their resistance can be varied, because the smooth muscle in their walls allows their diameter to be changed by bronchodilation or bronchoconstriction (**Table 4.1**).

- Bronchiole resistance is reduced by bronchodilation
- Bronchiole resistance is increased by bronchoconstriction

Two of the most common respiratory conditions, asthma and chronic obstructive pulmonary disease, are characterised by

Bronchiolar tone	
Bronchoconstriction	Bronchodilation
Parasympathetic stimulation at muscarinic acetylcholine receptors	Sympathetic stimulation at β_2 adrenergic receptors
Low airway carbon dioxide	Non-adrenergic, non-cholinergic innervation
Leukotrienes, histamine and bradykinin	

Table 4.1 Factors that cause bronchial constriction and dilation

inappropriate bronchoconstriction. The aims of treatment are to reduce inflammation (e.g. with inhaled steroids or montelukast, a leukotriene receptor antagonist) and to promote bronchodilation (e.g. with β_2-adrenergic receptor agonists).

Chronic obstructive pulmonary disease is characterised by irreversible small airway obstruction, and is almost always secondary to smoking. Chronic inflammation causes smooth muscle hyperplasia, increases mucus production, narrows airways and increases resistance to flow, with a marked decrease in airway pressure during expiration. Forced expiration results in a positive pleural pressure that exceeds airway pressure, resulting in airway collapse, cessation of airflow and obstruction during exhalation.

Gaseous exchange

Once air is inhaled, gaseous exchange occurs through the passive diffusion of gases between the alveoli and adjacent blood vessels, i.e. the pulmonary capillaries. In this way, blood transported from the heart to the lungs by the pulmonary arteries gains oxygen and loses carbon dioxide. The oxygenated, carbon dioxide-depleted blood is then carried back to the heart by the pulmonary veins.

The aim of gaseous exchange is to maintain respiratory gases in systemic circulation at partial pressures sufficient for metabolic needs.

Alveolar gases

Oxygen moves from the alveoli into pulmonary capillaries, and alveolar carbon dioxide moves in the opposite direction. These gases move across the respiratory membrane down their concentration gradients until their alveolar partial pressures equalise with the partial pressures at the ends of the pulmonary capillaries, where the pulmonary venous circulation begins.

The partial pressures of alveolar gases are almost stable throughout the respiratory cycle, for two reasons:

■ the volume reaching the alveoli in a normal breath is only about 350 mL of the 2.7 L FRC, the volume of air left in the lung after a normal exhalation
■ gases move extremely slowly in the alveoli, because of their large total cross-sectional area

Anatomical dead space – where gaseous exchange cannot occur – means that the partial pressures of gases leaving the lungs at the start of an exhalation are essentially the same as those in the atmosphere. In contrast, the partial pressures of gases expelled at the end of an exhalation are the same as those in the alveoli.

As air passes through the nose and upper airways, it becomes saturated with water vapour. This effect helps to avoid damage to the delicate cells of the alveoli from the inhalation of dry air.

The water vapour has a significant partial pressure of its own: roughly 6 kPa. The partial pressure of the water vapour reduces the partial pressures of the other gases relative to their values in dry air. Typical values are given in **Table 4.2**.

Alveolar carbon dioxide

The percentage of carbon dioxide in inspired air is almost zero (0.04%). Therefore virtually all the carbon dioxide in alveoli originates from the body, as a waste product of cellular respiration.

At the arterial ends of pulmonary capillaries, the PCO_2 is about 6 kPa. However, it is only 5 kPa in the alveoli. Therefore, carbon dioxide passively diffuses from the blood into the alveolar space, driven by the partial pressure gradient. By the end of the pulmonary capillary, P_aCO_2 has equalised with P_ACO_2.

The higher the rate of metabolic carbon dioxide production ($\dot{V}CO_2$), the higher the alveolar carbon dioxide. Ventilation removes the gas, because air moving into and out of the alveoli dilutes the alveolar carbon dioxide. Therefore:

$$P_ACO_2 \propto \dot{V}CO_2/\dot{V}_A$$

In this equation, P_ACO_2 is the partial pressure of carbon dioxide in the alveoli, and $\dot{V}_A$ is the alveolar ventilation (i.e. the volume of air reaching the alveoli in a given time period).

Plotting P_ACO_2 against $\dot{V}_A$ produces a slope known as the metabolic hyperbola (**Figure 4.11**). At a constant $\dot{V}CO_2$, $\dot{V}_A$ is the only factor influencing P_ACO_2 and, assuming normal gaseous exchange, P_aCO_2. Therefore P_aCO_2 can be used as a marker of the efficiency of ventilation.

By the time the blood has reached the venous ends of pulmonary capillaries, its PCO_2 will have equalised with that of the alveoli (i.e. P_ACO_2). After passing through the left side of the heart, this will enter the systemic arterial circulation. In this way, changes in ventilation directly affect the P_ACO_2 in the rest of the body.

■ Hyperventilation decreases PCO_2, causing respiratory alkalosis

Gas pressures		
Gas	Atmospheric pressure (kPa)	Alveolar pressure (kPa)
Carbon dioxide	0.05	5.5
Oxygen	21	13.5
Hydrogen	0	6.5
Nitrogen	80	75.5

Table 4.2 Partial pressures of gases in the atmosphere and in healthy alveoli

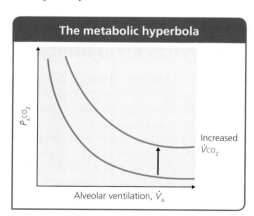

The metabolic hyperbola

Figure 4.11 The effect of changes in alveolar ventilation ($\dot{V}_A$), and increased carbon dioxide production ($\dot{V}CO_2$), on the partial pressure of arterial carbon dioxide (P_aCO_2).

- Impaired ventilation increases P_{CO_2}, causing respiratory acidosis

Alveolar oxygen

Oxygen enters alveoli from the air during breathing. Therefore the P_{O_2} in the alveoli, i.e. the P_AO_2, is proportional to the partial pressure of oxygen in the air and its rate of diffusion into the blood. If oxygen is inspired at a higher partial pressure, for example when supplementary oxygen is given, P_AO_2 is driven up.

Pulmonary capillaries arrive at the alveoli deficient in oxygen, because they carry blood from the systemic venous circulation. Oxygen from the alveoli enters the blood.

The higher the rate of oxygen use in cellular respiration ($\dot{V}_{O_2}$), and the lower the venous P_{O_2}, the greater the amount of oxygen leaving the alveoli. P_AO_2 decreases as alveolar oxygen is removed and its place is taken by carbon dioxide.

$$P_AO_2 \propto P_iO_2 - (\dot{V}_{O_2}/\dot{V}_A)$$

In this equation, P_iO_2 is the partial pressure of inspired oxygen.

Therefore as $\dot{V}_A$ increases, P_AO_2 approaches P_iO_2.

When the partial pressure of arterial oxygen (P_aO_2) is plotted against $\dot{V}_A$, the whole curve can be shifted by an increase in metabolic activity or a change in the partial pressure of inspired oxygen (**Figure 4.12**).

Respiratory quotient

The rate at which oxygen is replaced by carbon dioxide in the mix of alveolar gases is the respiratory quotient (RQ). It is the ratio between carbon dioxide production and oxygen intake:

$$RQ = \dot{V}_{CO_2}/\dot{V}_{O_2}$$

When pure carbohydrates are metabolised, one molecule of carbon dioxide is produced for each molecule of oxygen used. However, with fats or proteins, some oxygen is combined with hydrogen (and other atoms), so the RQ is < 1. For the average mixed western diet, the RQ is typically about 0.8.

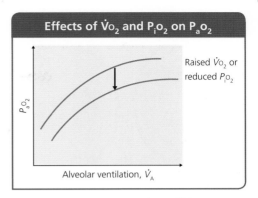

Effects of $\dot{V}_{O_2}$ and P_iO_2 on P_aO_2

Raised $\dot{V}_{O_2}$ or reduced P_iO_2

Alveolar ventilation, $\dot{V}_A$

Figure 4.12 As alveolar ventilation ($\dot{V}_A$) increases, the partial pressure of arterial oxygen (P_aO_2) increases. If the body's rate of oxygen use ($\dot{V}_{O_2}$) increases, or the partial pressure of inspired oxygen (P_iO_2) decreases, the curve shifts downwards, thereby reducing the ability of increasing $\dot{V}_A$ to increase P_AO_2.

Alveolar gas equation

We can use an estimate of alveolar P_{CO_2} (from expired carbon dioxide and ventilation rate or from arterial P_{CO_2}) along with knowledge of the RQ to estimate the P_AO_2 for a given inspired P_{O_2}. This is known as the alveolar gas equation, and a simplified form is:

$$P_AO_2 = P_iO_2 - (P_aCO_2 / RQ)$$

Therefore P_AO_2 can be calculated for a known partial pressure of arterial carbon dioxide (P_aCO_2), which is assumed to be equal to P_ACO_2. This equation can be used to calculate the alveolar–arterial P_{O_2} difference, which is useful clinically in the differential diagnosis of hypoxia.

Gaseous exchange in the lung

When gases move between the alveolar space and the blood in pulmonary capillaries, they pass through the four layers that comprise the alveolar diffusion barrier (**Figure 4.13**).

- The inner surface of each alveolus is lined by a small amount of alveolar (interstitial) fluid

The alveolar barrier

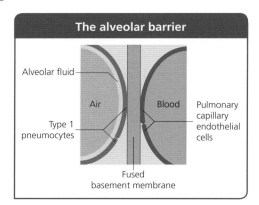

Alveolar fluid

Air   Blood   Pulmonary capillary endothelial cells

Type 1 pneumocytes

Fused basement membrane

Figure 4.13 The alveolar diffusion barrier is formed of four layers.

- This layer of fluid overlies type 1 pneumocytes (the alveolar epithelial cells that do not secrete surfactant)
- The layer of pneumocytes lies on the basement membrane of the alveolus, which is fused to the basement membrane of the adjacent pulmonary capillary
- The fused layer of basement membrane is next to a layer of endothelial cells

The diffusion capacity of the lung depends on the thickness of the barrier and the surface area available for gaseous exchange. Each of these factors may be affected by certain pathologies. For example, pulmonary fibrosis thickens the alveolar barrier, and emphysema reduces the surface area over which gases diffuse.

Determinants of rate of gaseous exchange

For a gas to pass through the alveolar barrier, it must go through a gaseous phase and a liquid phase before a phase of variable protein binding when it reaches the blood.

The rate of diffusion of an alveolar gas through the first of these phases is inversely proportional to its molecular weight (Graham's law); larger molecules move more slowly. Therefore oxygen – which has a molecular weight of 32 – diffuses through the alveolar space slightly more quickly than carbon dioxide, with a molecular weight of 44, does.

The movement of gas through the liquid phase depends on its partial pressure gradient

(Henry's law) and solubility coefficient (a measure of how readily it dissolves).

- Oxygen has a large partial pressure gradient across the alveolar barrier (5–13 kPa) but poor solubility in water
- Carbon dioxide has a smaller partial pressure gradient (6–5 kPa) but is highly soluble

Therefore, overall, carbon dioxide diffuses through the alveolar barrier 20 times faster than oxygen does.

Perfusion-limited gases

Under physiological conditions, oxygen and carbon dioxide are perfusion-limited gases. This means that their rate of exchange between alveoli and blood is limited by blood flow to the capillaries, and not by how readily they diffuse across the respiratory membrane. The alveolar and capillary partial pressures of each gas equalise during perfusion of the pulmonary capillaries (**Figure 4.14**). However, once equilibrium is reached at the venous ends of the pulmonary capillaries, no further diffusion of oxygen and carbon dioxide is possible.

An increase in the perfusion rate of pulmonary circulation increases the amount of gaseous exchange, as it provides more blood for

Perfusion- and diffusion-limited gases

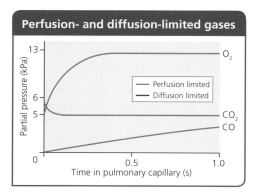

Partial pressure (kPa)

13 — ——— O_2

— Perfusion limited
— Diffusion limited

6 —
5 — ——— CO_2
        ——— CO

0   0.5   1.0
Time in pulmonary capillary (s)

Figure 4.14 The partial pressures of oxygen and carbon dioxide, as perfusion-limited gases, have fully equalised with their alveolar gas partial pressures by the time the blood reaches the venous end of the pulmonary capillary. In contrast, the partial pressure of carbon monoxide, a diffusion-limited gas, continues to increase as the blood travels the whole length of the vessel.

oxygen to pass into capillaries and for carbon dioxide to leave into the alveoli. Thus the rate of gaseous exchange is limited by the perfusion rate.

As an example, carbon dioxide is moderately soluble in water, so it dissolves in alveolar fluid to generate a partial pressure in the liquid phase. Carbon dioxide then diffuses through the rest of the alveolar barrier and into the blood in the pulmonary capillary. Only a small amount binds to proteins in the blood; almost all the carbon dioxide that diffuses through the alveolar barrier exerts a partial pressure in the blood. The result is full equilibrium at an early stage in the blood's transport along the length of the pulmonary capillary. Therefore in this case perfusion rate, not transport across the alveolar diffusion barrier, is the rate-limiting step.

Diffusion-limited gases

Gases with a high affinity for plasma proteins are diffusion-limited. This means that their rate of exchange is limited more by their rate of diffusion across the respiratory membrane, rather than blood flow through pulmonary capillaries, i.e. perfusion.

For example, carbon monoxide has a high affinity for haemoglobin, maintaining a low partial pressure (P_aCO_2) all along the capillary. Therefore carbon monoxide does not equilibrate by the end of the capillary, irrespective of blood flow. The exchange rate is limited by the diffusion rate.

Alveolar–arterial oxygen difference

In a normally functioning respiratory system, pulmonary venous Po_2 and P_AO_2 are equal. However, P_aO_2 in the systemic circulation is about 1 kPa lower than P_AO_2. This alveolar–arterial difference is a consequence of shunting and ventilation–perfusion ($\dot{V}/\dot{Q}$) mismatch (see page 124).

Shunting is the movement of blood from one side of the circulation to the other.

- **Left-to-right shunts** (e.g. in atrial septal defect) transfer blood from the systemic circulation to the pulmonary circulation; in the long term, these shunts can cause cardiac failure, because they increase blood flow in the pulmonary circulation
- **Right-to-left shunts** cause blood to pass from the systemic venous circulation back into the systemic arterial circulation, bypassing the lungs; the result is mixing of oxygenated and deoxygenated blood

There are two examples of right-to-left shunts, which reduce haemoglobin oxygen saturation of arterial blood:

- the bronchial arteries arise from the thoracic aorta to supply the conducting airways and drain into the pulmonary veins, i.e. back into systemic arterial circulation
- the Thebesian veins drain the myocardium of the left ventricle, depositing deoxygenated blood into the ventricle itself, mixing with oxygenated blood that enters systemic circulation

> **Pulmonary fibrosis is characterised by deposition of extracellular matrix in the interstitial space of lungs, thickening the diffusion barrier.** Eventually, this limits the movement of oxygen, the gas most susceptible to diffusion limitation, and chronic hypoxia develops. In severe cases, pulmonary fibrosis may impair ventilation to the point at which P_aCO_2 is increased.

Gas transport in blood

Blood carries oxygen to the tissues and carbon dioxide to the lungs. Various factors affect this transport.

Oxygen transport

Oxygen is transported in the blood in two ways: dissolved in plasma and bound to haemoglobin. At a partial pressure of only 13 kPa, the oxygen dissolved in blood would be insufficient to supply the body's tissues. Therefore they rely on haemoglobin for their oxygen supply.

About 98.5% of the oxygen in blood is bound to haemoglobin, enabling blood to be 'loaded' in the lungs and 'unloaded' in the tissues, thereby delivering oxygen to where it is most needed.

Blood oxygen levels are discussed as oxygen content and oxygen capacity estimated from blood samples:

■ the oxygen content is the total dissolved and haemoglobin-bound oxygen
■ the oxygen carrying capacity is the maximum amount of oxygen that can be carried by the measured amount of haemoglobin

Haemoglobin

Haemoglobin is a tetramer protein with four subunits. Each subunit comprises a polypeptide chain and a haem group; the latter binds oxygen reversibly. The subunits are linked by non-covalent bonds. There are four main types of subunit: alpha (α), beta (β), delta (δ) and gamma (γ). Different combinations of these subunits produce different types of haemoglobin.

The composition of different types of haemoglobin determines their function. Each subunit has a different oxygen affinity, affecting the overall affinity of the haemoglobin molecule. Fetal haemoglobin (HbF), for example, has a higher oxygen affinity than adult haemoglobin (HbA) in order to ensure the fetus' oxygen demands are met (**Table 4.3**).

■ HbA is the main adult haemoglobin and consists of two α and two β chains. The latter mean that HbA oxygen affinity varies according to the presence of 2,3-diphosphoglycerate (2,3-DPG)
■ HbA$_2$ contains two α and two δ chains. It normally has a minor role, but is important in compensating in individuals with β chain abnormalities
■ HbF consists of two α and two γ chains, conferring high oxygen affinity and exchange to fetal circulation in the placenta

Haemoglobin–oxygen dissociation curve

The coupling of oxygen to haem is driven by the partial pressure of oxygen dissolved in

Haemoglobins			
Characteristic	Haemoglobin A	Haemoglobin A2	Haemoglobin F
Proportion of total haemoglobin in an adult	98%	1%	1%
Proportion of total haemoglobin in a fetus	5–10%	0	90–95%
Globin chains	Two α chains	Two α chains	Two α chains
	Two β chains	Two δ chains	Two γ chains
2,3-Diphosphoglycerate binding	Binds 2,3-diphosphoglycerate to reduce oxygen affinity	Unable to bind	Unable to bind 2,3-diphosphoglycerate, so has a higher affinity for oxygen

Table 4.3 Examples of different types of haemoglobin

blood, i.e. P_aO_2. Each of the four haem groups may bind a molecule of oxygen to form oxy-haemoglobin. The binding is cooperative: the binding of an oxygen molecule to one haem facilitates the binding of another oxygen molecule to another haem. This property of haemoglobin is reflected by the sigmoidal shape of the haemoglobin–oxygen dissociation curve (**Figure 4.15**).

The haemoglobin–oxygen dissociation curve is a plot of haemoglobin saturation (as a percentage) against P_aO_2. Haemoglobin saturation (S_aO_2) is a measure of the amount of oxygen bound to haemoglobin in a sample, compared with the sample's oxygen capacity:

$$S_aO_2 \, (\%) = [(O_2 \text{ content} - \text{dissolved } O_2)/O_2 \text{ capacity}] \times 100$$

The consequence of cooperative binding is that when P_aO_2 is high (about 13 kPa), haemoglobin rapidly becomes almost fully saturated. This effect persists throughout the arterial system, even if tissue P_{O_2} decreases, because gas exchange cannot occur through arterial walls. However, as blood moves to the tissues, where tissue fluid P_{O_2} is substantially lower (4–8 kPa), oxygen dissociates more quickly and diffuses across the capillary membrane. In this way, oxygen is delivered efficiently to the most hypoxic tissues.

> Excessive breakdown of red blood cells (haemolysis) has various causes, including fragile red cell membranes, destruction by the immune system and intrinsic enzyme defects. Haemolysis has two effects: anaemia, with reduced oxygen-carrying capacity, and jaundice, resulting from increased bilirubin production. Treatment depends on the cause, but in severe cases patients require blood transfusions or immunosuppressants.

Curve shift and the Bohr effect

The haemoglobin–oxygen dissociation curve is shifted to the right or left by factors that influence the formation of oxyhaemoglobin. The curve is shifted to the right by characteristics of highly metabolically active tissues:

- increased carbon dioxide levels
- decreased pH
- increased temperature
- increased 2,3-DPG levels

Each of these factors promote the stability of deoxyhaemoglobin, so they are associated with the local release of oxygen and lower S_aO_2. An increase in carbon dioxide or a decrease in pH produces the Bohr effect (see **Figure 4.15**). This is a rightward shift in the haemoglobin-oxygen dissociation curve, reflecting reduced oxygen affinity, and is due to the effect of hydrogen ions (H$^+$) on haemoglobin.

2,3-DPG is a metabolic by-product of glycolysis, and its levels increase when cells are forced to use anaerobic metabolism. 2,3-DPG stabilises deoxyhaemoglobin by binding to haemoglobin α chains.

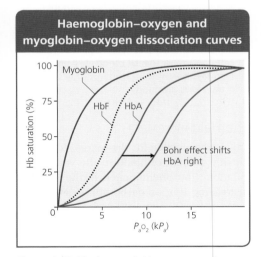

Haemoglobin–oxygen and myoglobin–oxygen dissociation curves

Figure 4.15 The haemoglobin–oxygen and myoglobin dissociation curves. The Bohr effect shifts the haemoglobin–oxygen dissociation curve to the right. Haemoglobin F has higher oxygen affinity than haemoglobin A, so its curve is set to the left. The myoglobin–oxygen dissociation curve is hyperbolic, reflecting its very high affinity for oxygen.

Myoglobin

Small amounts of this haem-containing molecule are present in highly metabolic tissues, particularly skeletal muscle.

Myoglobin binds only one molecule of oxygen, so cooperative of binding is not possible, and the myoglobin–oxygen dissociation curve is hyperbolic (**Figure 4.15**). Because myoglobin's affinity for oxygen is higher than that of haemoglobin, it draws oxygen from the blood and traps it in the muscle cells. Only at very low tissue Po_2 does myoglobin release its bound oxygen.

Haemoglobin F (fetal haemoglobin)

In the fetus, 98% of haemoglobin is HbF. The HbF tetramer comprises two α chains and two γ chains. The absence of α chains precludes the binding of 2,3-diphosphoglycerate, therefore haemoglobin F has a higher oxygen affinity than that of HbA. Consequently, the HbF–oxygen dissociation curve is permanently shifted to the left of that for HbA. This ensures the transfer of oxygen from the maternal circulation to HbF at the placental barrier.

Carbon dioxide transport

Carbon dioxide is carried in three ways:

- 90% as bicarbonate (HCO_3^-)
- 5% as dissolved carbon dioxide
- 5% bound to the amine groups of proteins, especially haemoglobin, as carbamino groups ($-NHCOO^-$)

The diffusion of dissolved carbon dioxide from tissues to blood is driven by a concentration gradient until its partial pressures achieve equilibrium. As the amount of carbon dioxide in the blood increases, it is used to form carbamino groups and bicarbonate.

In the lungs, dissolved carbon dioxide levels decrease as it diffuses into the alveoli. This process prompts the conversion of carbamino compounds and bicarbonate back to carbon dioxide. The reaction equilibrium shifts due to the low blood Pco_2, promoting loss of carbon dioxide from carbamino groups and conversion of bicarbonate back to carbon dioxide, which can then diffuse into alveoli.

This section focuses on the transport of carbon dioxide as bicarbonate, because this is form in which most of it is carried.

Carriage of carbon dioxide as bicarbonate

Carbon dioxide diffuses through the membranes of red blood cells; it then reacts with the water inside (**Figure 4.16**). This reaction is catalysed by carbonic anhydrase and forms carbonic acid, which dissociates rapidly into its constituent ions, i.e. bicarbonate and hydrogen ions:

$$CO_2 + H_2O \rightleftharpoons H_2CO_3 \rightleftharpoons HCO_3^- + H^+$$

Some of the hydrogen ions are buffered by binding to the amine groups of proteins, forming carbamino groups on haemoglobin molecules, for example. Bicarbonate leaves the red blood cells and passes into the plasma in exchange for chloride ions (Cl^-).

Anaemia is a decrease in the concentration of haemoglobin in the blood which reduces the oxygen-carrying capacity of blood. Despite a haemoglobin saturation of 100%, a patient with a haemoglobin concentration of 70 g/L has half the oxygen capacity of a patient with a normal concentration of haemoglobin (e.g. 140 g/L).

Anaemia is caused by reduced production of red cells, shortened red cell lifespan or loss of blood. Anaemia is frequently well tolerated but only when it develops gradually.

The Haldane effect

This is responsible for the increased carbon dioxide content of blood in the venous circulation. The phenomenon is the effect of decreasing P_aO_2 on carbon dioxide carriage by the blood (**Figure 4.17**).

The Haldane effect has two main causes:

- Deoxyhaemoglobin binds carbon dioxide as carbamino compounds more efficiently than oxyhaemoglobin does, thereby increasing the amount of carbon dioxide bound to haemoglobin
- Deoxyhaemoglobin is a weaker acid than oxyhaemoglobin, so it is better at

Carbon dioxide transport in the blood

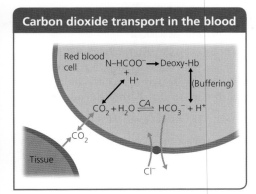

Figure 4.16 Carbon dioxide from cellular respiration is converted to bicarbonate and hydrogen ions by carbonic anhydrase (CA) in red blood cells. The hydrogen ions are buffered by the nitrogen (N$^-$) terminal ends of serum proteins such as haemoglobin (Hb).

The Haldane effect

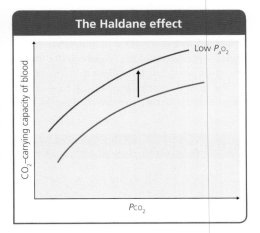

Figure 4.17 Deoxygenated blood has increased carbon dioxide–carrying capacity, which shifts the carbon dioxide dissociation curve vertically.

accepting hydrogen ions; this property promotes the generation of bicarbonate by carbonic anhydrase

The dissociation curve of carbon dioxide is essentially linear at physiological $P\mathrm{co_2}$, whereas that of oxygen is markedly non-linear. This gives the oxygen dissociation curve 'loading' and 'unloading' sections, whereas carbon dioxide dissociation is directly proportional to $P_a\mathrm{co_2}$. Also, the carbon dioxide content of blood is almost double that of oxygen:

- at a $P_a\mathrm{o_2}$ of 13 kPa, the oxygen content of blood is 150–200 mL/L
- at $P_a\mathrm{co_2}$ 5 kPa, its carbon dioxide content is 400–500 mL/L

This illustrates the importance of carbon dioxide transport as bicarbonate; it allows the transport of a large amount of cellular waste carbon dioxide whilst maintaining a relatively constant pH.

Role of the lungs in acid–base balance

Regulation of carbon dioxide, carbonic acid and bicarbonate in the lungs is crucial in the control of blood pH. Blood pH is discussed fully in Chapter 5.

Respiratory acidosis and alkalosis

Respiratory pathologies may cause acid–base abnormalities by altering $\dot{V}_A$, the amount of air reaching the alveoli.

- Hypoventilation decreases $\dot{V}_A$
- Hyperventilation increases $\dot{V}_A$

Conditions causing hypoventilation, such as chronic obstructive pulmonary disease, and inadequate ventilation relative to $\dot{V}\mathrm{co_2}$ cause a rightward shift along the metabolic hyperbola (**Figure 4.11**). The consequence is an increase in $P_a\mathrm{co_2}$, which promotes formation of carbonic acid, and thus hydrogen ions, by carbonic anhydrase. The excess hydrogen ions cause acidaemia (respiratory acidosis):

$$H_2O + \uparrow CO_2 \rightarrow \uparrow H^+ + HCO_3^-$$

Conversely, hyperventilation, for example as a result of pulmonary embolism and high altitude, causes a leftward shift along the metabolic hyperbola (see **Figure 4.11**). The consequent reduction in $P_a\mathrm{co_2}$ results in a decrease in hydrogen ions and therefore respiratory alkalosis:

$$H_2O + \downarrow CO_2 \rightarrow \downarrow H^+ + HCO_3^-$$

Measurements of blood pH, oxygen, carbon dioxide and bicarbonate are used to assess how well a patient is breathing, and whether or not respiratory support is required. For example, low pH accompanied by high carbon dioxide suggests inadequate ventilation, which requires ventilatory support, such as intubation and ventilation. Blood oxygen values are used to titrate oxygen therapy to demand, because measurement of oxygen saturation becomes less reliable at values < 93%.

Respiratory compensation for metabolic acidosis

If a non-respiratory pathology produces acid-aemia (a metabolic acidosis, e.g. in renal failure), the excess hydrogen ions combine with bicarbonate to form carbon dioxide:

$$H_2O + \uparrow CO_2 \leftarrow \uparrow H^+ + HCO_3^-$$

The increase in $P_a co_2$, together with the effect of low pH, stimulates an increase in $\dot{V}_A$ to help clear the excess carbon dioxide. pH normalises, because the respiratory system has compensated for the acidosis originating elsewhere.

Ventilation and perfusion

In respiratory physiology,

- ventilation is the movement of air into and out of the lungs, measured as $\dot{V}$, the volume of air per unit of time
- perfusion is the delivery of blood to the tissues of the body; it is usually expressed as $\dot{Q}$, the volume of blood per set weight of tissue per unit of time

$\dot{V}/\dot{Q}$ across the lung

Overall, the lung receives a larger volume of blood by perfusion (Q, 5 L/min) than the volume of air it receives by ventilation (V, 4 L/min). Therefore the $\dot{V}/\dot{Q}$ ratio is 0.8. However, ventilation and perfusion are not evenly distributed throughout the lung, because of the effects of gravity.

Ventilation

Ventilation is greater at the base of the lung; this tissue is more compliant than the apex and therefore receives 2.5 times more air. In other words, with each breath the lower part of the lung expands more than the upper part.

The apex of the lung is subject to the weight of the lung tissue beneath it, which pulls the lung away from the chest wall. Consequently, pleural pressure is more negative at the apex than at the base.

This means that the lung apex functions higher up on the compliance curve, as it is subjected to a distending - i.e. positive transmural – pressure at FRC (**Figure 4.18**). This is why the apex is less compliant than the base.

The greater compliance of the base of the lung enables it to take in more air than the apex

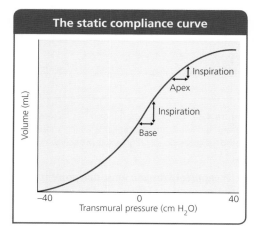

Figure 4.18 The static compliance curve shows how the volume of air moving into and out of the lungs changes with transmural pressure (the pressure inside the lung minus the pressure outside it). The apex is higher on the curve due to a more negative intrapleural pressure. The same increase in distending pressure during inspiration produces greater ventilation at the more compliant base of the lung compared with at the less compliant apex.

when a distending pressure is applied during inspiration, an effect that is illustrated when the values for the apex and base of the lung are plotted on the static compliance curve (static meaning in the absence of airflow).

Perfusion

Perfusion is also greater at the bases of the lungs than at their apices, with the base of each lung receiving 6 times more blood than the apex does.

The pulmonary vasculature is compliant and greatly influenced by gravity. These properties result in a higher hydrostatic pressure towards the lung bases and more capillaries are perfused than at the apex.

A plot of $\dot{V}$ against $\dot{Q}$ shows that, overall, the base receives disproportionately more perfusion and the apex more ventilation (**Figure 4.19**).

Effect on alveolar gases

The principles of the movement of alveolar gases discussed so far are based on a $\dot{V}/\dot{Q}$ of 0.8. However, $\dot{V}/\dot{Q}$ varies in different areas of the lung, and this variation influences airflow and gaseous exchange.

- At the apex, ventilation exceeds perfusion ($\dot{V}/\dot{Q} > 0.8$), which shifts the metabolic hyperbola leftwards (see **Figure 4.11**), resulting in reduced $P_A CO_2$ and increased $P_A O_2$
- At the base, perfusion exceeds ventilation ($\dot{V}/\dot{Q} < 0.8$), which results in carbon dioxide accumulation and a decreased supply of oxygen, i.e. $P_A CO_2$ is increased and $P_A O_2$ reduced

Physiological adjustment

Pulmonary arterioles and bronchioles are sensitive to changes in the partial pressures of gases in the airways, and they respond to try to correct the $\dot{V}/\dot{Q}$ ratio (**Table 4.4**). Consequently, blood is shunted towards well-ventilated areas and away from poorly ventilated areas.

These responses usually produce local changes; however, they may affect the entire lung under certain conditions. Under normal physiological conditions, the changes are adaptive, enabling efficient oxygenation of the blood by reducing blood flow in poorly ventilated areas. However, the effects can compound pathologies affecting the entire lung. For example, at high altitudes or in chronic hypoxic lung disease (e.g. emphysema), widespread pulmonary vasoconstriction causes pulmonary hypertension. This condition can lead to right-sided heart strain, and in the long term right-sided cardiac failure (cor pulmonale).

Another example is pneumonia, where infections and inflammatory infiltrate reduces the $\dot{V}/\dot{Q}$ ratio (**Figure 4.20**).

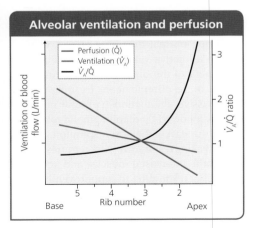

Figure 4.19 Alveolar ventilation and perfusion and their ratio at different levels of the lung.

Bronchiolar and pulmonary arteriolar responsiveness		
$\dot{V}/\dot{Q}$	Consequence	Response
Increased	Hyperoxia	Bronchoconstriction
	Hypocapnia	Vasodilation
Reduced	Hypoxia	Bronchodilation
	Hypercapnia	Vasoconstriction

Table 4.4 Response of bronchioles and pulmonary vasculature to local changes in ventilation/perfusion ($\dot{V}/\dot{Q}$) ratio

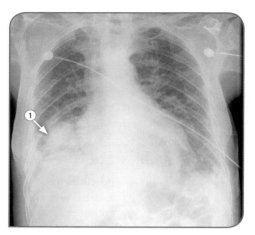

Pulmonary embolism causes a very high $\dot{V}/\dot{Q}$. The condition is almost always a consequence of embolisation of a large deep vein thrombosis from the pelvic veins into the pulmonary arteries. In the affected part of the lung, perfusion decreases to zero but ventilation continues, effectively creating alveolar dead space. Pulmonary embolism can cause potentially life-threatening severe hypoxia with back-pressure effects on the heart.

Figure 4.20 Chest X-ray showing a right lower zone pneumonia. Alveoli are filled with mucus, bacteria and inflammatory cells, which cause opacification on X-ray and a reduced ventilation/perfusion ratio. ① Pneumonic consolidation.

Control of breathing

Breathing patterns can be adjusted in response to changes both inside and outside the body.

Respiratory rhythm

Respiratory rhythm is controlled by both voluntary and involuntary mechanisms. The cerebral cortex can override the intrinsic control of inspiration and expiration for short periods, for example during speech. However, at all other times the respiratory cycle is under involuntary control, which determines:

- the initiation of inspiration and expiration
- the rate and depth of breathing

In this way, the body maintains optimal P_aO_2, P_aCO_2 and pH.

Neural centres

The primary centres for the control of respiration are in the medulla and pons of the brainstem. Dorsal and ventral groups of nuclei in the medulla interact with the pontine respiratory group and the medullary Bötzinger complex. Multiple connections between each of these centres provide the complex integration of stimulatory output to the phrenic nerve and intercostal muscles (**Figure 4.21**).

Input to respiratory nuclei comes from a number of sources. The nucleus tractus solitarius, a major integrating centre for the autonomic nervous system, communicates with the medullary respiratory centres.

During normal breathing at rest, inspiration is an active process brought about by movement of the diaphragm only, driven by activity in the phrenic nerve. Expiration is entirely passive; a reduction in phrenic nerve activity is followed by diaphragmatic relaxation before the start of the next inspiration.

Increasing respiratory work requires activation of the intercostal muscles and accessory muscles of respiration to support ventilation.

The Hering–Breuer reflex

The Hering–Breuer reflex is one mechanism contributing to the cessation of inspiration and the initiation of expiration. Slowly adapting stretch receptors in the small airways of the lung are activated as the lung expands. Afferent signals are then conveyed

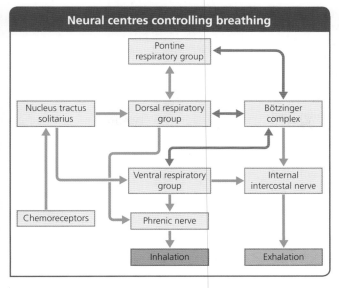

Figure 4.21 The key neural centres that control breathing. Green, excitatory connections; red, inhibitory connections.

to the nucleus tractus solitarius through the vagus nerve. The reflex output is a reduction in phrenic nerve activity.

Inhibition of the Hering–Breuer reflex can be demonstrated experimentally: severing of the vagus nerve (vagotomy) causes slow, deep inspiration.

Chemoreceptors

The main homeostatic role of the respiratory system is to keep blood gases (oxygen and carbon dioxide) and pH constant. This is dependent on the action of chemoreceptors, specialised nerve endings where a chemical stimulation is converted (or transduced) into an electrical signal. Their output allows ventilation to be matched to the body's requirements.

There are central receptors in the central nervous system, and peripheral chemoreceptors in the peripheries (**Table 4.5**).

Peripheral chemoreceptors

Peripheral chemoreceptors are present in the carotid body (innervated by the accessory nerve) and the wall of the aorta (innervated by the vagus nerve). They detect changes in arterial blood and are stimulated by:

- a decrease in P_aO_2
- an increase in P_aCO_2
- a decrease in pH (acidosis), regardless of the cause

The peripheral chemoreceptors are the only sites for response to hypoxia and metabolic acidosis.

Sensing of hypoxia

The carotid body is composed of modified neurons called glomus cells. Type 1 glomus cells are responsible for the transduction of chemical signals indicating hypoxia.

Chemoreceptors		
Characteristic	Central chemoreceptors	Peripheral chemoreceptors
Location	Medulla	Carotid body and aortic arch
Activating stimuli	Reduced cerebrospinal fluid pH (caused by increased P_aCO_2)	Reduced P_aO_2, increased P_aCO_2 and reduced serum pH
Overall response	Most of the response to carbon dioxide; normally dominant	All the response to oxygen and metabolic acidosis

P_aCO_2, partial pressure of arterial carbon dioxide; P_aO_2, partial pressure of arterial oxygen

Table 4.5 Comparison of the two types of chemoreceptor

These cells have an extremely high metabolic rate and therefore require a very high arterial blood flow. This extensive blood supply also means smaller changes in P_aO_2 are more easily detected by the glomus cells.

The exact mechanism by which type 1 glomus cells sense hypoxia remain unclear, but this results in the closure of potassium channels. The closure of these channels causes membrane depolarisation, which activates voltage-gated calcium channels. The resulting increase in intracellular calcium stimulates fusion of neurosecretory vesicles with the glomus cell membrane. The release of the transmitters stored in these vesicles initiates a signal that travels along the glossopharyngeal nerve.

Central chemoreceptors

Central chemoreceptors on the ventral surface of the medulla provide 80% of the body's overall response to carbon dioxide. They do this indirectly by responding to changes in the pH of the cerebrospinal fluid.

Carbon dioxide crosses into the cerebrospinal fluid (CSF), in which it dissolves spontaneously to form carbonic acid, which dissociates into bicarbonate and hydrogen ions. The blood–brain barrier is impermeable to ions, including hydrogen ions, so the pH of CSF is determined by P_aCO_2. When the central chemoreceptors detect an increase in CSF pH, they send signals to the brainstem respiratory centres to increase ventilation (**Figure 4.22**).

> **Patients with chronic hypercapnia, an excessive amount of carbon dioxide in the blood, develop tolerance to these higher levels.** Their central chemoreceptors no longer respond to increased carbon dioxide, because the import of serum bicarbonate neutralises cerebrospinal fluid pH.
>
> These patients rely on mild hypoxia to stimulate respiratory effort, so overtreatment of their mild hypoxia suppresses their respiratory effort. This results in severe hypoventilation and respiratory acidosis despite improved oxygen saturation values.

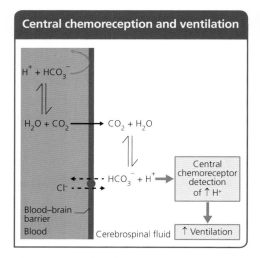

Central chemoreception and ventilation

Figure 4.22 Carbon dioxide crosses the blood–brain barrier. The resultant change in the pH of the cerebrospinal fluid is detected by central chemoreceptors. This effect stimulates an increase in alveolar ventilation.

Chronic hypercapnia

After long-standing ventilatory impairment, such as in COPD, the central chemoreceptor response to increased P_aCO_2 becomes blunted. High P_aCO_2 decreases cerebrospinal fluid pH. However, chronic exposure to carbon dioxide stimulates bicarbonate–chloride ion exchange over the blood–brain barrier. Bicarbonate is imported to buffer the excess hydrogen ions in the cerebrospinal fluid, but this reduces the body's response to P_aCO_2. Consequently, patients with chronic hypercapnia tolerate high P_aCO_2 and become much more reliant on P_aO_2 to stimulate breathing.

Overall response

Figures 4.23 and **4.24** show the body's responses to changes in P_aCO_2 and P_aO_2, respectively. Ventilation is much more sensitive to alterations in P_aCO_2 than it is to changes in P_aO_2. A small increase in P_aCO_2 causes a large, linear increase in $\dot{V}_A$. In contrast, the ventilatory response to a decrease in P_aO_2 is much more gradual, given the hyperbolic shape of the curve.

Changes in P_aCO_2, P_aO_2 and pH (arterial) are synergistic

- A decrease in P_aO_2 causes a leftward shift of the P_aCO_2–$\dot{V}_A$ curve (**Figure 4.25a**)
- An increase in P_aCO_2 or a decrease in pH causes an upward shift of the P_aO_2–$\dot{V}_A$ curve (**Figure 4.25b**).

Ondine's curse is an extremely rare condition arising from the loss of involuntary control of breathing. The unconscious control of ventilation is absent either because of a congenital abnormality or as a consequence of brain stem injury Patients rely on conscious effort for ventilation; without treatment, they develop respiratory arrest during sleep. Ondine was a water nymph who cursed her unfaithful mortal lover, making him forget to breathe when he fell asleep.

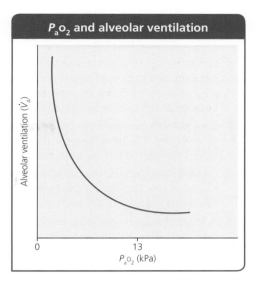

Figure 4.24 An increase in the partial pressure of arterial oxygen (P_aO_2) causes a gradual, hyperbolic decrease in alveolar ventilation ($\dot{V}_A$).

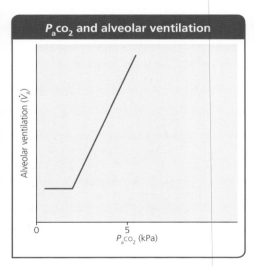

Figure 4.23 An increase in the partial pressure of arterial carbon dioxide (P_aCO_2) causes a sharp, linear rise in alveolar ventilation ($\dot{V}_A$).

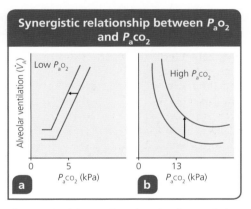

Figure 4.25 (a) Hypoxia makes alveolar ventilation ($\dot{V}_A$) more sensitive to changes in the partial pressure of carbon dioxide (P_aCO_2). (b) Hypercapnia makes $\dot{V}_A$ more sensitive to changes in the partial pressure of oxygen (P_aO_2).

Answers to starter questions

1. Lungs are soft structures consisting of elastic tissue with a tendency to collapse inwards. They are kept expanded by being connected to the chest wall by the pleurae. The pleurae lining the inside of the chest wall and the outside of the lung remain opposed because of the surface tension of the fluid between them.

2. Body tissues consume more oxygen and produce more carbon dioxide when active than when at rest. The more oxygen consumed, the lower the Po_2 of the tissue's interstitial fluid. The reduction in Po_2 promotes oxygen transfer from blood to tissue.

3. Carbon monoxide is a colourless, odourless gas with an extremely high affinity for haemoglobin. Therefore it prevents oxygen from binding to haemoglobin. The resulting tissue hypoxia (lack of oxygen) causes unconsciousness and cardiac arrest.

4. A series of nuclei in the pons and medulla initiate inspiration, stop inspiration and start expiration. They are influenced by the Hering–Breuer reflex, which detects lung stretch at the end of inspiration and acts to stop it. The duration of each breath also changes alongside the respiratory rate to maintain blood gases at optimum levels.

5. Chronic lung diseases (e.g. chronic obstructive pulmonary disease and pulmonary fibrosis) can cause chronic hypoxia. In an attempt to match the ventilation of alveoli, and the perfusion of blood to the alveolar capillaries [the ventilation ($\dot{V}$)/perfusion ($\dot{Q}$) ratio] pulmonary arterioles vasoconstrict. This increases pressure in the right side of the heart, and can eventually lead to right-sided heart failure (cor pulmonale).

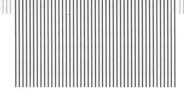

Chapter 5
Renal system

Starter questions

Answers to the following questions are on page 162.

1. What blood tests are used to check kidney function?
2. How is renal function sacrificed to preserve blood circulation?
3. Why do hyperkalaemia and acidosis present together?
4. Why might correcting low blood volume disrupt concentration control?
5. Why are so many drugs excreted by the kidney?

Introduction

The kidneys' central function is to filter blood of waste products and excrete them via urine. As part of this function, they monitor and regulate the blood's volume and electrolyte composition, which is crucial for the maintenance of blood pressure, pH and normal cellular function.

The kidneys are made up of around 1 million nephrons: tubular structures that filter the blood and then process the filtrate according to the body's needs. The vast majority of the filtered material is reabsorbed, with waste products and anything that is present in excess being lost into the urine. This homeostatic function is regulated by neuronal and hormonal inputs, in addition to intrinsic renal mechanisms.

Renal failure is often asymptomatic until very late stages, by which point there is multi-organ failure and significant immunosuppression. Failure necessitates dialysis: artificial replacement of kidney function to prevent toxicity and provide control of fluid balance in the body.

Case 4 Collapse, confusion and shortness of breath

Presentation

Carers find Enid, a 92-year-old lady, on the kitchen floor at 8 am. She is confused, coughing, short of breath and complaining of pain in her hip. She is thought to have fallen the previous night and been unable to get up. Enid lives in sheltered accommodation, is normally well, though she takes ramipril, an angiotensin converting enzyme (ACE) inhibitor, for heart failure, but has been coughing, pyrexial and largely bed-bound for the last 3 days.

She is taken by ambulance to the emergency department where the initial investigations show:

- A fracture in her left femur
- Lung consolidation seen on chest X-ray
- Initial blood tests demonstrate a creatinine of 373 μmol/L (normal range 70–150 μmol/L).

Analysis

It is common for elderly patients to have several concurrent and potentially compounding problems. Enid has pre-existing heart failure, and the coughing, temperature and X-ray evidence of consolidation suggest pneumonia, which may have led to confusion or delirium causing her to fall.

During her long period on the floor, blood loss from the fracture, dehydration due to inability to drink, and perhaps her heart failure have caused a reduction in effective circulating blood volume and therefore blood pressure. Her creatinine level suggests acute kidney injury (AKI, also called acute renal failure) from a reduction in kidney perfusion. Another factor may be her ACE inhibitor, which can reduce renal perfusion by decreasing glomerular capillary hydrostatic pressure.

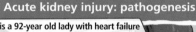

Acute kidney injury: pathogenesis

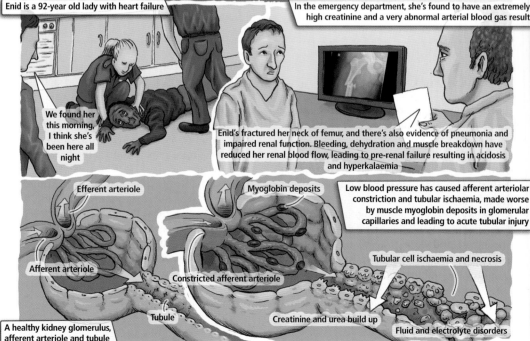

Enid is a 92-year old lady with heart failure

In the emergency department, she's found to have an extremely high creatinine and a very abnormal arterial blood gas result

We found her this morning, I think she's been here all night

Enid's fractured her neck of femur, and there's also evidence of pneumonia and impaired renal function. Bleeding, dehydration and muscle breakdown have reduced her renal blood flow, leading to pre-renal failure resulting in acidosis and hyperkalaemia

Efferent arteriole

Myoglobin deposits

Low blood pressure has caused afferent arteriolar constriction and tubular ischaemia, made worse by muscle myoglobin deposits in glomerular capillaries and leading to acute tubular injury

Tubular cell ischaemia and necrosis

Afferent arteriole

Constricted afferent arteriole

Tubule

Creatinine and urea build up

A healthy kidney glomerulus, afferent arteriole and tubule

Fluid and electrolyte disorders

Case 4 *continued*

Further case

Additional blood tests show:

- CK (creatine kinase): 11,500 IU/L (normal range 25–170 IU/L),
- K^+ (potassium ions): 6.5 mmol/L (normal range 3.5–5.0 mmol/L)
- pH: 7.23 (normal range 7.35–7.45)
- HCO_3^- 16 mmol/L (normal range 24–30 mmol/L.

Enid undergoes urgent surgical repair of her femur and is treated with intravenous antibiotics for pneumonia. Her ACE inhibitor is withheld and she is given intravenous fluid to compensate for fluid loss. After several days of supportive treatment she begins to improve; her creatinine comes down to 180 μmol/L and her metabolic acidosis (low pH and low HCO_3^-) resolves.

Further analysis

Her fracture, and the length of time she spent lying on the floor, appears to have caused significant breakdown in her muscle (rhabdomyolysis), leading to significantly raised creatine kinase, a muscle cell enzyme released into the blood when cells are damaged. The other blood tests indicate AKI and loss of renal function: acidosis as H^+ (hydrogen) ions are not excreted; hyperkalaemia as K^+ is not excreted.

Hyperkalaemia also occurs with muscle breakdown as it is released from damaged cells.

Enid is given intravenous fluid to improve her blood pressure and the perfusion of her organs, and her nephrotoxic medication (ramipril) is stopped. Her hyperkalaemia will resolve spontaneously as renal function returns, although giving bicarbonate to help her acid–base disturbance will also help cells to take up potassium, thus reducing the levels in the blood.

Kidney structure and function

The kidneys are two bean-shaped organs 8–12 cm long, which lie against the posterior wall of the abdomen. They are described as retroperitoneal, because the peritoneum only covers them anteriorly, rather than enclosing them. They span the vertebrae from T12 to about L3: the right kidney is lower than the left, as the liver pushes it down during development. The lateral border of each is convex, whereas the medial side has an indentation called the hilum. This is where the renal artery enters, and the renal vein and ureters exit. Although human kidneys have a smooth outer profile, they are made up of a number of lobes: this structure is evident in the renal papillae (the individual medullary components of each lobe) which can be seen when the kidney is cut in coronal section.

An outer (cortical) region can be identified, with the inner (medullary) region divided into a number of pyramids, whose points form the papillae (**Figure 5.1**). Along with structural tissue, kidneys consist of vascular and tubular elements that are closely intertwined.

Renal circulation

Kidneys are highly vascular, reflecting their main function in processing the blood, and receive almost 20% of resting cardiac output (about 1 L/min). This greatly exceeds the metabolic needs of the kidney.

Arterial circulation

The renal artery enters the kidney at the hilum. After dividing into five segmental

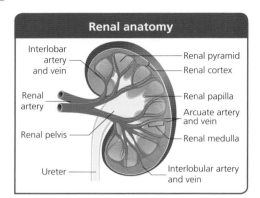

Renal anatomy

Interlobar artery and vein
Renal pyramid
Renal cortex
Renal artery
Renal papilla
Arcuate artery and vein
Renal pelvis
Renal medulla
Ureter
Interlobular artery and vein

Figure 5.1 Gross anatomy of the kidney. The origin of the kidney as a set of lobes can be seen in the papillae of the inner medullae, and in the vasculature which shows a lobar arrangement. However, the cortical tissue of the different lobes merge to form a smooth outline. Blood vessels, nerves and the ureter pass into and out of the kidney via the renal hilum on the medial aspect of the kidney.

arteries, it branches into interlobar arteries which run along the sides of the renal pyramids. Interlobar arteries then divide to form arcuate arteries at the junction of the medulla and cortex: these run along the corticomedullary boundary.

Interlobular arteries arise from the arcuate arteries, and run through the cortex towards the surface of the kidney. They supply afferent arterioles that enter the glomeruli at the beginning of each nephron. Glomerular capillaries are the site of filtration: some fluid from the blood leaves the capillaries and enters the nephron, while the remainder, including all the cellular components of the blood and virtually all the plasma proteins, pass into the efferent arteriole and go on to supply the peritubular capillaries. This represents a portal system: two sets of capillaries in series. This is crucial to reabsorbing filtered material back into the blood.

Some of the peritubular capillaries form hairpin loops, which run down into the medulla and out again, in parallel with the loops of Henle. These are the vasa recta (**Figure 5.10**): blood flow through these is limited to the bare minimum required for tissue

survival, so in contrast to the cortical regions, where there is a plentiful blood supply, the inner medulla can easily become ischaemic.

Venous circulation

Peritubular capillaries feed blood back into the renal vein via a sequence of venules and veins, running alongside the equivalent arteries but in the opposite direction through the same sequence of structures. Ultimately the blood drains to the inferior vena cava via the renal vein.

Tubular elements

After filtration out of the glomerular capillaries, fluid enters Bowman's capsule, the first part of the nephron and the functional unit of the kidney (**Figure 5.2**). Each nephron is a tube made up of a simple epithelium and is about 5 cm long (including the collecting duct segment, which is embryologically distinct from the rest). The tubule varies in diameter from about 15 μm to about 60 μm as it passes through different regions. Different nephrons merge to form collecting ducts of about 200 μm in diameter, before they form the ducts of Bellini where the final urine drains into the renal calyces. As filtered fluid passes through the nephron it is extensively processed: more than 99% of salt and water is reabsorbed while other material is secreted into the fluid.

The glomeruli, proximal convoluted tubules, distal convoluted tubules and the early parts of the collecting ducts lie in the cortex, while the loop of Henle runs down into the medulla before returning to the cortex, and the collecting duct runs down to empty out of the papillary tip. About 80% of nephrons are cortical: their glomeruli lie near the surface of the kidney and they have only short loops of Henle (with no thin ascending section) that only run down into the outer medulla. The remaining 20% of (juxtamedullary nephrons) have their glomeruli lying deep in the cortex and much longer loops of that run down into the inner medulla.

The nephron

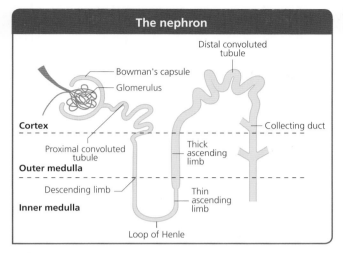

Distal convoluted tubule

Bowman's capsule

Glomerulus

Cortex

Collecting duct

Proximal convoluted tubule

Thick ascending limb

Outer medulla

Descending limb

Thin ascending limb

Inner medulla

Loop of Henle

Figure 5.2 The general structure of a nephron.

The renal pelvis

The medullae of each lobe narrow to a point (the papilla) out of which the ducts of Bellini drain. Wrapped around this is funnels made of connective tissue that catches the urine: the minor calyces. They drain into larger funnels, the major calyces, which drain into the pelvis of the kidney. From here, the urine passes to the ureter.

Renal processes

The production of the tubular fluid from the blood and its gradual conversion into the urine depends on three processes:

- **Filtration**: blood is 'sieved' by the glomerular filtration membrane to form an initial filtrate
- **Reabsorption**: substances move from the tubular filtrate back into the blood
- **Secretion**: substances are transported from blood or interstitial fluid into the tubular fluid.

Excretion is the irreversible removal of a substance from plasma, and occurs when the above processes result in the substance entering the renal pelvis as a component of urine.

Filtration

The glomerulus is the site of filtration where fluid is filtered out of the blood across a specialised barrier into Bowman's space, from where it can flow into the nephron. During its passage along the renal tubules the exact constitution of the filtrate is adjusted according to the body's needs to produce the final urine.

Glomerular structure and function

The afferent arteriole supplies a knot of glomerular capillaries, which are enclosed within a 'balloon' at the start of the renal tubule – Bowman's capsule (**Figure 5.3**). These capillaries provide a large surface area. Approximately 20% of plasma entering via the afferent arterioles is filtered across the glomerular filtration membrane; the rest enters the efferent arteriole and passes to the peritubular capillaries.

The vascular tone of the efferent arteriole maintains a constantly high hydrostatic pressure in the glomerular capillary bed that drives filtration in the glomerulus. Fluid (including water, sugars, and salts) is forced out

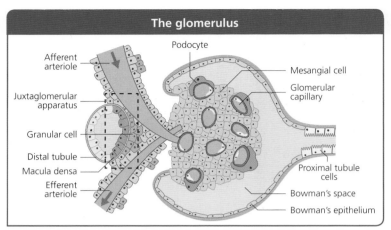

The glomerulus

- Afferent arteriole
- Podocyte
- Mesangial cell
- Glomerular capillary
- Juxtaglomerular apparatus
- Granular cell
- Distal tubule
- Macula densa
- Efferent arteriole
- Proximal tubule cells
- Bowman's space
- Bowman's epithelium

Figure 5.3 A glomerulus, fed by afferent, and drained by efferent, arterioles. The juxtaglomerular apparatus, which is involved in tubuloglomerular feedback, is shown with part of the distal part of the same nephron.

of the capillaries – a process called ultrafiltration – and collects in Bowman's space.

Support cells

The glomerular capillaries are encased by podocytes (the visceral epithelial cells of Bowman's capsule), so called because they project processes which branch to form tiny 'feet' which interdigitate (like interlocking fingers) as they wrap over the capillaries. Podocyte processes secrete a dense layer of basement membrane around the glomerular capillaries; both the processes and basement membrane help support the capillaries. The knot of capillaries is also supported by mesangial cells that sit between the capillaries, which are contractile (influencing glomerular capillary blood flow) and can maintain the structure of the glomerulus. They also have a phagocytic role of defence and repair.

Glomerular filtration membrane

There are three structures between glomerular capillary blood and the filtrate in Bowman's capsule that form the glomerular filtration membrane (**Figure 5.4**):

- Capillary endothelial cells
- Specialised basement membrane
- Podocyte cell foot processes.

Glomerular capillaries are fenestrated, i.e. there are holes through the endothelial cells,

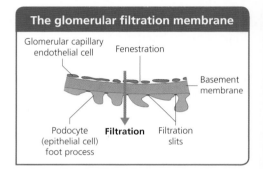

The glomerular filtration membrane

- Glomerular capillary endothelial cell
- Fenestration
- Basement membrane
- Podocyte (epithelial cell) foot process
- **Filtration**
- Filtration slits

Figure 5.4 The glomerular filtration membrane is formed of the fenestrated capillary endothelium, negatively-charged basement membrane and slit pores between podocyte foot processes.

through which smaller molecules, ions and water can pass freely. The endothelial cells sit on an unusually thick, negatively charged basement membrane, which helps to repel (negatively charged) plasma proteins by its charge and physical presence.

Finally, podocytes have pedicels, or foot processes, which interdigitate with each other as they encircle the capillaries. Slit diaphragms between these processes act as a further barrier to the passage of proteins. Overall, the barrier allows free filtration of molecules smaller than about 7 kDa, and prevents passage of molecules larger than about 70 kDa. Diseases that damage this sensitive membrane, such as diabetes or glomerulonephritis, can allow larger molecules to pass through.

Factors determining ultrafiltration

In the circulation of fluid in most systemic capillary beds, tissue fluid is secreted at the arterial end of the bed and most of the fluid is then reabsorbed at the venous end. Fluid movement across the capillary walls determined by filtration pressures: the balance between oncotic, osmotic and hydrostatic pressure (Starling's forces, page 86). In the glomerular capillaries the hydrostatic pressure is much higher and more constant, leading to a larger amount of fluid being forced out.

> **Diabetes and hypertension damage the glomerular filtration membrane increasing permeability and allowing proteins to enter the filtrate and urine.** This accelerates membrane damage and impairs renal function. Detecting even small amounts of albumin in the urine is a sensitive indicator of diabetic and hypertensive renal disease.

Glomerular filtrate

Glomerular filtrate is similar to plasma except for the absence of proteins larger than 70 kDa. The proteins left in the plasma, that leave the glomerulus and travel to the peritubular capillaries, increase the oncotic pressure of the blood, helping to draw the fluid absorbed from the renal tubules back into the peritubular capillaries.

Filtration pressures

The high hydrostatic pressure in the glomerular capillaries is maintained by the resistance posed by the efferent arterioles, which maintains high filtration pressure along the entire length of the capillaries (**Figure 5.5**).

10 mmHg of hydrostatic pressure in Bowman's space opposes ultrafiltration, but is necessary to drive fluid movement through the nephron. Normally, there is no oncotic pressure in Bowman's space, as the filtrate contains no proteins. However, capillary oncotic pressure rises towards the end of the capillary as the relative amount of protein – blocked from leaving – concentrates as fluid leaves the capillary.

The overall filtration pressure, i.e. the balance of these filtration pressures, determines the rate at which fluid moves across the glomerular membrane; the glomerular filtration rate (GFR):

$$GFR = k_f (\text{forces favouring filtration} - \text{forces opposing filtration})$$
$$GFR = k_f (P_{cap} + \pi_{BC}) - (P_{BS} + \pi_{cap})$$

Where k_f is a filtration coefficient, P is hydrostatic pressure, π oncotic pressure, cap represents the glomerular capillaries and

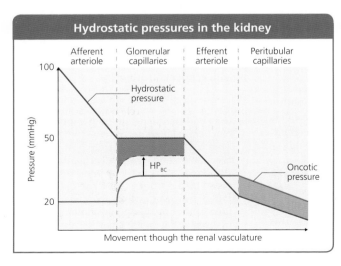

Hydrostatic pressures in the kidney

Figure 5.5 Hydrostatic pressures throughout the renal vasculature. Glomerular ultrafiltration (fluid leaving capillaries) is shaded dark blue and tubular reabsorption (fluid entering capillaries) shaded red. The effect of the hydrostatic pressure in Bowman's capsule is indicated at the level of the glomerulus. Note how the resistance of the efferent arterioles keeps pressure high in the glomerular capillaries, favouring filtration, and low in the peritubular capillaries, favouring reabsorption. HP_{BC}, hydrostatic pressure in Bowman's capsule.

BS represents Bowman's space. Since π_{BC} should be 0 – i.e. there is no oncotic pressure in Bowman's capsule – we can see that the main driver for filtration is the hydrostatic pressure in the capillaries, while the rise in oncotic pressure as fluid leaves acts as a counterbalancing force.

Glomerular filtration rate (GFR)

If we assume the kidneys receive 1 L/min of blood and that blood has a cell content (i.e. haematocrit) of 40%, then the renal plasma flow is 600 mL/min. Twenty per cent of this is then filtered through the glomerular membrane, i.e. GFR is normally around 120 mL/min for a 70 kg man. GFR is an important element of kidney function and is used clinically to assess kidney function and screen for and monitor renal disease.

GFR is tightly regulated by mechanisms that adjust the glomerular hydrostatic pressure, the main determinant of filtration rate.

> **GFR decreases by approximately 1 mL/min/yr** due to age-related degeneration.

Estimating GFR

GFR is quantified by clearance measurements that measure how quickly an injected substance is cleared from the blood by the kidney, or estimated by comparing plasma and urine levels of creatinine, a naturally occurring metabolite.

Clearance measurements

This method measures the volume of plasma cleared of a substance in a given time, usually a minute. The clearance of a substance reflects whether the substance is filtered at the glomerulus, and/or reabsorbed or secreted by the tubules.

To reflect the rate of glomerular filtration accurately, the substance must be freely filtered in the glomerulus, but not metabolised, reabsorbed or secreted by the tubules. This means that its level in the urine (compared to the plasma) directly reflects the rate of filtration. Inulin is suitable and the most commonly used substance. It is not made by the body, but can be infused intravenously to give a constant plasma level and the rate of its appearance in the urine can be measured.

The GFR is calculated by comparing plasma and urine concentrations of the substance, and the rate of urine production, e.g. for substance X:

$$C_x = \frac{U_x \times V}{P_x}$$

Where U_x and P_x are the urinary and plasma concentration of X and V represents the urine flow in mL/min.

Substances that are not freely filtered (e.g. plasma proteins) or are filtered freely but subsequently reabsorbed in the tubules (e.g. glucose) should have a clearance very close to 0. Conversely, a clearance higher than the actual GFR implies it is being actively secreted in the tubules, as is the case for many drugs.

Creatinine clearance

Measuring inulin clearance is the most accurate measure of GFR, but it is too impractical for regular clinical use. GFR is more commonly estimated by comparing the concentration of creatinine – a small nitrogenous compound produced by muscle breakdown – in the urine and plasma. Its level in plasma is influenced by muscle mass and exercise, but it is freely filtered and there is minimal absorption/secretion in the tubules.

Once measurements have been obtained, different formulae are then used to calculate estimated GFR (eGFR), in the context of age, weight, gender and ethnicity.

> **Urea and creatinine are both important biochemical markers of renal function.** Urea is a waste product from protein breakdown and is normally cleared by the kidney. If renal function decreases, blood urea nitrogen (BUN) can become raised. However, unlike creatinine, urea cannot be used to estimate GFR accurately as it is significantly reabsorbed in the tubules.

Regulation of glomerular filtration

Homeostatic mechanisms keep GFR constant despite relatively wide changes in systemic blood pressure and flow rates. There are two main mechanisms: the myogenic reflex, and tubuloglomerular feedback. Both do this by causing vasoconstriction or vasodilatation of the afferent and efferent arterioles to alter hydrostatic pressure in the glomerular capillaries (**Table 5.1**), the main determinant of GFR.

Myogenic reflex

The myogenic reflex is an intrinsic property of vascular smooth muscle (page 83). When increased blood pressure stretches the arteriole, there is a reflex constriction of its muscle (**Figure 3.14**). This occurs in both afferent and efferent arterioles, and prevents renal blood flow from increasing when blood pressure does. Since afferent constriction will reduce, and efferent constriction will increase GFR, the overall effect on GFR is modest.

Tubuloglomerular feedback mechanism

The tubuloglomerular feedback mechanism has a more significant effect on GFR. It coordinates a response of the renal, endocrine and autonomic nervous systems to changes in salt concentration in the distal convoluted tubule (DCT). This system is based on the physical proximity of the DCT to the glomerulus of the same nephron.

The juxtaglomerular apparatus

The macula densa is made up of specialised cells in the DCT that lie adjacent to the glomerulus of the same nephron (**Figure 5.3**). These cells are part of the juxtaglomerular apparatus, which also includes extraglomerular mesangial cells and granular cells in the wall of the afferent arteriole.

Salt concentrations in the DCT are monitored by the macula densa so that an increase causes a contraction of the afferent arteriole, reducing GFR. Conversely, a decrease in DCT salt concentration leads to a decrease in afferent arteriolar tone, increasing GFR and the release of renin from the granular cells, which indirectly increases tubular salt reabsorption.

Renin-angiotensin-aldosterone system

The release of renin activates the renin-angiotensin-aldosterone system (RAAS; see page 152) and the production of the hormones angiotensin II and aldosterone.

Angiotensin II has many effects, the common result of which is to increase the systemic blood pressure. Systemically, angiotensin II increases total peripheral resistance (TPR) and therefore mean arterial blood pressure (mABP). Within the kidney, it causes intense vasoconstriction of the efferent arteriole and moderate constriction of the afferent arteriole

Effects of changes in afferent and efferent arteriolar tone		
	Vasoconstriction	Vasodilatation
Afferent arteriole	Reduced glomerular capillary HP	Increased glomerular capillary HP
	Increased vascular resistance	Reduced vascular resistance
	Decreased RBF and GFR	Increased RBF and GFR
Efferent arteriole	Increased glomerular capillary HP	Reduced glomerular capillary HP
	Reduced peritubular capillary HP	Increased peritubular capillary HP
	Increased vascular resistance	Reduced vascular resistance
	Increased GFR but decreased RBF	Increased RBF but decreased GFR

Table 5.1 The upstream and downstream effects of tone changes in the afferent and efferent arterioles. HP, hydrostatic pressure; mABP, mean arterial blood pressure; RBF, renal blood flow; GFR, glomerular filtration rate.

which increases hydrostatic pressure in the glomerular capillaries and therefore the GFR. Aldosterone increases salt in the distal tubule and collecting duct, which supports the circulating plasma volume and helps to stop blood pressure decreasing.

> **Glomerulonephritis (inflammation of glomeruli) usually presents with proteinuria – protein in the urine – or haematuria – blood in the urine – with or without renal failure.** Causes include systemic immune diseases, where antibody–antigen complexes deposit in the glomerular filtration membrane and stimulate an inflammatory response that damages the filter.

Tubular functions

The glomerular filtrate passes through the renal tubules on the way to the renal pelvis, where it then drains into the ureters and bladder. Along the way, there is variable reabsorption of ions and nutrients back into the blood to prevent their loss, and the filtrate is concentrated to preserve water as needed.

Tubular structure and function

As fluid leaves the glomerulus, it enters the proximal convoluted tubule. It then passes into the loop of Henle, which runs down into the medulla before returning to the cortex, passing by its own glomerulus and becoming the distal convoluted tubule. Its last section

is the collecting duct, which runs through the medulla, draining urine into the renal pelvis. From there, urine drains via the ureters to the bladder.

Tubular sections

Each tubular section has specialised functions that alter filtrate constituents, transferring substances between the tubular lumen and the peritubular capillaries that run alongside the nephron (**Table 5.2**). Tubular reabsorption is the movement of water and solutes out of the tubules and into peritubular capillaries; secretion is the opposite. Most reabsorption occurs in the proximal convoluted tubule (PCT) and DCT.

Nephron function		
Component	Function	
Glomerulus	Ultrafiltration of blood to form filtrate in Bowman's capsule	
Proximal convoluted tubule	Reabsorbs 65% Na^+ and H_2O, essentially all glucose and amino acids, PO_4^{3-} and HCO_3^-	Secretes weak acids & bases including drugs
Loop of Henle	Establishes the hyperosmolar medullary interstitial gradient	About 20% of filtered water is absorbed in the dTL, and about 25% of filtered salt will be absorbed in the TAL
Distal (convoluted) tubule	Na^+ and Ca^{2+} reabsorption	Further reabsorption and secretion of K^+/H^+
Collecting duct	Principal cells: ADH-dependent water reabsorption and aldosterone-dependent reabsorption of Na^+ and secretion of K^+/H^+	Intercalated cells: acid–base regulation and K^+ excretion

Table 5.2 Functions of the different sections of the renal nephron. ADH, antidiuretic hormone.

Proximal convoluted tubule

The PCT absorbs 65% of Na^+ (sodium ions) and water, some PO_4^{3-} (phosphate ions) and HCO_3^- (bicarbonate) and virtually all the glucose and amino acids. There is also active secretion of both weak acids and bases, including many drugs.

Loop of Henle

The loop of Henle is a hairpin loop that descends into the renal medulla before returning to the cortex. This arrangement allows a process called counter current multiplication, which is dependent on the different characteristics of the two limbs of the loop. In the descending limb, water permeability is high allowing the fluid to become more concentrated, while in the thick ascending limb there is active transport of salt out of the tubular fluid into the medullary interstitium. The salt accumulates to generate a high osmolality in the inner medullary interstitium. This medullary gradient is then exploited by the last section of tubule – the collecting duct – to concentrate the filtrate as it passes back through the medulla on its way to the pelvis.

Distal convoluted tubule

The DCT is primarily involved in the hormone-regulated reabsorption of Na^+ and Ca^{2+}, as well as K^+ secretion. It is also the section where filtrate is monitored by the juxtaglomerular apparatus as a part of the tubuloglomerular feedback system regulating GFR (see page 139).

Collecting duct

The collecting duct is where the final determination of the urine concentration occurs. There is water reabsorption regulated by the action of antidiuretic hormone (ADH), a posterior pituitary hormone secreted in response to increased plasma osmolarity, and salt reabsorption, regulated by the steroid hormone aldosterone.

There are two types of collecting duct epithelial cells: principal cells, which make up about 2/3rds of the cells in the cortex and increase in relative abundance as the collecting duct passes down into the medulla, are the sites of aldosterone and ADH action and hence salt and water reabsorption. Intercalated cells are responsible for acid–base regulation. There are two main types; α intercalated cells secrete protons into the urine (partly in exchange for K^+) and return bicarbonate to the circulation, β cells have the opposite action, excreting bicarbonate and releasing protons into the blood.

> Acute kidney injury (AKI, or acute renal failure) is most commonly caused by renal hypoperfusion – due to a drop in blood pressure, caused by either heart failure or a decrease in circulating volume, in dehydration or blood loss. If ischaemia continues, AKI progresses to acute tubular necrosis (ATN), the death of tubular cells. If this occurs, kidney function does not return to normal when renal perfusion pressure is restored, and patients may require a long period to recover.

Tubular reabsorption

Reabsorption involves the movement of substances from the lumen into tubular cells, out of the cells and into the lateral intercellular space, and finally into the peritubular capillaries. At the same time, water is drawn either through the cells or between them (paracellularly) by the osmotic gradient resulting from solute transport. Some substances (such as chloride ions) get left behind in the tubule and can then flow passively down their concentration gradient through the tight junctions between the cells, which are particularly leaky in this epithelium.

The blood in the peritubular capillaries is enriched in plasma proteins, which were not filtered with the fluid in the glomerulus. Consequently, there is an unusually high oncotic pressure here. This, combined with the low hydrostatic pressure after the blood has flowed through the efferent arterioles, means the Starling forces in this region strongly favour the movement of fluid out of the interstitium into the blood (**Figure 5.5**). This helps to take up the large amounts of fluid being reabsorbed from the PCT.

Tubular transport of ions

The concentrations of Na^+ and K^+ in the extracellular fluid are crucial for determining the resting membrane potential of cells, which is required for normal cellular function. Their homeostasis is therefore essential for all cellular metabolism and life and is largely maintained by the kidneys. Most reabsorption of ions and other valuable solutes– and secondary water reabsorption – occurs in the PCT.

Exploiting the sodium gradient

Na^+/K^+-ATPase pumps on the basolateral membrane of PCT cells use energy from ATP hydrolysis directly to pump Na^+ out of the cell and K^+ into the cell. These pumps represent the key energy-consuming process of the whole tubule, accounting for over 75% of all ATP used. As a consequence, the intracellular sodium ion concentration is much lower than it is outside. When Na^+ are allowed to move down the gradient energy is released, this is be used to move other substances up a concentration gradient: secondary active transport (see page 19). This Na^+-linked cotransport is used to secrete and reabsorb various substances in the tubules (**Figure 5.6**), and is also how net Na^+ reabsorption occurs, since Na^+ typically enters cells across the apical membrane and leaves across the basolateral membrane.

> The SGLT-2 glucose cotransporter of the PCT is renal-specific and therefore a potential target for drugs which lower plasma glucose levels in type 2 diabetes. Canagliflozin uses this mechanism to improve glycaemic control, decrease body weight and lower blood pressure, as water osmotically follows 'trapped' glucose into the urine.

Na^+/Glucose cotransporters

One major example is the SGLT2 Na^+-linked cotransporter that reabsorbs glucose from the proximal tubule. SGLT2 proteins on the apical membrane of the PCT cells combine the transport of Na^+ travelling down its gradient with a glucose molecule, which can be carried up its concentration gradient into the cells. These reabsorb 98% of glucose in the filtrate; the similar SGLT1 transporter (which takes 2 Na^+ ions, so can work against a bigger glucose gradient) reabsorbs the rest just before the loop of Henle. Without them vast

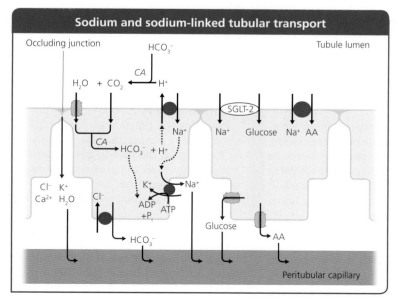

Sodium and sodium-linked tubular transport

Occluding junction

Tubule lumen

HCO_3^-

CA

$H_2O + CO_2 \longleftarrow H^+$

SGLT-2

Na^+ Na^+ Glucose Na^+ AA

CA

$HCO_3^- + H^+$

Cl^- K^+

Ca^{2+} H_2O Cl^- $K^+ \longrightarrow Na^+$

ADP ATP
$+P_i$

Glucose

HCO_3^- AA

Peritubular capillary

Figure 5.6
Mechanism for reabsorption of Na^+ in the proximal tubule and how it is coupled to tubular transport of other substances. AA, amino acid. Active pumping of Na^+ out of cells on the basolateral side provides a driving force for Na^+ entry on the apical surface, bringing other substrates with it. CA, carbonic anhydrase. SGLT-2, sodium-glucose linked transporter 2.

amounts of energy would be lost as glucose in the urine – glycosuria. The same cotransporter is involved in glucose gut absorption (see page 217).

> **In uncontrolled diabetes mellitus plasma glucose is high** and the tubular fluid contains more glucose than the transport system can handle. Glucose is therefore lost in the urine, making it sweet, giving glycosuria its name.

Water reabsorption

Reabsorption of Na^+ and other solutes generates an osmotic gradient that drives the reabsorption of water from filtrate. Water can pass nearly freely through the PCT due to aquaporin-1 (AQP-1) water channels in both apical and basolateral membranes of the cells. About 80% of the reabsorbed water moves through the cells; the rest moves paracellularly through leaky tight junctions. Overall, about two-thirds of all filtered water is reabsorbed in the PCT.

Hydrogen ions and bicarbonate

The Na^+/H^+ exchanger pumps hydrogen ions (H^+, i.e. protons) into the tubular lumen in exchange for Na^+, to reabsorb needed Na^+ and secrete excess acid – a waste product of metabolism. Most of this activity occurs in the PCT.

Carbonic anhydrase

The protons secreted in exchange for Na^+ interact with HCO_3^- ions to form carbonic acid. Carbonic anhydrase in the brush border breaks this down to CO_2 and water, which can then diffuse into the cells. Once there, intracellular carbonic anhydrase converts them back to carbonic acid, which dissociates to release protons to be pumped back out and bicarbonate to return to the circulation.

Bicarbonate

HCO_3^- is transported across the basolateral membrane on an anion exchanger, usually in exchange for Cl^- (**Figure 5.6**). Thus the net effect is to transport $NaHCO_3$ (sodium bicarbonate) back to the bloodstream. HCO_3^- is the main buffer in the extracellular fluids and is crucial in maintaining their acid–base balance.

Potassium ions

K^+ is the main intracellular cation, important along with Na^+ in maintaining the resting membrane potential of all cells. Accordingly, plasma K^+ concentration is closely regulated between 3.5–5.5 mmol/L and even small changes outside this range can have severe effects on cardiac function. Most of the filtered potassium is absorbed as it passes along the nephron and homeostasis is achieved by potassium secretion in the collecting duct under the control of aldosterone.

Proximal convoluted tubule

In the PCT there is passive, mainly paracellular, reabsorption of K^+. More is reabsorbed in the loop of Henle via $Na^+/K^+/2Cl^-$ (NKCC2) cotransporters, but much of this K^+ recycles passively back into the tubule to allow this transporter to continue functioning.

Distal convoluted tubule and collecting duct

After PCT reabsorption, K^+ is secreted in the DCT and early collecting duct via renal outer medullary K^+ channels (ROMK) in principal cells and absorbed by an H^+/K^+-ATPase in the α intercalated cells. The rate of this is determined by:

- **Aldosterone** increasing the rate of secretion: this is the main regulatory element. Hyperkalaemia is a strong stimulus for aldosterone release.
- **K^+ concentration** in the tubular cells: a raised intracellular $[K^+]$ increases the driving force for secretion.
- **Flow rate**: increased tubular flow rate increases Na^+ reabsorption, which increases the electrical gradient favouring K^+ secretion. High flow also maintains the concentration gradient for K^+ secretion since there is less time for K^+ to accumulate.

- **Acidity**: H^+ and K^+ are exchanged by H^+/K^+-ATPase. Furthermore, secretion of one reduces the electrical gradient for secretion of the other. Therefore acidosis promotes hyperkalaemia, and vice versa.

Calcium ions

The concentration of calcium ions (Ca^{2+}) in the extracellular fluid is critical for the normal function of excitable tissues, and muscle in particular. It is also used as a signalling molecule by many cells. Calcium ions are reabsorbed throughout the nephron. In the PCT this is largely passive and parallels the movement of salt and water. There is also paracellular reabsorption in the thick ascending limb of the loop of Henle driven by the electrical gradient and cation-selective permeability of the tight junctions.

However, the DCT is the main site of plasma Ca^{2+} regulation. Here, parathyroid hormone (PTH) increases the rate of reabsorption, via apical Ca^{2+} channels, basolateral Ca^{2+}-ATPase and a Na^+/Ca^{2+}-exchanger.

Chloride ions

Chloride (Cl^-) is the main anion in the extracellular fluid and is needed to provide an electrical balance for the Na^+ and K^+ ions. Reabsorption in the PCT is mainly paracellular: as other solutes and water are absorbed, the concentration of chloride ions rises, providing a concentration to drive its passive reabsorption into the peritubular interstitium. Cl^- can also move transcellularly via anion exchangers (see page 212).

More is reabsorbed in the loop of Henle, where it enters cells on the Na^+/K^+/$2Cl^-$ co-transporter in the apical membrane and leaves via CLC channels on the basolateral membrane. This is similar in the DCT, but chloride enters via the Na^+/Cl^- cotransporter (NCC). In the collecting duct there is some paracellular reabsorption driven by the absorption of Na^+, which sets up an electrical gradient.

Phosphate ions

Phosphate is a major intracellular anion and is a constituent of bone. The concentrations of calcium and phosphate in blood are close to those required to cause precipitation. This allows them to bind together in the formation of bone. Therefore the concentrations of Ca^{2+} and PO_4^{3-} have to be tightly regulated in a coordinated way. Around 80% of filtered PO_4^{3-} is reabsorbed in the PCT via co-transport with Na^+. This is negatively regulated by parathyroid hormone (PTH) such that increased PTH (which will increase plasma Ca^{2+}) promotes PO_4^{3-} loss in the urine.

> **Na^+-linked transport of sugars and amino acids** across cell membranes allows these precious molecules to be absorbed in the intestine and reabsorbed in renal tubules, even in low concentrations. They can move against their concentration gradient as transport is linked to the energy-supplying Na^+ movement.

Magnesium

Blood concentration of magnesium (Mg^{2+}) must be closely maintained because it is required for the normal function of many enzymes and for the stability of proteins. To keep the body in homeostasis, most filtered Mg^{2+} is reabsorbed. Around 80% of filtered Mg^{2+} is reabsorbed in the thick ascending limb of the loop of Henle, where it moves paracellularly driven by the electrical gradient set up by chloride reabsorption. There is minor passive reabsorption in other regions.

Tubular transport of amino acids

Amino acids are the building blocks of proteins and some also function as neurotransmitters or can be metabolised into energy pathways. About 43 g of more than 25 types of amino acid are filtered from plasma each day, but almost all are reabsorbed by the end of the PCT.

Like glucose, amino acids are reabsorbed by apical Na^+-amino acid cotransporters in the PCT. There are about seven types of these, each with a different affinity for different amino acids and, as with glucose, basolateral transport is via passive transporters and these

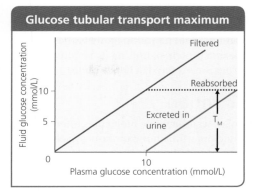

Glucose tubular transport maximum

Figure 5.7 The transport maximum (T_M) principle for reabsorption of glucose. Once the filtered glucose level rises above T_M, glucose begins to appear in the urine.

systems can become saturated. This is the concept of tubular maximum (T_M). For example, if the T_M for glucose is exceeded, despite the maximum rate of reabsorption, glucose would still appear in the urine (**Figure 5.7**). The same principle of T_M can be applied to amino acids.

Tubular transport of urea

Urea is a potentially toxic waste product of protein breakdown. Surprisingly, 60% of filtered urea is reabsorbed and only 40% is excreted. Excreting more would cause excessive water loss due to urea's osmotic effect. Despite this, the nephron has a concentrating mechanism that means a significant amount of urea can be excreted without excessive water loss.

Glomerulus and the proximal convoluted tubule

Urea freely crosses the glomerular filtration membrane. Around 50% of filtered urea is freely reabsorbed in the PCT, as it follows the osmotic gradient from the concentrating filtrate into the diluting capillary blood.

Loop of Henle and the distal convoluted tubule

The loop of Henle has some permeability to urea and the medullary interstitium has a high urea concentration, so some moves back into the tubular fluid. This means there may actually be more urea in the tubular fluid entering the DCT than was originally filtered. The thick ascending limb, DCT and cortical collecting duct are largely impermeable to urea, so it is concentrated in the filtrate as water is reabsorbed.

Collecting duct

ADH causes an increase in UT-A urea transporter proteins and aquaporin channels (see page XX) on the apical membrane of medullary collecting duct epithelium. UT-A vastly increases membrane permeability to urea and allows urea to flow back out of the tubule and into the interstitium. This reduces the osmotic diuretic effect of urea in the filtrate and concentrates the urine.

Urea 'trapping'

Essentially, urea circulates by diffusion between the medullary sections of the loop of Henle, the interstitium and the collecting duct, i.e. it is 'trapped' in the medulla. This contributes to the high osmolarity of the medullary interstitium that is essential for concentrating urine and avoiding excessive water loss in the collecting duct.

Both urea and creatinine diffuse freely across the glomerular filtration membrane, but only urea is affected by tubular activity. A decrease in blood flow (hypoperfusion) to the kidneys decreases GFR and the renal response is to retain as much fluid as possible; possibly increasing plasma urea far more than creatinine. Therefore, prerenal causes of acute kidney injury, mostly due to hypoperfusion, lead to a more markedly raised urea than creatinine.

Tubular secretion

Some blood substances enter the filtrate by active tubular cell secretion. They are usually substances with excessive levels or that are toxic. Secretion can occur in addition to, or instead of, glomerular filtration. Some drugs are also actively secreted.

Hydrogen ion secretion

Normal metabolism and exercise result in the accumulation of acid in the body (and blood). The kidney deals with this by secreting hydrogen ions in both the proximal tubule, where the Na^+/H^+ exchanger secretes H^+ in exchange for Na^+ reabsorption, and in the collecting duct, where α intercalated cells secrete H^+. Together these result in the net secretion of about 70 mM of H^+ each day.

> **The tubules secrete H^+ to counter acid produced from metabolism.** In acute renal failure, this secretion fails and acid accumulates in the blood causing acidaemia.

Ammonium ion secretion

During respiratory compensation for acidosis, bicarbonate is lost from the body, so more needs to be generated to maintain homeostasis. Glutamine metabolism in the proximal tubule generates two molecules of ammonia, which are excreted into the urine as ammonium ions and two bicarbonate ions that are returned to the blood. The ammonium ions in the tubular fluid act as a buffer, helping to excrete protons (from other acids) without lowering the pH of the urine too much. Lowering the pH of the urine too much would disrupt the equilibrium of the other reactions and transport process.

Potassium ion secretion

Potassium is secreted in the collecting duct. Absorption of Na^+ through ENaC generates a lumen-negative potential. This provides a driving force for potassium to leave the principal cells through ROMK channels.

Drug excretion

Excretion is the irreversible loss of a substance from the plasma out of the body. Many drugs are excreted in the urine, either by filtration, if they or a metabolite are water-soluble and polar, or by active tubular secretion.

Drug excretion – like the excretion of any molecule - is influenced by its size, concentration, renal handling and whether it binds plasma proteins, limiting its filtration. Other drugs are excreted in hepatic bile.

Filtration

Polar, water-soluble molecules filter freely at the glomerulus but cannot passively diffuse through tubular cells back into the capillaries. This is why many drugs are metabolised by the liver to sulphate, glucuronic acid or glycine conjugates: conjugation makes them soluble and polar and enhances renal excretion. Non-polar molecules tend to be readily reabsorbed and so tubular handling depends on pH, as this affects the dissociation of acidic and basic molecules.

> **Aspirin is a weak acid, so is uncharged in urine with a normal pH (mildly acidic).** It diffuses out of the tubular fluid into cells and is not well excreted. When bicarbonate is infused, urine become alkaline and aspirin loses protons, causing it to be trapped and excreted in the urine.

Active tubular secretion

Many drugs are actively secreted by tubular cell transporters, particularly in the PCT. These transporters show little specificity and can be saturated at relatively low plasma drug concentrations. Examples include organic anion transporters (OATs) and permeability-glycoproteins (P-gp).

Organic anion transporters

OATs are found on the basolateral membrane of PCT epithelial cells. An example is OAT-1, which secretes a wide variety of small hydrophilic anions (typically weak acids) into the cell in exchange for dicarboxylate. Substrates include ACE_{is}, non-steroidal anti-inflammatory drugs (NSAIDs), diuretics and prostaglandins, as well as antibiotics such as penicillin. These anions then cross the apical membrane on anion exchangers, typically for chloride. There are also organic cation transporters (OCTs) on the basolateral membrane for the export of weakly basic molecules.

Permeability-glycoproteins

P-gp on the apical membrane secretes a wide variety of molecules, including steroids, digoxin, doxorubicin and vinblastine. They are an ancient cellular defence, also found in intestinal, brain and liver cells.

> **Chronic renal failure is associated with a massive reduction in drug excretion:** therefore much smaller doses of some drugs need to be given to avoid toxicity.

Concentration of urine

In the glomerulus and PCT water is able to follow the movement of solutes freely from the lumen into tubular cells, resulting in isotonic filtrate in the PCT. However, if an isotonic urine was excreted excessive amounts of water would be lost and we would need to drink almost continuously. To avoid this the kidney generates a much more concentrated urine by setting up a large osmotic gradient in the medullary interstitium that extracts water osmotically from the collecting duct as it passes through the medulla (**Figure 5.8**).

Loop of Henle

The loop of Henle (**Figure 5.2**) lies between the PCT and DCT, and starts and ends in the cortex with a hairpin loop that runs down into the renal medulla. About 80% of nephrons have short loops that only reach the outer medulla, but 20% are juxtamedullary nephrons with glomeruli close to the corticomedullary boundary and long loops that descend into the inner medulla.

The osmotic gradient is created by counter-current mechanisms of the tubular fluid and blood flow.

Counter-current mechanisms

Counter-current mechanisms use the flow of fluid in opposite directions through structures to maximise the exchange of things between them. In the kidney there are two such systems:

- **Countercurrent multiplication**: in the loop of Henle, the descending and ascending limbs work together using active transport to generate an osmotic gradient. This is needed for water reabsorption in the collecting duct.
- **Countercurrent exchange**: the capillaries in the medulla (vasa recta) also form hairpin loops, but the exchange between them and the interstitium is purely passive and cannot contribute to generation of the gradient. It minimises the damage that

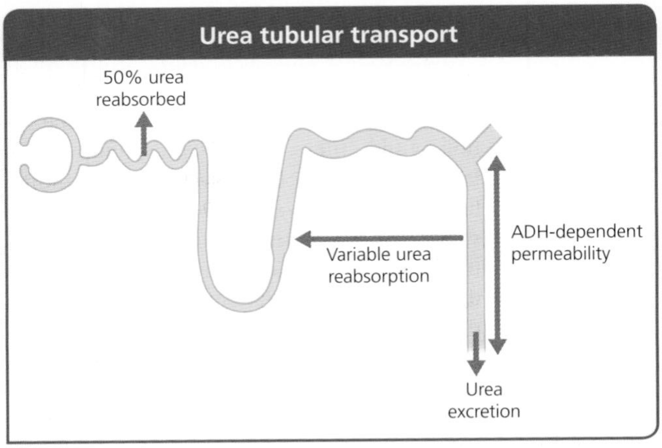

Urea tubular transport

50% urea reabsorbed

Variable urea reabsorption

ADH-dependent permeability

Urea excretion

Figure 5.8 Reabsorption and excretion of urea throughout the nephron. In the collecting duct, it is reabsorbed under the control of antidiuretic hormone (ADH).

would otherwise occur due to blood flow through it.

> **Osmolarity** is a measure of solute concentration expressed as the number of osmoles of solute per litre of solution. Osmolarity measures the concentration of an osmotic solution; when solutions expand with increasing temperature, osmolarity decreases.
>
> **Osmolality** is solute concentration defined as the number of osmoles of solute per kilogram of solvent so osmolality measures the concentration of particles in a fluid. The volume of a solvent does not change with pressure or temperature, so it is relatively easier to determine than osmolarity.

Limbs of the loop of Henle

The loop of Henle consists of a descending thin limb that is highly permeable to water and an ascending limb that is virtually impermeable to water. The ascending limb has thin and thick parts (**Figure 5.9**), though

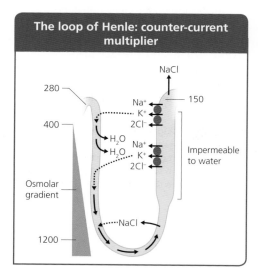

Figure 5.9 The loop of Henle functions as a counter-current multiplier to take hyperosmolar solution to the deepest parts of the medulla, leaving hypo-osmolar tubular fluid in the distal tubule. This is the basis of the tubule subsequently generating concentrated urine in the collecting duct. All values are in mOsm/kg H_2O.

short-loop nephrons lack a thin ascending section.

The thick ascending tubular cells are rich in mitochondria. They have plentiful Na^+/K^+ ATPase (and chloride channels) on the baso-lateral membrane and $Na^+/K^+/2Cl^-$ — cotrans-porters on the apical membrane. Tubular cells pump salt very actively out of the tubule, but are almost perfectly impermeable to water: as a consequence they can generate an osmotic gradient of around 200 mOsm/Kg of water be-tween the lumen and the interstitium. By con-trast, there are very few mitochondria in the thin ascending limbs of the inner medulla: the multiplication process in this region must use a mechanism that is not yet well understood.

Salt flows out of the tubule into the cells on the cotransporter, driven by the sodium gradi-ent into the cell. Sodium is pumped out by the Na^+/K^+ ATPase, while chloride leaves passively via its channels. Potassium recycles back into the lumen (via ROMK channels), so that the process doesn't stall because of the lack of K^+. Since water can't follow the salt (Na^+ and Cl^-) the tubular fluid becomes more dilute while the interstitial fluid becomes more concen-trated.

> **Tonicity** is the difference in osmotic pressure between two solutions separated by a semi-permeable membrane; a hypertonic solution has a higher concentration of solute(s) and draws water from the relatively hypotonic one.

Raised interstitial osmolality draws water out of the fluid in the descending thin limb increasing the solute concentration of the tu-bular fluid. There is also some influx of salt from the interstitium into the descending limb: the net consequence is to increase the solute concentration of the tubular fluid. As this more concentrated fluid flows round into the lower part of the ascending limb it allows the pumping mechanism there to start from a higher baseline meaning the interstitium can be made more concentrated. This causes fluid in the descending limb to become more con-centrated, and so on. The process is described as countercurrent multiplication because the pumps at each level are 'preparing the ground' for those deeper in the medulla: multiplying their effect. While a concentration gradient of about 200 mOsm can be generated at each level, a total gradient about 5 times that great can be generated overall (**Figure 5.9**).

> **Loop diuretics (e.g. furosemide) are powerful diuretics used to treat pulmonary oedema in heart failure.** They inhibit the $Na^+/K^+/2Cl^-$ cotransporter in the loop of Henle, preventing it from increasing the tonicity of the medullary interstitium. The salt that remains in the tubule holds onto water osmotically so with decreased tonicity in the medullary interstitium there is less ADH-dependent water reabsorption in the collecting duct and more urine is produced.

Counter-current multiplication

The loop increases the osmotic gradient in the medullary interstitium, from isotonic with plasma (around 290 mOsm/kg H_2O) in the cortex to 1000 mOsm/kg H_2O or more at the papillary tip, the deepest part of the medulla. A further consequence of this mechanism is that filtrate leaves the thick ascending limb markedly hypotonic – around 100 mOsm/kg H_2O.

Remember the context: the filtrate is constantly flowing, the descending and ascending limbs doing so in opposite directions and the vasa recta peritubular capillaries are also counter-current. In between the tubules and capillaries is the interstitial fluid.

Summary of mechanism

A simple way to consider the counter-current mechanism is:

1. The descending limb lets out water but no solutes
2. The thick ascending limb does not let out water and pumps out solutes
3. This increases interstitial osmolality, drawing water out of the descending limb
4. This increases solute concentration of the fluid entering the ascending limb, leading to more pumping of solutes out
5. This increases interstitial osmolality....and back to 3.

The loop of steps 3 to 5 is what multiplies the hypertonicity of the interstitium.

Vasa recta

The vasa recta are the capillaries that supply the loop of Henle and have the potential to dilute the hypertonic medullary interstitium. They are arranged in a hairpin loop so they act as a counter-current exchange system. Like other capillaries, they are freely permeable to small solutes and water.

As blood flows down the descending limb of the vasa recta, passing through an interstitium with ever higher osmolality, it equilibrates with the interstitium (**Figure 5.10**), i.e. water leaves and solutes enter. Then, as blood ascends and the interstitium around it becomes progressively more dilute, the solutes leave and pass back into the interstitium while water is taken up. This is an entirely passive process so there is always some 'lag' in plasma osmolality relative to the interstitial osmolality.

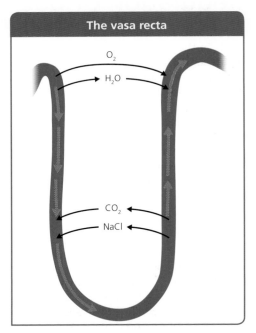

The vasa recta

Figure 5.10 The vasa recta capillaries mirror the loop of Henle, allowing free diffusion of substances between ascending and descending limbs. One side effect of this is that much of the oxygen bypasses the deep medulla, putting it at risk of ischaemia.

The osmotic gradient generated by the loop of Henle is somewhat lessened by this.

Gas exchange

An unfortunate side effect of the vasa rectal hairpin counter-current exchange is that it also affects respiratory gases, with CO_2 concentrating and recycling in the medulla and O_2 remaining in the cortex. Combined with what is already a limited blood supply, this leaves the medulla vulnerable to ischaemia when supply is limited further.

The urinary tract

The final product of the nephrons is urine, deposited by collecting ducts at the renal papillae into the renal pelvis.

The transitional epithelium that lines the ureters, bladder and superior urethra is impermeable to water and salts due to its keratin protein content. Therefore no water or salt reabsorption occurs after the collecting ducts.

> **Hypoxic medullary interstitial cells produce prostaglandins (PGs) to vasodilate local arterioles and increase their blood supply. This impairs urinary concentrating capacity, as relatively increased blood flow 'washes out' the** hypertonic environment, but it prevents the tissue becoming too ischaemic. PGs also reduce Na^+/K^+ ATPase activity, to limit energy and oxygen consumption. NSAIDs block PG production and can interfere with this delicate balance and lead to papillary necrosis, where the inner medullary tissues die due to hypoxia.

Regulation of body fluid volume

The kidneys, by their effect on water and Na^+ levels in the blood, have a large role in the regulation of fluid compartment volumes and constituents (see page 30).

As Na^+ is the main solute in extra-cellular fluid (ECF), it is the main determinant of ECF volume. A rise in total Na^+ results in hyperosmolality, which increases ADH and thirst. Thus the net effect of Na^+ intake is to increase ECF, while the effect of Na^+ loss is to reduce ECF since water will be lost to compensate for any hyponatraemia.

Hormones of sodium homeostasis	
Hormones promoting Na^+ reabsorption	Hormones promoting Na^+ excretion
Angiotensin II	Atrial natriuretic peptide
Aldosterone	Brain-type natriuretic peptide
Cortisol	
Oestrogens	C-type natriuretic peptide

Table 5.3 The main hormones affecting Na^+ reabsorption and excretion (i.e. natriuresis).

Hormonal regulation

Na^+ and water homeostasis are regulated by various hormones that increase or decrease Na^+ and water reabsorption in the renal tubules (**Table 5.3**). However, the main hormonal system controlling effective circulating volume (ECV), and therefore total body water is the renin–angiotensin–aldosterone system (RAAS). This is because changes in osmolality cause rapid changes in antidiuretic hormone (ADH), so any change in osmolality causes loss or retention of water (thirst will increase water intake if required).

Osmoregulation

Osmoregulation is the homeostatic regulation of the osmotic pressure of body fluids. It is largely a function of the ADH system, which controls the variable reabsorption of water in the collecting duct.

Plasma osmolality

Plasma osmolality is closely regulated around 285–295 mOsm/kg H_2O. As the osmolality increases above this, water moves out of cells causing them to shrink, while a reduction in osmolality causes cell swelling. This is associated with cellular dysfunction, particularly in the central nervous system (CNS).

Antidiuretic hormone

The main ADH in humans is arginine vasopressin, a peptide hormone that can act at two receptors: V_1 and V_2 (**Table 5.4**).Without ADH, the apical side of the collecting duct is virtually impermeable to water, resulting in dilute urine as no water is reabsorbed. At its maximum effect, via V_2 receptors, ADH allows filtrate to approach the tonicity of the medullary interstitium, greatly concentrating urine and retaining water in the body.

Antidiuretic hormone release

ADH is synthesised by magnocellular neurons in the supra-optic (SON) and paraventricular (PVN) nuclei in the hypothalamus, and is transported in vesicles along the axons of the nuclei to the posterior pituitary. They are released into the bloodstream by exocytosis, primarily in response to an increase in plasma osmolality (**Figure 5.11**). Osmosensory neurons in the organum vasculosum of the lamina terminalis (OVLT) of the hypothalamus begin to shrink in the hyperosmolar environment, stimulating ADH release by the magnocellular neurons.

V_2 receptor binding

Collecting duct tubular cells have V_2 receptors on their basolateral membranes. These are G protein-coupled receptors, and ADH binding causes an increase in intracellular cyclic adenosine monophosphate (cAMP), a second messenger molecule that conveys and amplifies the signal inside the cell (see page 22). In the case of ADH, the increased cAMP results in activation of protein kinase A, which phosphoryl atesaquaporin-2 (AQP2) channels and causes their transfer from intracellular vesicles into the apical membrane (**Figure 5.12**) to allow the passage of water across the apical plasma membrane. Water then leaves the cell through other aquaporins (3 and 4) on the basolateral membrane.

Antidiuretic hormone effect

The absence of ADH results in a large volume of dilute urine (up to 20 L/day, <100 mOsm/kg H_2O).In the presence of maximal ADH, the

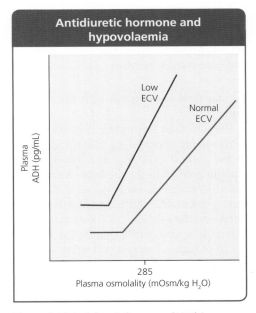

Figure 5.11 Antidiuretic hormone (ADH) is released in direct proportion to plasma osmolality, but the relationship is sensitised in the presence of hypovolaemia, i.e. with a low effective circulating volume (ECV).

ADH-receptors		
	Vasopressin-1 receptor	Vasopressin-2 receptor
Location	Vascular smooth muscle cell	Collecting duct principal cell
Secondary messenger	$PIP_2 \rightarrow$ increase Ca^{2+}	$G_s \rightarrow AC \rightarrow$ increase cAMP
Effect	Smooth muscle contraction	AQP2 channels into apical membrane
Function	Vasoconstriction	Water reabsorption in collecting duct

Table 5.4 Comparison of vasopressin receptors V1 and V2. ADH, antidiuretic hormone.PIP_2, phosphatidylinositol 4,5-bisphosphate; G_s, stimulatory heterotrimeric G protein. AC, adenylate cyclase. cAMP, cyclic adenosine monophosphate.

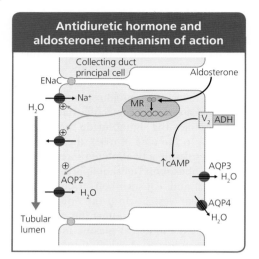

Antidiuretic hormone and aldosterone: mechanism of action

Figure 5.12 Antidiuretic hormone (ADH) and aldosterone action on collecting duct tubular cells. ADH binds V2 receptors on the basolateral membrane and increases vesicular transport of aquaporin-2 (AQP2) channels to the apical membrane, allowing water to flow out of the tubular fluid. Water leaves basolaterally via AQP3 and AQP4 channels, which are permanently present in the membrane. Aldosterone, a steroid hormone, binds intracellular mineralocorticoid receptors (MR) to increase the number and activity of basolateral Na^+/K^+-ATPase and apical Na^+ (ENaC) and K^+ (ROMK) channels, increasing Na^+ reabsorption and K^+ secretion.

tubular fluid equilibrates with the interstitium.

Because fluid leaving the loop of Henle is so hypotonic, much of the water is absorbed in the cortical collecting duct reducing the amount going into the medulla. Water is reabsorbed progressively in the medullary collecting duct and, with maximal ADH effect, filtrate reaches around 1200 mOsm/kg H_2O. This results in a small volume (as little as 0.5 L) of highly concentrated urine, and the reabsorption of water in excess of solute dilutes the plasma.

Thirst

Renal water reabsorption can only stop a water deficit getting worse; once plasma osmolality exceeds about 295 mOsm/kg H_2O there is an increasingly strong sensation of thirst, usually leading to the intake of additional water. This is controlled by the hypothalamus with a separate group of osmoreceptors, also found in the OVLT and subfornical organ (SFO). They sense plasma osmolality and angiotensin II and activate the median preoptic nucleus of the hypothalamus.

> **Head injury, sepsis, malignancy and heart failure can all present with excessive secretion of ADH.** The resulting excessive water reabsorption dilutes plasma solutes causing hypo-osmolality and hyponatraemia. Severe hyponatraemia causes reduced consciousness and seizures. Treatment is by fluid restriction or, in severe cases with ADH antagonists.

Renin–angiotensin–aldosterone system

The renin–angiotensin–aldosterone system is a multi-organ hormonal system that regulates body fluid volume, and therefore blood pressure. It involves the liver, kidneys, lungs, adrenal glands, hypothalamus, pituitary gland as well as the sympathetic nervous system. When active its end result is the tubular reabsorption of salt and the vasoconstriction of systemic arterioles.

Initiation – renin

Renin is a protease enzyme. It is released by granular cells in the wall of the afferent arteriole into the bloodstream. These cells are a part of the JGA, and are stimulated by events indicating a reduced ECV:

- Reduced afferent arteriolar wall stretch
- Reduced Na^+ delivery to the macula densa (the 'glomerulo-tubular feedback' mechanism, see page 139)
- Activation of β-adrenoreceptors on granular cells by the sympathetic nervous system.

The sympathetic drive stimulation for renin release is initiated by baroreceptors in the heart and great vessels

Circulating renin cleaves angiotensinogen, a globulin protein made by hepatocytes and secreted into the blood to produce angiotensin I, which is rapidly converted to angiotensin II by angiotensin-converting enzyme (ACE, **Figure 5.13**) in the lungs, kidneys and elsewhere in the body.

Effect - angiotensin II

Angiotensin II is a potent vasoconstrictor of all arterioles in the body, which increases total peripheral resistance and therefore mean arterial blood pressure. Importantly, in the kidney, angiotensin II constricts the efferent arteriole much more than the afferent. This helps to maintain glomerular capillary hydrostatic pressure and maintain GFR. Angiotensin II also:

- Binds to type 1 angiotensin II receptors on PCT cells, activating basolateral Na^+/K^+-ATPase transporters, causing an increase in the rate of Na^+ and water reabsorption
- Enhances ADH release by increasing the sensitivity of the osmoreceptors to osmotic and volaemic stimuli, increasing ADH-dependent water reabsorption
- Stimulates aldosterone release from the zona glomerulosa in the adrenal cortex. Aldosterone is a steroid hormone that increases salt reabsorption in the distal tubule.

These actions all tend to maintain circulating volume. Aldosterone also reduces salt losses in the colon and in sweat, further helping to protect body fluid balance.

> **Angiotensin-converting enzyme inhibitors (e.g. ramipril and lisinopril) are a group of blood pressure lowering drugs** that block the conversion of angiotensin I to angiotensin II, the most active product of the renin-angiotensin-aldosterone system (RAAS). They reduce patient mortality in heart disease, chronic kidney disease, stroke and peripheral vascular disease, particularly in those also affected with diabetes.

Aldosterone

Aldosterone is a mineralocorticoid steroid hormone produced in the zona glomerulosa of the adrenal cortex. It exerts an important effect on blood pressure by increasing Na^+ reabsorption in the DCT and collecting duct.

Aldosterone release

It is released in response to:

- Angiotensin II (as part of the RAAS)
- High plasma K^+
- Low plasma Na^+- although this is rare, since the ADH system normally corrects

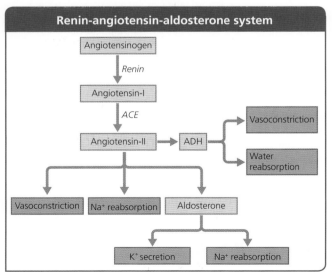

Figure 5.13 The renin-angiotensin-aldosterone system of blood pressure homeostasis involves enzymes of the liver, lung and kidney with actions on peripheral arterioles and the kidney. ACE, angiotensin-converting enzyme. ADH, antidiuretic hormone

this rapidly, by allowing water loss until plasma Na⁺ returns to normal.

Aldosterone actions on the tubule

Aldosterone raises plasma [Na⁺] and blood pressure, and decreases plasma [K⁺]. The mechanism by which aldosterone can control both Na⁺ and K⁺ is still unclear, but probably represents it having different effects in the CDT and collecting duct.

Aldosterone binds to intracellular mineralocorticoid receptors in cells of the DCT and collecting duct, causing increased transcription of genes for an enzyme, serum and glucocorticoid-regulated kinase (SGK), which causes more ENaC and ROMK channels to be inserted into the apical membrane, and the basolateral Na⁺/K⁺-ATPase pumps to be more active. It later increases production of Na⁺/K⁺-ATPase and apical channels themselves. This effect increases Na⁺ reabsorption, which will increase intravascular volume. Dietary salt intake will supplement this, returning the total body salt and ECV to normal.

Aldosterone also increases the cell surface expression of apical ROMK channels in collecting duct principal cells and reduces secretion of H⁺ in exchange for K⁺ in intercalated cells. Both of these actions reduce plasma K⁺.

Natriuretic hormones

Atrial and b-type natriuretic peptides (ANP and BNP, respectively) are hormones that antagonise the RAAS and decrease blood pressure.

Natriuretic peptide release

They are released mainly by cardiomyocytes in response to excessive stretch. ANP is released by the atria and BNP by the ventricles. The main effect comes from ANP release from the atria, which are stretched when venous return to the heart is high, normally reflecting an increased effective circulating volume.

Natriuretic peptide receptors

NPs bind to natriuretic peptide receptors (NPRs), which are themselves guanylate cyclases, found on:

- Vascular endothelial cells
- Glomerular mesangial cells
- Medullary collecting duct cells
- There are also NPRs in the lung and adipose tissue

Binding leads to elevated levels of the secondary messenger cyclic guanosine monophosphate (cGMP). In medullary collecting duct cells, NPR binding blocks apical Na⁺ channels from opening.

Action

ANP and BNP are both potent vasodilators that decrease systemic vascular resistance. In the kidney, they:

- Decrease Na⁺ reabsorption by the renal tubules, i.e. they oppose the effect of aldosterone
- Increase GFR by mesangial cell relaxation, afferent arteriole dilation and efferent arteriole constriction
- Increase blood flow in vasa recta to dilute the medullary interstitium
- Inhibit renin secretion

Raised levels of natriuretic peptides are indicators of heart failure. When the heart is failing to pump sufficient blood, cardiomyocyte stretch continues to activate release of ANP and BNP. BNP is a more useful clinical indicator, as its half-life in the plasma is twice that of ANP.

Interaction of volume and osmoregulation

The control of fluid volume and osmolality are closely intertwined as they directly affect each other:

- **ADH release** is stimulated by increased plasma osmolality to cause a reduction in plasma osmolality and limit decreases in intravascular volume
- **Aldosterone release**, in contrast, is stimulated by decreased circulating volume to cause an increase in tubular Na^+ retention

These two systems need to interact to control both circulating volume and total body Na^+.

Osmoreceptor sensitivity

Volume and osmoregulation are partly integrated by an important supplementary effect of intravascular volume on ADH release. If the volume falls substantially, the osmoreceptor response is increased so that at any given plasma osmolality there will be more ADH release. In effect, the body accepts a suboptimal osmolality to defend circulating volume when conditions are critical. Conversely, in hypertension the body will accept a modest hypernatraemia in order to lower the circulating volume (**Table 5.5**).

For example, if a patient becomes hypovolaemic with hyperosmolality secondary to dehydration, the combination of ADH and RAAS is likely to correct both their volume status and osmolality.

In contrast, a patient who suffers a haemorrhage will be hypovolaemic with normal

Interaction of osmoregulation and volume regulation	
Stimulus for ADH release	Effect
Hyperosmolality with hypovolaemia	Normo-osmolality with euvolaemia
Hyperosmolality with normovolaemia	Normo-osmolality with hypervolaemia
Normo-osmolality with hypovolaemia	Hypo-osmolality with normovolaemia

Table 5.5 The disruption volume status or plasma osmolality by ADH, dependent on stimulus for release. ADH, antidiuretic hormone.

osmolality. Release of ADH in this circumstance will help to correct volume status, but will result in hypo-osmolality. Since aldosterone is also released, salt retention will gradually correct this returning the circulating volume to normal.

> **Conn's syndrome is primary aldosteronism caused by aldosterone-secreting tumours in the zona glomerulosa of the adrenal cortex.** Over-secretion of aldosterone by the adrenal glands is diagnosed by a plasma aldosterone: renin ratio over 30. Symptoms include hypertension, chronic headaches and muscle cramps and weakness due to electrolyte imbalances.

Acid–base balance

The level of acid in the blood can greatly affect the conformation of macromolecules and the efficiency of biochemical reactions in all cells and body fluids, so the maintenance of blood (and other fluid) pH of between 7.35 and 7.45 is important. Outside of this range, excess acid (acidosis) or alkali (alkalosis) can quickly impair or derange many physiological processes.

Principles of acid–base balance

Acid–base balance is constantly challenged by the production of acid from metabolism of carbon (i.e. carbonic acid, formed when CO_2

dissolves in water) and other substances converted to non-volatile acids (e.g. sulphuric acid and phosphoric acid).

pH and acidity

Concentrations of H^+ vary across such a wide range of concentrations that a log scale is used:

$$pH = -\log_{10}[H^+]$$

For example, the hydrogen ion concentration in the stomach might be 10 mM (pH 2), while in the blood it is around 40 nM (pH 7.4). Slightly counterintuitively, a high pH represents a low hydrogen ion concentration and vice versa.

Buffers

The body has three main buffer systems that keep pH within the physiological range:

- Bicarbonate/carbonic acid system
- Protein in cells and the plasma, including haemoglobin in erythrocytes
- Different phosphate ions (HPO_4^{3-} and $H_2PO_4^{2-}$) act as a buffer system

Because of the high concentration of bicarbonate ions in the extracellular fluid (25 mM) and because CO_2 (and so carbonic acid) can be rapidly removed by the lungs, the bicarbonate system is the most important in limiting acidosis or alkalosis.

Chemical buffers

An acidic compound is one that produces free H^+ when dissolved in water:

$$HA \rightleftharpoons H^+ + A^-$$

Where HA is an acid (e.g. carbonic acid) that dissociates to give H^+ and A^-, the conjugate base (e.g. HCO_3^-).

The strength of the acid determines to what extent it dissociates and, therefore, the concentration of free H^+ in a solution. A mixture of a weak - and therefore only partly dissociated - acid and its conjugate base form a buffer: a solution that will tend to minimise changes in H^+.

If H^+ ions are added to a buffer they will tend to associate with the conjugate base, converting it to the acid form and reducing the number of H^+ ions in solution. If H^+ ions are removed, some of the acid will break down, creating more.

The Henderson–Hasselbalch equation

The Henderson–Hasselbalch equation describes the pH of a system based upon the relative concentrations of HA and A^-:

$$pH = pKa + Log_{10} ([A^-] / [HA])$$

Where pKa is a measure of the degree of dissociation of HA into its ions when in solution. Therefore, when considering a single weak acid:

$$pH \propto [A^-] / [HA]$$

This means changes in pH are proportional to the relative concentration of the base and its acid.

Bicarbonate buffering system

Plasma pH is influenced by the interaction of a number of buffer systems, including PO_4^{3-} and plasma proteins that can bind H^+ ions.

Bicarbonate is a very effective buffer system because it has two linked equilibria affecting the carbonic acid concentration:

$$H_2O + CO_2 \rightleftharpoons H_2CO_3 \rightleftharpoons H^+ + HCO_3^-$$

The consequence of this is an increase in buffering power: if H^+ is buffered by bicarbonate, forming carbonic acid. Some of this will break down to form CO_2 and water, but the CO_2 will be exhaled. Thus, there is very little rise in carbonic acid concentration as acid is neutralised by the system. Since the bicarbonate concentration is very large compared to the hydrogen ion concentration (almost 1 million fold higher), and won't change much in buffering a short-term acid load, the ratio of bicarbonate to carbonic acid also won't change much and pH will remain very close to the required level.

A 34-year-old woman presents to the emergency department with severe left-sided abdominal pain. The pain is intermittent, with intense bursts lasting 5–10 minutes. A CT scan demonstrates a ureteric calculus impacted at the left ureterovesical junction.

Urinary tract stones (nephrolithiasis if in the kidney, urolithiasis anywhere in the tract) are mineral collections that form in the renal pelvis, most commonly due to precipitation of calcium phosphate.

They are best visualized on CT, though many appear on X-ray or ultrasound.

They present anywhere from renal pelvis to bladder but commonly lodge at three sites of ureteral narrowing:

- The junction of the renal pelvis and start of the narrow ureter
- Where the ureter passes over the iliac blood vessels
- At the ureterovesical junction.

Carbonic anhydrase

The first phase of the reaction is catalysed by carbonic anhydrase so that it occurs rapidly in the blood. Carbonic anhydrase is found in all cells, but its key locations in regulating blood acid–base balance are in erythrocytes where it carries out the reactions just described, and in the renal tubule where it is central in the reabsorption and synthesis of bicarbonate (see page 158).

The second phase of the reaction is a simple acid dissociation reaction that requires no catalyst.

Equilibration

Any change in the concentration of any of the system's substrates will cause a shift in the equilibria. For example, adding more acid (i.e. H^+) will use up bicarbonate and 'push' the reaction to the left, generating more CO_2 and water, but maintaining a relatively constant concentration of H^+.

Compensation

In addition to the rapid buffering capacity of the bicarbonate system, there are additional mechanisms of compensation; means of pH change that depend on the body not being an entirely closed system. For example, excess CO_2 produced in the previous example can be exhaled out of the system by lung ventilation, shifting the reaction further to the left. Similarly, the kidney can compensate for acidaemia by excreting H^+, or for alkalaemia by excreting HCO_3^-. This is the basis of respiratory and renal compensation. Typically, respiratory compensation occurs fast (within minutes) but because it depends on an acid-stimulated increase in ventilation that abates as the acidosis resolves it is always incomplete. Furthermore, it progressively depletes the plasma bicarbonate. In contrast, the kidneys act more slowly (hours or even days), but because they can generate new bicarbonate metabolically they can return the body to its optimum state.

Calculating plasma pH

If we apply the Henderson–Hasselbalch equation to the bicarbonate buffer reaction then we derive:

$$pH \propto [HCO_3^-] / [H_2CO_3]$$

$$pH \propto [HCO_3^-] / [Paco_2]$$

Therefore, we can see that plasma pH is determined primarily by the ratio between HCO_3^- and $Paco_2$. In practice it is very difficult to measure the concentration of H_2CO_3, so $Paco_2$ can be used in its place. As discussed on page 116, ventilation controls $Paco_2$, whereas the renal tubules can control HCO_3^-.

A simplified version of the Henderson–Hasselbalch equation for the bicarbonate buffer system allows us to calculate plasma pH knowing the HCO_3^- concentration and the $Paco_2$:

$$pH = 6.1 + Log_{10}([HCO_3^-]/(0.03 \times Paco_2))$$

Note that this version of the equation assumes a $Paco_2$ expressed in mm Hg, though nowadays most blood-gas analysers use kPa.

Tubular control of acid–base balance

The bulk of bicarbonate reabsorption and proton secretion occurs in the proximal tubule, while the final, regulated processes occur in the intercalated cells of the collecting duct.

Proximal convoluted tubule

Tubular cells in the PCT are able to secrete H^+ and effectively use it to reabsorb filtered HCO_3^-. However, if the H^+ secreted into the lumen is picked up by another buffer, such as filtered organic anions or phosphate groups, it is lost in the urine. This effectively generates new HCO_3^-, since the intracellular H^+ was generated as carbonic acid. This HCO_3^- can then be released into the bloodstream.

Cells of the PCT can also break down glutamine to α-ketoglutarate. This generates two molecules of NH_3 that can diffuse into the tubular lumen and pick up protons to become NH_4^+, simultaneously making two new HCO_3^- available for transport into the bloodstream (**Figure 5.14**).

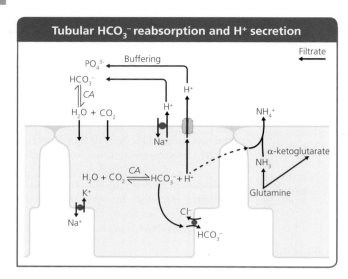

Figure 5.14 Mechanisms of HCO_3^- reabsorption and synthesis, and H^+ secretion in renal proximal tubular cells.

Collecting duct

The intercalated cells in the collecting duct control both H^+ and HCO_3^- secretion and absorption, and therefore have an important role in preventing both acidosis and alkalosis.

α-Intercalated cells

α-Intercalated cells secrete H^+ and reabsorb HCO_3^-.

Hydrogen ion secretion

α-Intercalated cells have H^+ ATPase and H^+/K^+ ATPase pumps on their apical membrane, both of which increase H^+ secretion. H^+/K^+ ATPase pumps H^+ into the lumen in exchange for K^+, and are therefore also important for K^+ regulation. Their expression and activity rise in hypokalaemia and contribute to hypokalaemia-associated alkalosis, as acid secretion is increased.

Activity of both pumps increases during systemic acidosis, while high aldosterone levels, by increasing Na^+ reabsorption in the principal cells, favours excretion by the H^+ ATPase. The H^+ secreted by these pumps is derived from carbonic acid generated within the cell, so again new HCO_3^- is released into the bloodstream. These active pumps can generate much bigger pH gradients than the Na^+/H^+ exchanger in the proximal tubule can work against, and allow us to acidify the urine in the collecting ducts to as low as pH 4.

Bicarbonate reabsorption

α-Intercalated cells also have Cl^-/HCO_3^- exchangers on their basolateral membrane, which export the bicarbonate into the bloodstream.

β-Intercalated cells

β-Intercalated cells secrete HCO_3^- into the urine and H^+ into the blood. They have transporters similar to those in the α-intercalated cells, but with the opposite arrangement (H^+ ATPase on the basolateral membrane, with an anion exchanger on the apical membrane).

Bicarbonate production

The generation of new HCO_3^- in the kidney, mainly by the proximal tubule cells, is an important part of the body's acid–base homeostasis in order to counterbalance loss of bicarbonate due to exhalation of CO_2.

Acid–base abnormalities

A normal blood pH of 7.35–7.45 reflects a ratio of HCO_3^- : $PaCO_2$ of approximately 20:1. Acidosis occurs if there is a fall in HCO_3^- or a rise in $PaCO_2$, whereas alkalosis occurs if there is a rise in HCO_3^- or a fall in $PaCO_2$. After determining blood pH, abnormalities are classified according to whether the cause is due to metabolic or respiratory problems (**Table 5.6**).

Acid–base abnormalities		
	Acidosis pH <7.4	Alkalosis pH >7.4
Respiratory	$Paco_2$ high	$PaCO_2$ low
	Caused by hypoventilation (e.g. COPD exacerbation)	Due to hyperventilation (e.g. panic attack)
	Renal compensation: increased proton secretion and HCO_3^- synthesis	Renal compensation: HCO_3^- loss
Metabolic	HCO_3^- low	HCO_3^- high
	Causes: renal failure, DKA, sepsis	Causes: vomiting, hypokalaemia
	Respiratory compensation: hyperventilation to lower $Paco_2$	Minimal respiratory compensation: potentially some respiratory depression
	Renal compensation (if not due to renal failure): increased proton secretion and HCO_3^- synthesis	Renal compensation: HCO_3^- loss

Table 5.6 Acid–base abnormalities. COPD, chronic-obstructive pulmonary disease. DKA, diabetic ketoacidosis.

Principles

Three principles of acid–base balance are important to understand abnormalities:

1. The Henderson–Hasselbalch equation - the buffering relationship between H^+ and CO_2, catalysed by carbonic anhydrase:

$$H^+ + HCO_3^- \rightleftharpoons H_2O_3 \rightleftharpoons H_2O + O_2$$

2. pH compensation – the lungs and kidneys manipulate the body's levels of CO_2 and HCO_3^-, respectively

3. The four acid–base states are defined by blood pH, HCO_3^- and $Paco_2$:
   i. Respiratory acidosis (due to CO_2 retention)
   ii. Respiratory alkalosis (due to hyperventilation and CO_2 deficit)
   iii. Metabolic acidosis (due to excess acid ingestion or production, or failure of the kidneys to excrete acid)
   iv. Metabolic alkalosis (due to excess acid loss (e.g. vomiting) or alkali ingestion (e.g. antacids) (**Figure 5.15**)

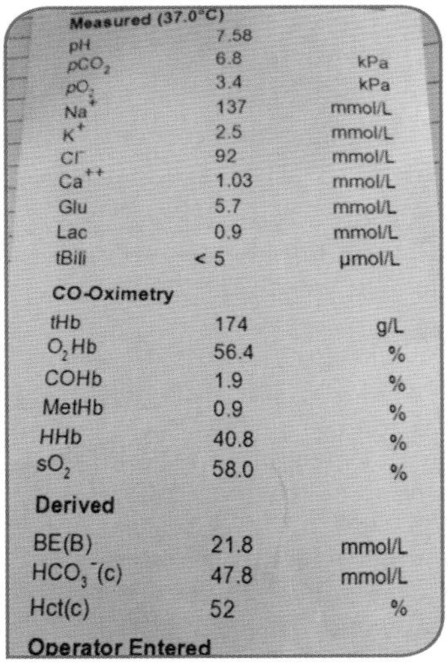

Measured (37.0°C)		
pH	7.58	
pCO₂	6.8	kPa
pO₂	3.4	kPa
Na⁺	137	mmol/L
K⁺	2.5	mmol/L
Cl⁻	92	mmol/L
Ca⁺⁺	1.03	mmol/L
Glu	5.7	mmol/L
Lac	0.9	mmol/L
tBili	< 5	µmol/L
CO-Oximetry		
tHb	174	g/L
O₂Hb	56.4	%
COHb	1.9	%
MetHb	0.9	%
HHb	40.8	%
sO₂	58.0	%
Derived		
BE(B)	21.8	mmol/L
HCO₃⁻(c)	47.8	mmol/L
Hct(c)	52	%
Operator Entered		

Figure 5.15 Venous blood gas results showing a severe, chronic metabolic alkalosis secondary to hypokalaemia. Hypokalaemia promotes loss of H^+. The markedly raised HCO_3^- demonstrates that this is chronic.

Clinical terms of blood pH can be confusing:

- Acidaemia and alkalaemia describe abnormal arterial blood pH (<7.35 or >7.45, respectively)
- Acidosis and alkalosis refer to the metabolic processes that may lead to acidaemia and alkalaemia.

They are, however, commonly used interchangeably.

pH compensation

When one organ system failure results in an acid base abnormality, the lungs and kidneys will aim to compensate in order to bring plasma pH back to normal. For example, impaired lung ventilation causes $Paco_2$ to rise and a respiratory acidosis develops. To compensate, the kidneys will increase HCO_3^- reabsorption and generation to bring the ratio of HCO_3^- to $Paco_2$ and the pH back towards normal.

Respiratory compensation involves a change in ventilation to increase or decrease $Paco_2$, and has a quick effect starting within a few minutes. Renal compensation adjusts HCO_3^- reabsorption and generation and takes several days to fully develop.

pH correction

Compensation is slightly different to correction of a pH abnormality. Correction refers to restoration of normal acid–base balance, whereas compensation allows the pH to be nearer normal despite abnormally high or low HCO_3^- or $Paco_2$. In other words, there is still an underlying problem (such as CO_2 retention), but this is being balanced by another (excess HCO_3^-) in order to keep pH close to normal.

Diagnosis

The Davenport diagram (**Figure 5.16**) shows the interrelationship between plasma pH, HCO_3^- and $Paco_2$. By comparing a patient's parameters with the chart, it is possible to get an idea of the type of disease causing the problem and whether it is likely to be of very recent onset, or whether there has been time for substantial compensation to occur.

> **Diabetic ketoacidosis is a non-renal metabolic acidosis.** Insulin deficiency means plasma glucose cannot be utilized by cells, which switch to lipolysis (fat breakdown) causing accumulation of acidic ketones. This ketoacidaemia uses up buffering HCO_3^- stimulating the kidneys to synthesise more. Ketoacidosis stimulates peripheral chemoreceptors, increasing ventilation to reduce $Paco_2$, which results in **Kussmaul breathing,** a clinical sign of metabolic acidosis, with deep, sighing breaths.

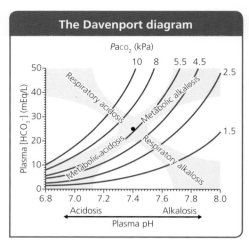

Figure 5.16 The Davenport diagram aids diagnosis of acid–base disorders by plotting plasma pH, HCO_3^- concentration and the arterial partial pressure of CO_2, The latter two are direct determinants of pH and their proportions indicate whether the cause is metabolic or respiratory. By plotting a set of values on the diagram it is easy to see what the primary defect was and what level of compensation has occurred, giving some indication of the duration of the underlying problem.

Micturition

Micturition (urination) is the voiding of urine from the urinary bladder. Filling of the bladder occurs passively as urine drains from the kidney. Relaxation of the bladder wall is under local reflexive and autonomic control, until a muscular tension is reached initiating reflexive contraction of the bladder, although this is under a voluntary override, allowing voiding to be delayed.

peristalsis–wave-like contractions of smooth muscle in the ureter wall - into the urinary bladder. The bladder is a muscular, hollow organ in the anterior pelvis (**Figure 5.17**). Its wall is expandable and has three flexible layers:

- An outer fibrous serosa
- The detrusor smooth muscle
- A transitional epithelium on the inside.

Ureters and bladder

Urine drains from the collecting ducts into the renal pelvis and ureters, where it is moved by

Detrusor muscle

The detrusor responds to local reflexes but is also influenced by autonomic innervation.

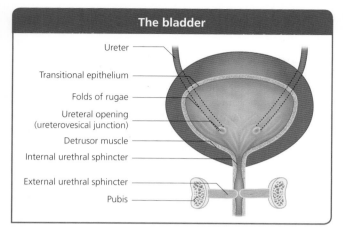

The bladder

- Ureter
- Transitional epithelium
- Folds of rugae
- Ureteral opening (ureterovesical junction)
- Detrusor muscle
- Internal urethral sphincter
- External urethral sphincter
- Pubis

Figure 5.17 The urinary bladder.

It contracts in response to parasympathetic stimulation and relaxes under sympathetic activation. It contracts spontaneously when the bladder becomes full.

The detrusor is thickened at the neck of the bladder, and forms the internal urethral sphincter. Where the urethra passes through the pelvic floor, the external urethral sphincter, a ring of skeletal muscle, can compress it. Both sphincters are important in control of urinary flow, allowing continence.

Bladder mucosa

The rugae are folds of bladder mucosa epithelium lining the bladder. This folding allows for increased capacity as the bladder fills. Transitional epithelium is so called as it can consist of a single to many layers of cells depending on its degree of contraction or expansion.

> **People with upper motor neurone (UMN) damage in the spinal cord, such as from spinal injuries, may lack voluntary bladder control.** The bladder becomes relatively hypertonic, with more frequent contractions, emptying spontaneously and frequently with small amounts of urine. Patients also lose awareness that their bladder is full, so reflex contractions become too strong to be overcome by voluntary control.

Control of micturition

The inflation of the bladder, as well as the urge and the action of passing urine is initiated and controlled by mechanoreceptors in its wall and urethral flow receptors, both of which supply afferent neurons to a reflex arc in the spinal cord, with efferent neurons running back to bladder muscles.

Stretch and flow receptors

Mechanoreceptors in the detrusor are activated by stretch, and form a positive reflex arc with sacral parasympathetic motor nerves that supply the detrusor. Initially, their activation leads to a progressive relaxation of detrusor fibres. The flow receptors in the proximal urethra detect the passage of urine.

Storage phase

The bladder is designed to store a maximum of about 200–500 mL of urine with almost no increase in internal pressure, though its total capacity may reach 1L. It increases its capacity by:

- Bladder stretch activation of the reflex arc that inhibits the detrusor, promoting relaxation
- Layers of transitional epithelium slide over each other with expansion until a single layer forms
- The bladder mucosal rugae unfold as it fills.

As the bladder continues to fill, increasing stretch receptor activations leads to an increase in spontaneous detrusor contractions. Eventually, internal pressure in the bladder begins to rise and detrusor reflex depolarisations become more frequent; this is felt as the urge to pass urine.

Voiding phase

Initiation of micturition – in individuals with sufficient descending inhibition of reflexes, i.e. full upper motor neuron function – is under voluntary control, though the exact mechanism of initiation is unclear.

There is voluntary relaxation of the external urethral sphincter via the pudendal nerve, to allow urine flow in the urethra. The detrusor contracts forcefully under the control of parasympathetic motor nerves. Sympathetic stimulation to the internal urethral sphincter is reduced, which causes its relaxation. This flow is detected by urethral receptors, which further activates the parasympathetic motor neurones for detrusor contraction.

Answers to starter questions

1. The estimated glomerular filtration rate (eGFR) is used to give an estimate of the rate that fluid is filtered in the kidney. Creatinine is used as a measure of GFR because it is freely filtered but not reabsorbed. Its production depends on age, ethnicity and muscle mass, so a formula for eGFR is used to calculate what a patient's normal rate should be. Urea also rises with deteriorating renal function but it is disproportionately affected by dehydration in comparison to creatinine and undergoes significant reabsorption, so cannot be used to estimate GFR.

2. The kidney normally receives around 20% of the resting cardiac output. If blood pressure is low, and perfusion of critical organs such as the brain is compromised, the renal arterioles will constrict (because of sympathetic drive). This reduces the blood flow to the kidney and supports the perfusion of other organs. However, the consequence is greatly reduced renal function: glomerular filtration will fall dramatically, and parts of the kidney may become ischaemic, leading to acute kidney injury (renal failure) if sustained.

3. Potassium and acid secretion both occur in the collecting duct, and secretion of one tends to lower secretion of the other. The α-intercalated cells express an H^+/K^+-ATPase, which secretes H^+ into the urine in exchange for K^+, thus reducing the excretion of potassium. Conversely, K^+ secretion from the principal cells into the urine reduces the electrical gradient for H^+ secretion, leading to acid being retained in the body. Similarly, very rapid secretion of H^+ during an acidosis will impair K^+ secretion, tending to lead to hyperkalaemia.

4. Plasma osmolality (blood concentration) is controlled by antidiuretic hormone (ADH) which regulates water reabsorption in the collecting duct. However, ADH is also released in severe hypovolaemia (low blood volume) with normal plasma osmolality, preventing water loss but at the expense of causing hypo-osmolality.

5. Most drugs will be filtered at the glomerulus, and pass into the urine, although this is limited for drugs which bind substantially to plasma proteins. In addition, many drugs are actively secreted into the proximal convoluted tubule in the kidney. For some, e.g. diuretics such as furosemide and thiazides, this is beneficial because it allows them to act. For others, e.g. penicillin, it shortens their half-life and means more frequent doses need to be taken. In some cases the drug impairs renal function, either because it reaches toxic concentrations within the nephron or because it precipitates and blocks the nephron.

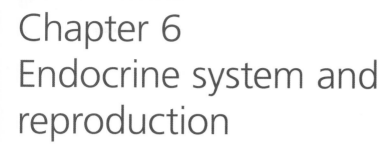

Chapter 6
Endocrine system and reproduction

Starter questions

Answers to the following questions are on page 191.

1. Why are the hypothalamus and pituitary the 'masters' of the endocrine system?
2. Why can removing the thyroid cause low calcium levels?
3. Why does adrenal insufficiency cause skin hyperpigmentation?
4. What determines the length of a menstrual cycle?
5. When does sperm production stop?

Introduction

In contrast to the nervous system, which exerts targeted control by direct innervation, the endocrine system allows the simultaneous control of multiple, distant tissues. It does this by producing substances called hormones that are distributed via the bloodstream and affect their target organs. The hormones have complex effects on different organs and influence processes such as growth, metabolic activity and cellular secretions. To maintain homeostasis, all endocrine systems are subject to feedback from end-organs that alters the secretion of the hormones acting on them.

A number of hormones are involved in the action of the reproductive system. This system produces haploid gametes (ovum and sperm), which fuse to form an embryo. Understanding the events that take place in the developing fetus is key to understanding a number of pathologies that can present even up to adulthood.

Case 5 Excessive thirst and frequent urination

Presentation

John, a 12-year-old boy, presents to the emergency department very unwell. His mother says he has had flu for a few days but has become progressively worse, with vomiting and drowsiness. John appears thin and very dehydrated (sunken eyes and loss of skin elasticity). His blood pressure is 78/58 mmHg, his blood sugar is 23.4 mmol/L, his blood pH is 7.13 and there are ketones in his urine when tested by dipstick.

John's mother says that he has been passing urine more frequently and drinking more fluids lately. There is no family history of diabetes and John has previously been well.

Analysis

This is a classical presentation of type 1 diabetes mellitus with diabetic ketoacidosis (**Figure 6.1**). Type 1 diabetes mellitus is an autoimmune condition caused by the destruction of the β cells in the pancreas, which produce insulin. This results in an absolute deficiency of insulin (in contrast to type 1 diabetes where there is a relative deficiency of insulin). There may be a gradual onset of hyperglycaemia, manifesting as polyuria (an increased volume and frequency of passing urine) and polydipsia (excessive thirst) due to the osmotic action of glucose in urine (see page 145). An intercurrent illness can precipitate an acute presentation of type 1 diabetes mellitus with DKA; here the influenza virus infection has increased the body's requirement for insulin.

Diabetic ketoacidosis occurs when there is a lack of the insulin-mediated suppression of ketone production (see page 233). In high concentrations, the two main ketones, β-hydroxybutyrate and acetone are acidic and cause acidosis. Patients are often very unwell with severe

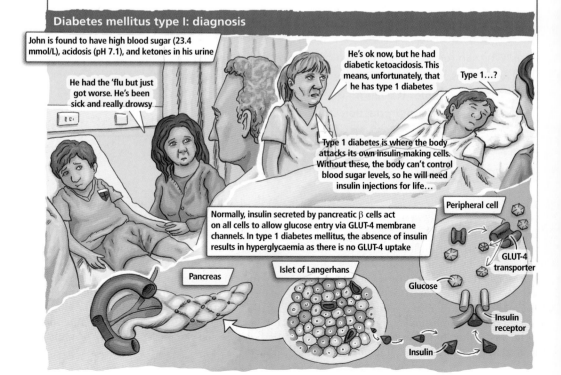

Diabetes mellitus type I: diagnosis

John is found to have high blood sugar (23.4 mmol/L), acidosis (pH 7.1), and ketones in his urine

He had the 'flu but just got worse. He's been sick and really drowsy

He's ok now, but he had diabetic ketoacidosis. This means, unfortunately, that he has type 1 diabetes

Type 1...?

Type 1 diabetes is where the body attacks its own insulin-making cells. Without these, the body can't control blood sugar levels, so he will need insulin injections for life...

Normally, insulin secreted by pancreatic β cells act on all cells to allow glucose entry via GLUT-4 membrane channels. In type 1 diabetes mellitus, the absence of insulin results in hyperglycaemia as there is no GLUT-4 uptake

Peripheral cell

GLUT-4 transporter

Pancreas

Islet of Langerhans

Glucose

Insulin receptor

Insulin

Case 5 *continued*

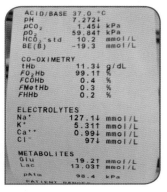

Figure 6.1 Arterial blood gas results for a patient with severe diabetic ketoacidosis. The patient is acidotic, hyperglycaemic, hyperventilating (causing low CO_2) and has low HCO_3^-. In addition, part of the acidosis will be due to their hugely raised lactate. This patient was receiving high-flow oxygen at the time.

dehydration (due to urinary losses) at the point of presentation.

Further case

John is given intravenous fluid and then, 1 hour later, intravenous insulin is started. His condition improves, but he requires intravenous potassium replacement to treat the hypokalaemia that is caused by the insulin. Once he has recovered from the acute event, John and his mother are counselled on the need for lifelong insulin injections.

Further analysis

First, the dehydration must be corrected by administering fluids which also helps correct the acidosis. Insulin is then administered intravenously for rapid, reliable delivery. Because insulin activates the cellular Na^+/K^+ pump, which carries potassium ions (K^+) intracellularly, patients are at risk of developing dangerous hypokalaemia. The resolving acidosis may further increase this risk because, as the level of hydrogen ions (H^+) in the plasma falls, the cells tend to release H^+, and K^+ are taken into the cells in exchange (see page 144).

The treatment of type 1 diabetes mellitus requires lifelong subcutaneous insulin administration as β cell function will never recover. Patients are highly insulin sensitive (unlike patients with type 2 diabetes) and have absolute insulin deficiency, so hypoglycaemic agents (e.g. metformin) are not useful because they require the presence of insulin to work.

Case 6 Painless lump in right breast

Presentation

Sally, an otherwise fit 38-year-old woman, presents to her general practitioner with a painless lump in her right breast. The lump is firm and there is puckering of the overlying skin, but the lump can be moved freely over the chest wall. Sally states that her mother died of breast cancer at 52 years of age and her sister underwent a bilateral mastectomy for ductal carcinoma when she was 43.

Analysis

Breast cancer is the most common cancer in women, and its incidence increases with age. Sally's presentation of a firm, painless lump that is relatively immobile is highly suggestive of breast cancer. Puckering of the skin or fixture of the lump to the chest wall increases the risk that the lump is malignant.

Sally's case is slightly atypical because most breast lumps in patients under the

Case 6 *continued*

age of 50 years are benign. For example, fibroadenomas are smooth, rubbery lumps that move easily.

Sally's strong family history of young-onset and bilateral breast cancer is worrying. It raises the suspicion that there may be an underlying genetic mutation causing the familial trend of malignancy.

Further case

Sally is referred to the breast clinic where she undergoes a 'triple assessment': clinical examination, mammography and biopsy. She is diagnosed with a high-grade locally advanced ductal carcinoma with no signs of metastasis. She has a mastectomy and begins adjuvant treatment with chemotherapy and hormone therapy.

Sally and her family attend a clinical genetics service where they are tested for genetic causes of familial breast cancer. Sally and her sister are found to have a germline mutation (in all DNA of cells) in the *BRCA1* gene.

Further analysis

Cancer is a genetic disease and its development is influenced by environmental factors. It is often characterised by:

■ Mutations that inactivate tumour suppressor genes, which normally prevent the uncontrolled growth of cells
■ Gain-of-function mutations in oncogenes, which promote cell growth

These leads to changes that include a loss of control over the cell cycle, the replication of abnormal DNA, an increased DNA mutation rate and resistance to apoptosis (see page 15).

The vast majority of cancers are 'sporadic', i.e. they result from mutations in tumour suppressor genes or oncogenes that are acquired during life rather than being inherited. There are, however, a few familial cancer syndromes that are caused by the inheritance of a mutated tumour suppressor gene, which is present in all the cells.

BRCA1 gene

BRCA1 is a tumour suppressor gene that is involved in several cell-cycle checkpoints (see page 15) and in the repair of damaged DNA. Both copies of *BRCA1* in a cell must become mutated for its action to be completely lost. *BRCA1* mutations are inherited in an autosomal dominant manner. If one copy has already been inherited in a mutated form, only one sporadic mutation has to occur in the other (normal) copy of *BRCA1* for a cancer to start developing; the cancer presents thus at an earlier age than it would if a mutated copy had not been inherited.

Breast cancer is typically treated with surgery, followed by adjuvant chemotherapy and hormone therapy for at least 5 years. Patients with a *BRCA* germline mutation may be offered a prophylactic bilateral mastectomy (before signs of cancer develop) to reduce their risk of developing breast cancer, which would otherwise be almost 100%.

Pituitary gland

The pituitary gland secretes a variety of hormones with many different functions. It controls several other glands through the action of these hormones. A complete loss of pituitary function is devastating and would not be compatible with life, as it is needed for regulation of normal metabolism and fluid balance.

Structure and function

The pituitary is a pea-sized gland that sits at the base of the brain in the sella turcica of the sphenoid bone. It lies immediately beneath the hypothalamus and is connected to it by the pituitary stalk (the infundibulum), which is key to the pituitary's function (**Figure 6.2**). The pituitary is divided into two parts, which are anatomically and functionally distinct: the anterior and posterior pituitary gland.

Anterior pituitary

The anterior pituitary (adenohypophysis) is derived from the roof of the pharynx (derived from ectoderm). It is composed of several types of densely packed epithelial cells, each type synthesising one of six peptide hormones. These anterior pituitary hormones are all controlled by hormones secreted from the hypothalamus, which travel down the pituitary stalk and influence the production of anterior pituitary hormones via a portal blood system (two sets of capillaries in series, joined by an arteriole).

Posterior pituitary

The posterior pituitary (neurohypophysis) can be considered to be an extension of the brain. It forms as a downgrowth from the hypothalamus. It is composed of the axons and terminal boutons (secretory process) of neuronal cells that are situated in the hypothalamus. The posterior pituitary hormones are synthesised in the cell bodies of the hypothalamic neurones and travel down their axons to the posterior pituitary, where they are stored before controlled release into the bloodstream.

Anterior pituitary hormones

The six anterior pituitary hormones are described in **Table 6.1**.

Growth hormone

Growth hormone is released by somatotrophs in response to growth hormone-releasing hormone (GHRH). The release of growth hormone is suppressed by somatostatin (**Figure 6.3**). Both GHRH and somatostatin are produced by the hypothalamus.

Growth hormone binds to cellular growth hormone receptors. These receptors produce signals in the cells by activating the enzyme tyrosine kinase. This mediates the acute actions of growth hormone, which are sometimes

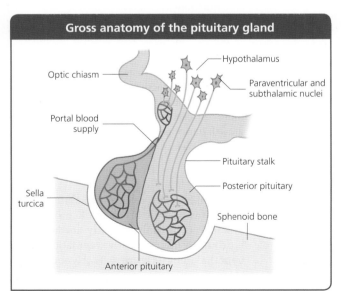

Gross anatomy of the pituitary gland

Optic chiasm

Hypothalamus

Paraventricular and subthalamic nuclei

Portal blood supply

Pituitary stalk

Posterior pituitary

Sella turcica

Sphenoid bone

Anterior pituitary

Figure 6.2 Gross anatomy of the pituitary gland demonstrating its position within the sphenoid bone, its connection to hypothalamus and its close proximity to the optic chiasm.

Anterior pituitary hormones		
Hormone	Hypothalamic control	Action
Adrenocorticotrophic hormone (ACTH)	Corticotrophin-releasing hormone increases ACTH	Adrenal hyperplasia and increased adrenal cortex hormones
Luteinising hormone (LH)/follicle-stimulating hormone (FSH)	Gonadotropin-releasing hormone (GnRH) increases LH and FSH	Sex steroid production and gamete maturation
TSH (thyroid-stimulating hormone)	Thyrotropin-releasing hormone (TRH) increases TSH	Increased tri-iodothyronine/thyroxine production
Growth hormone (GH)	Growth hormone-releasing hormone (GHRH) increases GH Somatostatin inhibits GH	Soft tissue growth Catabolism Metabolic regulation
Prolactin (PRL)	Dopamine inhibits PRL release TRH increases PRL release	Lactogenesis and suppression of GnRH release

Table 6.1 Hormones released by the anterior pituitary gland and their control by the hypothalamus

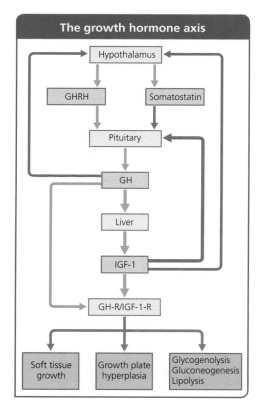

Figure 6.3 The growth hormone (GH) axis. The majority of its action and negative feedback is mediated by insulin-like growth factor 1 (IGF-1), which is produced by the liver. GHRH, growth hormone-releasing hormone; R, receptor.

described as anti-insulin or diabetogenic. However, the majority of actions of growth hormone are mediated by insulin-like growth factor-1 (IGF-1), a hormone released by the liver in response to growth hormone stimulation. IGF-1 also provides most of the negative feedback that limits the release of growth hormone.

Together, IGF-1 and growth hormone have the following actions:

- Stimulate the growth of soft tissues
- Promote proliferation at the growth plate of the bones
- Increase lipolysis, glycogenolysis and gluconeogenesis (diabetogenic effects, i.e. increase blood sugar)

In children, prior to fusion of the skeletal growth plates, the main action of growth hormone is to promote skeletal growth. In adults, GH has a more complex metabolic role (see above); adult growth hormone deficiency causes central adiposity with a lack of lean tissue.

Prolactin

Lactotrophs cells release prolactin: a hormone involved in breast milk production. Prolactin is the only pituitary hormone that is primarily under negative regulation by the hypothalamus (**Figure 6.4**). Hypothalamic

Control of prolactin

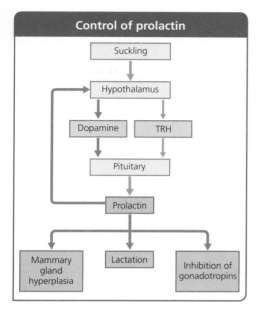

Figure 6.4 Control of prolactin. The release of dopamine from the hypothalamus negatively influences pituitary prolactin release. TRH, thyrotropin-releasing hormone.

dopamine suppresses prolactin release; therefore, a reduction in dopamine secretion causes a rise in serum prolactin.

Like growth hormone, prolactin binds to a tyrosine kinase-associated receptor. Stimulation of this receptor causes mammary gland hyperplasia and lactation. Oestradiol (see page 182) enhances the actions of prolactin on the breast.

The strongest stimulus for prolactin secretion is suckling. This sends signals via an afferent pathway that acts on the arcuate nucleus in the hypothalamus to suppress dopamine release and therefore increase prolactin release. Thyrotropin-releasing hormone (TRH) has a minor role in promoting prolactin release. It is thought to be responsible for the raised prolactin level that is associated with hypothyroidism (see page 173).

The neural signals that reach the hypothalamus from suckling also lead to the suppression of gonadotropin (LH/FSH) release. This is one of the key mechanisms that mediates lactational amenorrhoea, whereby women who are breastfeeding do not have normal ovulatory cycles and are consequently infertile (provided certain criteria are met).

Posterior pituitary hormones

Antidiuretic hormone (ADH, or vasopressin) and oxytocin are closely related peptide hormones that share seven of their nine amino acids. They are synthesised in the supraoptic and paraventricular nuclei of the hypothalamus, and are released by neurosecretion from the posterior pituitary.

Antidiuretic hormone

ADH is synthesised and released primarily in response to hypothalamic hyperosmolality. The ADH then acts on the distal tubules in the kidneys to promote water reabsorption, which corrects of the high osmolality. ADH is discussed further on page 151.

Oxytocin

Oxytocin is released during suckling (**Figure 6.5**). This activates afferent neurones that increase the synthesis of oxytocin by the hypothalamus and its release via the posterior pituitary. The oxytocin then causes contraction of the myoepithelial cells in the mammary ducts, leading to the expulsion of breast milk.

Oxytocin release is also increased during labour by distension of the cervix (the

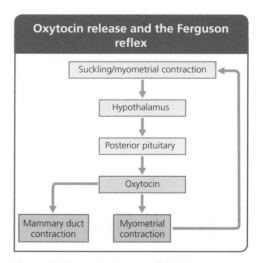

Figure 6.5 Oxytocin release and the Ferguson reflex. Myometrial contraction causes a positive feedback loop that stimulates oxytocin release.

Ferguson reflex) or uterine mechanoreceptors. The oxytocin then promotes contraction
of the uterine muscle (the myometrium). This
is a good example of a positive feedback loop.
Oxytocin release also occurs after stimulation
of the uterine mechanoreceptors.

> **Acromegaly is caused by excess
> secretion of growth hormone in adults,
> after fusion of the bony growth
> plates has occurred,** usually due to a
> benign pituitary tumour (adenoma)
> of the somatotrophs. Excess growth
> hormone causes an insidious increase
> in soft tissue growth; patients may
> notice gloves or hats no longer fit. It
> also causes type 2 diabetes, accelerated
> cardiovascular disease and an increased
> risk of colorectal cancer. If the pituitary
> adenoma grows upwards out of
> the sella turcica, it compresses the
> optic chiasm, resulting in bitemporal
> hemianopia (loss of vision in the outer
> half of both visual fields) (see page 250).

Thyroid gland

The thyroid gland secretes thyroxine (T_4) and
tri-iodothyronine (T_3), which are hormones
needed for normal metabolic activity, growth
and brain function. A lack or excess of thyroid hormones causes patients to become
unwell with a catalogue of different signs and
symptoms (as described below).

Structure and function

The thyroid is a brown gland that surrounds
the trachea at the level of C3–C4. It is formed
of two lateral lobes united by an isthmus,
which passes anterior to the trachea (**Figure
6.6**). It is composed of:

- **Follicles,** which are lined by follicular
  cells and contain colloid in their centre.
  Colloid is a proteinaceous fluid that
  contains thyroglobulin (the precursor to
  thyroid hormones). The follicular cells
  produce the hormones tri-iodothyronine
  (T_3) and thyroxine (T_4), which are
  essential for numerous metabolic
  processes
- **Parafollicular or C cells,** which are
  interspersed between the follicles
  (**Figure 6.7**). These produce the hormone
  calcitonin, which lowers the serum
  calcium level (see page 181)

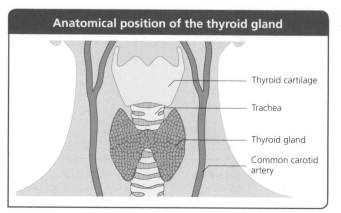

Anatomical position of the thyroid gland

Thyroid cartilage

Trachea

Thyroid gland

Common carotid
artery

Figure 6.6 Anatomical position of
the thyroid gland.

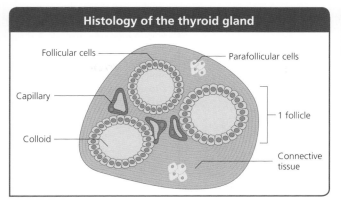

Figure 6.7 Histology of the thyroid gland. Parafollicular cells are interspersed between follicles that contain colloid.

Embedded within the posterior surface of the thyroid are the parathyroid glands. These release parathyroid hormone (PTH), which increases serum calcium levels.

T_3 and T_4

The thyroid hormones, T_3 and T_4, are amino acid-based hormones that cause changes in gene transcription to influence a variety of processes; for example, the basal metabolic rate (amount of energy the body uses), lipid and carbohydrate metabolism, cognitive function, and sympathetic nervous activity.

Hypothalamic-pituitary-thyroid axis

The hypothalamus and pituitary act together to regulate the secretion of the thyroid hormones (**Figure 6.8**). The hypothalamus produces TRH, which stimulates the release of TSH from the pituitary gland. TSH increases the production of T_3 and T_4 at every level of the synthetic pathway (described below), as well as causing follicular cell hyperplasia (therefore more cell to produce T_3 and T_4).

Thyroid hormone synthesis

The thyroid hormones are formed from the amino acid tyrosine and iodine (**Figure 6.9**).

In the initial step, the follicular cells synthesise thyroglobulin (a large protein containing multiple tyrosine residues) in their rough endoplasmic reticulum. The thyroglobulin is then moved through the Golgi apparatus

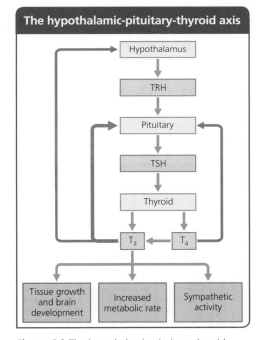

Figure 6.8 The hypothalamic-pituitary-thyroid axis. Most of the action and negative feedback is mediated by tri-iodothyronine (T_3), formed from the peripheral conversion of thyroxine (T_4). TRH, thyrotropin-releasing hormone; TSH, thyroid-stimulating hormone.

before being exported into the thyroid follicles for storage. In addition, the follicular cells actively take up iodine, from the blood, and secrete it into the follicles for the next stage of the process.

The colloid in the follicles also contains thyroid peroxidase, an enzyme that iodinates the

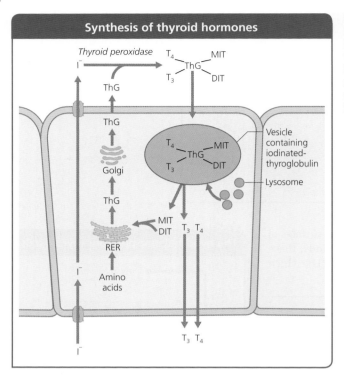

Synthesis of thyroid hormones

Figure 6.9 Synthesis of thyroid hormones. Thyroid peroxidase leads to the iodination of thyroglobulin (ThG) in the follicle lumen. DIT, di-iodothyronine; MIT, monoiodothyronine; RER, rough endoplasmic reticulum; T_3, tri-iodothyronine; T_4, thyroxine.

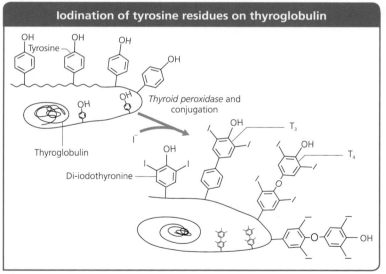

Iodination of tyrosine residues on thyroglobulin

Figure 6.10 Iodination of tyrosine residues on thyroglobulin by thyroid peroxidase, followed by conjugation to produce triiodothyronine (T_3) and thyroxine (T_4) residues.

tyrosine residues of the thyroglobulin. Each tyrosine can be iodinated at two sites. Two iodotyrosine residues then undergo a rearrangement, called conjugation, which results in the formation of an iodothyronine residue. This can be iodinated in three or four places (**Figure 6.10**).

Next, the iodinated thyroglobulin is endocytosed into vesicles in the follicular cells, and these vesicles then fuse with lysosomes in the cell. The proteolytic enzymes from the lysosomes cleave the iodothyronine groups, resulting in a mixture of monoiodothyronine, di-iodothyronine, T_3 and T_4. Monoiodothyronine and di-iodothyronine are transported back into the rough endoplasmic reticulum for recycling, whereas the T_3 and T_4 are secreted into the blood.

Hypothyroidism

A clinical deficiency of thyroid hormone activity produces a constellation of signs and symptoms, including fatigue, a feeling of cold, weight gain, bradycardia and hair loss. The most common cause in developed countries is the autoimmune condition Hashimoto's thyroiditis. However, iodine deficiency is a major cause worldwide. In the setting of iodine deficiency, patients can present with huge goitres (visible enlargement of the thyroid) as feedback from the low level of T_4 increases the production of TSH, causing the gland to proliferate to try and increase its activity.

T_3 and reverse T_3 (rT_3)

The follicular cells secrete a mixture of about 90% T_4 and 10% T_3; however, T_3 provides 90–95% of the biological action and exerts most of the negative feedback to control the secretion of TSH and TRH. T_4 is converted into T_3 to give biological effect. T_3 is produced from T_4 in the liver by the removal of iodine (deiodination). The liver then releases T_3 into the circulation to be transported to the tissues.

The position of the iodine residues on the inner and outer rings of the T_3 molecule determines whether it is active (T_3) or inactive (rT_3). Usually, around 50% of T_4 is deiodinated on the outer ring, leading to active T_3; however, if deiodination occurs on the inner ring, rT_3 is generated. In states of high T_3 demand (e.g. severe infection), the balance between T_3 and rT_3 balance shifts towards the active form, and when T_3 requirements are low, the balance shifts towards the inactive form.

Mechanism of action of T_3

T_3 diffuses from the bloodstream into the cells and binds to a receptor on the nucleus. This in turn binds to a thyroid response element that is present in some genes and acts as a transcription factor. As a result, there is an increased synthesis of proteins that mediate the actions of T_3. These produce:

- Increased metabolic rate
- Normal development and growth of the brain
- Increased sympathetic neural activity

Graves' disease is the most common cause of thyrotoxicosis (the clinical result of increased levels of T_3) in young people. It is an autoimmune condition mediated partly by production of antibodies that bind to and activate TSH receptors. Patients present with anxiety, weight loss, tachycardia and diarrhoea. Graves' disease also causes swelling in the periorbital tissues, potentially compressing the optic nerve and causing blindness.

Endocrine pancreas

The pancreas is an organ in the abdomen; it has both exocrine and endocrine functions. It secretes several hormones, including insulin which is needed for normal glucose, fat and protein metabolism. Reduced or absent action of insulin characterises diabetes mellitus.

Structure and function

The pancreas lies retroperitoneally in the abdomen and is located posterior to the stomach. In addition to having an endocrine role, it is an exocrine gland due to its role in digestion (see page 223).

Interspersed between the pancreatic exocrine glands are clusters of endocrine cells: the islets of Langerhans (**Figure 6.11**). These are composed of three main cell types, each secreting a different peptide hormone (**Table 6.2**). The β cells are located at the centre of islets and are much more numerous than the peripheral α cells.

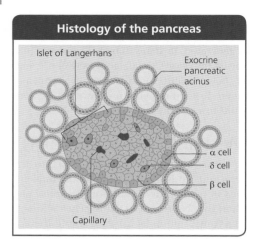

Histology of the pancreas

Islet of Langerhans

Exocrine pancreatic acinus

α cell

δ cell

β cell

Capillary

Figure 6.11 Islets of Langerhans are surrounded by exocrine pancreatic tissue. The blood flows from the centre of the islet out to the periphery.

α Cells

These cells secrete glucagon in response to hypoglycaemia and in the fasting state. Glucagon is a catabolic hormone, i.e. a hormone that signals breakdown of large molecules into smaller ones. It is one of the main hormones signalling hepatic breakdown of glycogen to glucose, thereby antagonising the action of insulin and helping to maintain an energy supply during fasting (see Chapter 7 for further details on postprandial and fasting states).

Glucagonoma

Tumours of pancreatic α cells are relatively rare, but they can present insidiously with excess glucagon production. Typically, they are found in elderly men who suddenly develop type 2 diabetes but show weight loss rather than obesity. The excess glucagon promotes hyperglycaemia, but as there is no insulin deficiency, patients do not develop ketoacidosis (only a small amount of insulin is needed to stop ketone production). A severe, progressive skin rash also suggests that a tumour is present. If the tumour is surgically removed, 85% of patients survive at 5 years.

β Cells

The β cells are responsible for the production of insulin, the main anabolic hormone (anabolic hormones signal the synthesis of large macromolecules from smaller ones, e.g. triglycerides from fatty acids). It is key to the pathogenesis of diabetes. Insulin's actions are discussed below.

δ Cells

The δ cells produce the hormone somatostatin. This has a number of effects on the gastrointestinal tract, for example suppressing the secretion of other hormones such as gastrin, cholecystokinin, vasoactive intestinal peptide and histamine.

Insulin

Insulin is a peptide hormone produced from the cleavage of pre-proinsulin to proinsulin, and then by loss of the C chain of proinsulin to give insulin (**Figure 6.12**). The production of C peptide is therefore used as a marker of endogenous insulin synthesis.

Insulin secretion follows two patterns (**Figure 6.13**). First, there is a basal, constitutive

\multicolumn{5}{c}{**Hormones of the islets of Langerhans**}				

Cell	Hormone	Receptor type	Secondary messenger	Function
α Cell	Insulin	Tyrosine kinase	Insulin–receptor substrates	Anabolism, lowers blood glucose
β Cell	Glucagon	G-protein-coupled receptor	$G_s \rightarrow AC \rightarrow$ increase cAMP, and $PIP_2 \rightarrow$ increase Ca^{2+}	Catabolism, raises blood glucose
δ Cell	Somatostatin	G-protein-coupled receptor	$G_i \rightarrow AC \rightarrow$ reduced cAMP	Suppression of multiple hormones, e.g. vasoactive intestinal peptide, gastrin

Table 6.2 Hormones produced by the islets of Langerhans and their mechanisms of action

Insulin synthesis

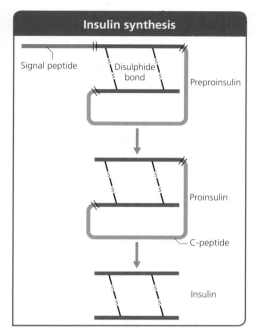

Figure 6.12 Insulin synthesis. Cleavage of pre-proinsulin to proinsulin. The C peptide chain is then released to produce insulin.

(continuous, irrespective of stimuli) secretion of insulin, regardless of the serum glucose level. Second, there is a release of insulin that has been stored during the postprandial (fed) state. This is released in response to:

- High serum glucose levels
- Carbohydrate in the small intestine – mediated by the incretin system (see below)

A greater release of insulin is seen if protein is ingested along with the carbohydrate.

Actions of insulin

The actions of insulin are:

- Increased glucose uptake by fat and muscle
- Inhibition of gluconeogenesis, glycogenolysis, lipolysis and proteolysis
- Increased glycogenesis, lipogenesis and proteogenesis

The insulin receptor has a tyrosine kinase domain, which phosphorylates insulin receptor substrate-1 (IRS-1, a separate protein) along with other proteins. Phosphorylated IRS-1 causes the incorporation of the glucose transporter GLUT-4 into cellular membranes, resulting in an increased uptake of glucose from the serum. IRS-1 also triggers a kinase chain that alters which genes the cell transcribes, moving it towards an anabolic state.

> **Hypoglycaemia is exceptionally rare in healthy people.** Causes include liver failure, drugs, alcohol and insulinomas, rare tumours caused by a proliferation of β cells in the islets of Langerhans. Patients typically present with episodes of light-headedness or with feeling sweaty and unwell between meals, with resolution of symptoms after eating.

Mechanism of secretion

Pancreatic β cells express the relatively low-affinity GLUT-2 transporter. Thus, a rise in serum glucose leads to an increased rate of glucose uptake into the pancreatic cells. This in turn increases the rate of glycolysis, leading to elevated concentrations of ATP (**Figure 6.14**). The uptake of amino acids after

Insulin release throughout the day

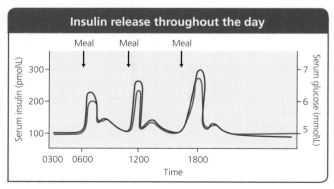

Figure 6.13 Insulin release throughout the day. A meal causes a peak in insulin release (red) to match a small rise in blood glucose (blue). Basal insulin release occurs even during the postprandial phases.

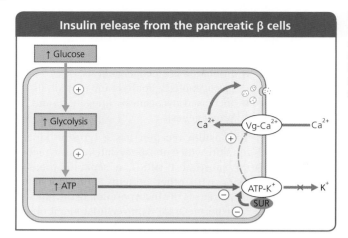

Figure 6.14 Insulin release from the pancreatic β cells. Increased ATP causes closure of the ATP-sensitive K⁺ channels, resulting in membrane depolarisation and Ca^{2+}-mediated insulin release. SUR, sulphonylurea receptor.

a high-protein meal can have a similar effect.

The raised intracellular ATP causes the closure of ATP-sensitive K⁺ channels in the membranes of the β cells that are constitutively open. This causes β-cell depolarisation, which activates voltage-gated calcium ion (Ca^{2+}) channels. The resulting Ca^{2+} influx stimulates the fusion of the insulin storage granules with the cell surface membrane. In this way, insulin is secreted.

Linked to the potassium channels are receptors that can bind to sulphonylureas, which are hypoglycaemic drugs. Binding of sulphonylureas closes the potassium channels and thus increases insulin secretion.

Incretin system

Independent of the above mechanism, insulin is released in response to small bowel intraluminal carbohydrate, a reaction that is mediated by the incretin system (**Figure 6.15**). When carbohydrates are detected in the gut lumen, L-cells in the duodenum and jejunum release glucagon-like peptide-1 (GLP-1). This enters the bloodstream, where much of it is degraded by the enzyme dipeptidyl peptidase-4. The remaining GLP-1 binds to a G-protein-coupled receptor (present on target cells), causing:

■ Increased insulin release
■ Suppression of glucagon release
■ Increased satiety
■ Slowed gastric emptying

John, a 78-year-old man, is admitted to hospital with central crushing chest pain and is diagnosed with a myocardial infarction. His blood glucose is 17.2 mmol/L. He is obese and hypertensive, but has no other known medical conditions.

Type 2 diabetes mellitus presents incidentally very commonly. It is characterised by insulin resistance, therefore tissues require higher serum concentrations of insulin to produce the same effect. Initially, the pancreas compensates by increasing production of insulin, but tissue resistance eventually exceeds the maximum rate of insulin production, leading to symptoms of diabetes.

Type 2 diabetes mellitus almost always occurs in the presence of central obesity. Visceral adipocytes are very insulin resistant and have a high spontaneous rate of lipolysis. This, together with other features of the 'metabolic syndrome' (hypertension and a raised cholesterol level), predispose to atherosclerotic cardiovascular disease.

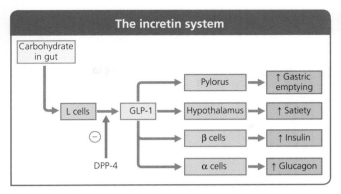

The incretin system

Figure 6.15 The incretin system. The majority of the glucagon-like peptide-1 (GLP-1) is broken down by the enzyme dipeptidyl peptidase-4 (DPP-4) before it can have any effect.

Adrenal glands

The adrenal glands are located in the abdomen on top of the kidneys. They secrete steroid hormones that are needed for: control of body salt (and water) content, metabolism of carbohydrates and fats, and normal sexual function. Complete loss of adrenal function is incompatible with life, causing Addison's syndrome (see below).

Structure and function

The two adrenal glands are pyramidal yellow-brown glands that overlie the superior poles of the kidneys. They are composed of an inner medulla and an outer cortex, which is divided into three layers (**Figure 6.16**).

Adrenal cortex

The adrenal cortex manages the secretion of steroid hormones, with each of its three layers producing a different group of steroids. The three layers are functionally distinct due to the expression of different enzymes in the steroid synthesis pathway (**Figure 6.17**). The structure of all the steroid hormones is based upon cholesterol, with the first, and rate-limiting step, being the conversion of cholesterol into pregnenolone. The pregnenolone is then actively imported into the smooth endoplasmic reticulum.

Zona glomerulosa

The zona glomerulosa secretes mineralocorticoids, primarily aldosterone. Aldosterone causes the renal reabsorption of sodium and water, with a loss of potassium into the urine. This process is controlled by the renin–angiotensin–aldosterone system, and independently by the serum potassium concentration (see page 152).

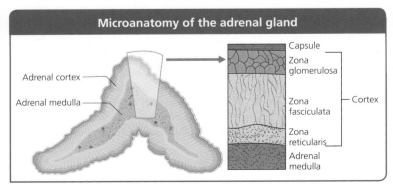

Microanatomy of the adrenal gland

Figure 6.16 Microanatomy of the adrenal gland. The adrenal cortex is divided into three functionally different layers: zona glomerulosa, zona fasciculata and zona reticularis.

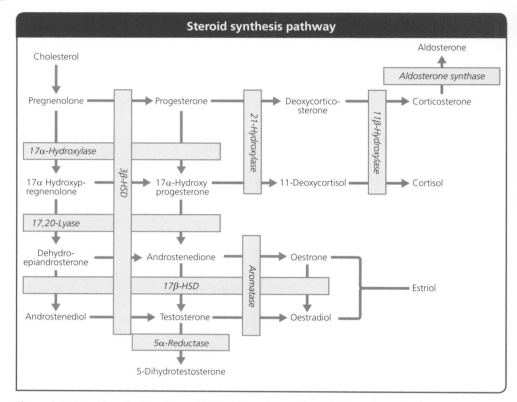

Figure 6.17 Steroid synthesis pathway. All steroids are formed from cholesterol. HSD, hydroxysteroid dehydrogenase.

Zona fasciculata

This layer produces glucocorticoids, most importantly cortisol. Cortisol has a variety of metabolic actions, as described below.

Zona reticularis

The zona reticularis produces a proportion of the body's sex steroids (mainly androgens, which are converted peripherally into dehydroepiandrosterone [DHEA], oestrogens and testosterones). In adults, this represents a modest fraction of sex hormone production compared with that occurring in the ovaries or testes. In men, secretion by the adrenal gland is of little importance. In women, however, it remains the main source of androgens and is important in maintaining muscle mass and libido.

Adrenal medulla

The adrenal medulla acts in harmony with the sympathetic nervous system. It can be considered as representing postganglionic sympathetic neurones that are secreting into the bloodstream rather than into a synapse.

The medulla is composed of enterochromaffin cells, derived from neural crest cells, which synthesise catecholamines from tyrosine. The enterochromaffin cells are directly innervated by preganglionic sympathetic neurones and release noradrenaline (norepinephrine) and adrenaline (epinephrine) when they are activated. Unlike sympathetic neurones, enterochromaffin cells produce 80% adrenaline and 20% noradrenaline (sympathetic neurones secrete 90% noradrenaline and 10% adrenaline). This represents only a minor part of the effect of the sympathetic nervous system, and it is possible to survive without an adrenal medulla. However, the adrenal glands and sympathetic nervous system have complementary roles as different adrenoreceptors respond differently to adrenaline and noradrenaline (see Chapter 2).

Glucocorticoids

Glucocorticoids are steroid hormones secreted by the adrenal cortex zona fasciculata. They cause transcriptional effects on a variety of metabolic processes; therefore, they are essential for life. Glucocorticoids and mineralocorticoids have a similar structure and slightly overlapping functions. Mineralocorticoids are only concerned with salt and water reabsorption and potassium excretion, whereas glucocorticoids have other metabolic roles. Glucocorticoids can weakly bind to mineralocorticoid receptors and therefore glucocorticoids also have an effect on salt and water reabsorption.

Hypothalamic–pituitary–adrenal axis

The hypothalamic–pituitary–adrenal axis controls the production of glucocorticoids by the zona fasciculata (**Figure 6.18**). The hypothalamus secretes corticotrophin-releasing hormone in response to psychological or physical stress, and in turn the corticotrophin-releasing hormone in turn increases the production of ACTH by the anterior pituitary. This causes an upregulation of the enzymes involved in steroid synthesis in the adrenal cortex, and hyperplasia of the epithelial cells of the cortex.

The majority of the negative feedback is mediated by cortisol at the level of the pituitary gland.

ACTH synthesis

ACTH is produced from a large precursor molecule, pro-opiomelanocortin. As pro-opiomelanocortin is cleaved in the anterior pituitary to give ACTH, melanocyte-stimulating

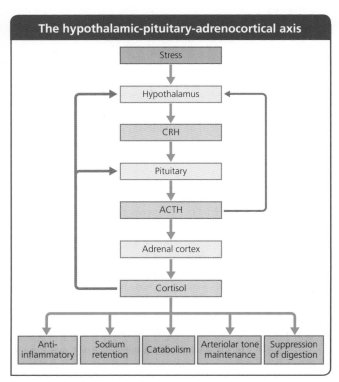

Figure 6.18 The hypothalamic-pituitary-adrenocortical axis. Cortisol from the zona fasciculata provides most of the negative feedback at the pituitary. ACTH, adrenocorticotrophic hormone, CRH, corticotrophin-releasing hormone.

hormone is also cleaved from pro-opiomela-nocortin.

Cortisol

As a steroid hormone, cortisol is able to diffuse through the cell membranes to bind to a nuclear receptor. The cortisol–receptor unit associates with other proteins to form a transcription factor complex, which transcribes various proteins that account for the actions of cortisol:

- Anti-inflammatory
- Sodium (and indirectly water) retention
- Insulin antagonism (catabolism)
- Fetal maturation
- Maintenance of arteriolar tone

- Reduced muscle mass
- Increased bone resorption

Addison's disease most frequently occurs secondary to autoimmune disease. However, it was originally described as tuberculosis-mediated destruction of the adrenal gland. Primary adrenal failure manifests as weight loss, fatigue, hypotension and electrolyte imbalance (hyperkalaemia with hyponatraemia). Patients may also have hyperpigmentation, as more melanocyte-stimulating hormone is secreted as a by-product when the loss of cortisol-mediated negative feedback causes increased ACTH production.

Parathyroid glands and calcium regulation

The parathyroid glands in the neck secrete parathyroid hormone, which acts to maintain (increase) serum Ca^{2+} levels. Their absence causes hypocalcaemia (low Ca^{2+} in the blood), which leads to muscle spasms and heart rhythm abnormalities.

Structure and function

The parathyroid glands are four small glands, each the size of a grain of rice, that are located on the posterior surface of the thyroid. Each lobe of the thyroid is associated with one superior and one inferior parathyroid gland. The parathyroids are composed of densely packed chief cells, which produce PTH, and larger oxyphil cells, whose function is unknown.

Serum calcium regulation

A stable serum calcium concentration is crucial to maintaining the functioning of all the excitable tissues, and severe abnormalities cause cardiac arrhythmias due to the role of Ca^{2+} in action potentials. The serum concentration is thus maintained within tight limits. The plasma level of calcium is controlled by the interaction of the gut and kidney responses to PTH, calcitonin and vitamin D.

The majority of the calcium in the body is stored in the form of hydroxyapatite, a calcium–phosphate compound that is bound to osteoid in bone. This serves as a potential source for replenishing the serum calcium pool.

About half of the calcium in the plasma is bound to albumin, and it is only the free, unbound (ionised) component that is available to interact with the cells. Therefore, total plasma calcium levels must always be considered in the light of the plasma albumin concentration, and an 'adjusted calcium' figure is calculated each time calcium is measured, taking this into consideration.

Parathyroid hormone

The chief cells express calcium receptors that can sense the blood concentration of Ca^{2+}. If these sense a fall in Ca^{2+} level, the chief cells are stimulated to release PTH, which acts to raise the serum calcium level (**Figure 6.19**). PTH is a small peptide hormone, which binds to a G-protein-coupled receptor (on target cell surfaces) and acts on several tissues, with the following results:

- Osteoclast activity is increased, resulting in bone resorption and hence the release of calcium

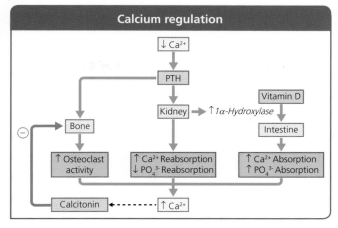

Calcium regulation

Figure 6.19 Calcium regulation. Parathyroid hormone (PTH) is released in response to hypocalcaemia and acts in conjunction with vitamin D to raise the Ca^{2+} level. Calcitonin antagonises the action of PTH on the osteoclasts. PO_4^{3-}, phosphate ion.

- Renal tubular reabsorption of calcium is increased, while the reabsorption of phosphate is decreased
- There is an increased renal expression of the enzyme 1α-hydroxylase, which synthesises vitamin D

Vitamin D

Vitamin D is predominantly synthesised in the skin from 7-dehydrocholesterol in response to ultraviolet light (**Figure 6.20**). It is also ingested in dairy products, although in much smaller amounts than can be produced by exposure to sunlight.

The vitamin D ingested or produced in response to sunlight is not, however, synthesised in its active form. Instead, it must undergo two hydroxylation reactions. First, the enzyme 25-hydroxylase, which is constitutively expressed in the liver, produces 25-(OH)-D$_3$ from vitamin D (7-cholecalciferol). Second, there is rate-limiting step is the α-hydroxylation of vitamin D, which occurs in the renal tubules and is under the control of PTH. This causes production of the active compound 1,25-(OH)-D3.

As a steroid, vitamin D binds to an intracellular receptor that promotes the transcription of genes to produce proteins that:

- Increase the gastrointestinal uptake of calcium and phosphate
- Maintain bone mineralisation

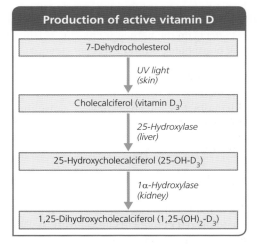

Production of active vitamin D

7-Dehydrocholesterol

UV light (skin)

Cholecalciferol (vitamin D$_3$)

25-Hydroxylase (liver)

25-Hydroxycholecalciferol (25-OH-D$_3$)

1α-Hydroxylase (kidney)

1,25-Dihydroxycholecalciferol (1,25-(OH)$_2$-D$_3$)

Figure 6.20 The production of active vitamin D requires two activating hydroxylation reactions; the 1α-hydroxylation in the kidney is the rate-limiting step.

Effect on bone

If calcium concentrations are low, vitamin D increases the uptake of calcium from the gastrointestinal tract, but does not cause the resorption of osteoid to release calcium. If the serum calcium level is normal, vitamin D also aids in the deposition of hydroxyapatite onto bone collagen. If, however, there is hypocalcaemia, vitamin D does not prevent PTH-mediated bone resorption. Vitamin D will help mineralise bones (provided that normal levels are present), but maintenance of Ca^{2+} by PTH is more important.

If the primary deficiency is of vitamin D deficiency rather than calcium, the bones are undermineralised (as seen in rickets in children, or osteomalacia in adults, which differ due to fusion of growth plates during adolescence). The bones contain adequate collagen, but this is not hardened by formation of osteoid. If the vitamin D deficiency is severe enough to cause hypocalcaemia, secondary hyperparathyroidism may result (due to the negative feedback loop).

A raised serum PTH concentration is diagnostic of hyperparathyroidism. In primary hyperparathyroidism, the excess PTH is usually caused by a benign adenoma and results in bone resorption and hypercalcaemia. This causes renal stones, weakness, constipation and neuropsychiatric disturbances. Treatment is usually surgical removal of the parathyroid glands, followed by lifelong calcium supplementation.

Calcitonin

Calcitonin is released from the C cells of the thyroid in response to a rise in plasma calcium level. It acts to lower the plasma calcium level, mainly by inhibiting osteoclast-mediated resorption of the bones. It also has modest effects on the kidney, increasing calcium and phosphate excretion. It is not essential to life, so patients who have undergone thyroidectomy do not routinely require calcitonin replacement. Tumours of C cells secreting calcitonin may, but do not always, cause clinically significant hypocalcaemia.

Medullary thyroid carcinoma

Tumours of the C cells are a rare cause of thyroid cancer. Medullary thyroid carcinoma (MTC) results in an excessive secretion of calcitonin so patients present with features of hypocalcaemia, including tingling lips, muscle weakness and cramps. MTC can be familial and in some cases forms part of multiple endocrine neoplasia syndrome, in which patients develop several endocrine tumours in different organs.

Female reproductive system

The female reproductive system comprises anatomical components (e.g. ovaries, Fallopian tubes, uterus) and hormones (e.g. GnRH, LH, FSH, oestrogen), which together produce ova (the female gametes) and provide a uterus capable of carrying a fetus to delivery.

the ovaries. These lie in close proximity to the opening of the Fallopian tubes, which connect the abdominal cavity and the uterus (**Figure 6.21**). The hormones are produced in the ovarian follicles, which are collections of cells surrounding a single ovum. Both the follicle and the ovum must undergo maturation (processes known as folliculogenesis and oogenesis, respectively) before ovulation can occur.

Structure and function

The female reproductive system undergoes cycles to produce an ovum approximately once a month from the ovaries, at the same time ensuring that the endometrium is suitable for implantation should fertilisation occur. This is a complex series of events that depends on coordination by the endocrine system to provide an optimal timing of events.

The majority of female sex steroids (oestrogens and progesterone) are produced by

Hypothalamic–pituitary–ovarian axis

Unlike most other feedback loops discussed in this chapter, the hypothalamic–pituitary–ovarian axis can display positive or negative feedback, depending on phase of the menstrual cycle (**Figure 6.22**).

LH, released from the anterior pituitary, promotes oestrogen production in the ovaries.

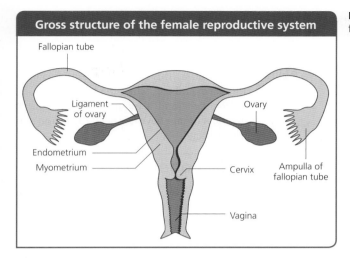

Figure 6.21 Gross structure of the female reproductive system.

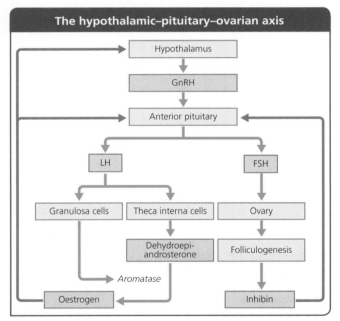

Figure 6.22 The hypothalamic–pituitary–ovarian axis. The granulosa cell enzyme aromatase is required to make oestrogens from theca cell androgens. DHEA, dehydroepiandrosterone; FSH, follicle-stimulating hormone; GnRH, gonadotropin-releasing hormone; LH, luteinising hormone.

To do this, LH acts on the theca interna cells of the ovarian follicle to increase the synthesis of DHEA (and androstenedione which is essentially interchangeable with DHEA in this process). These diffuse through the follicle's basement membrane and enter the granulosa cells. LH also stimulates the upregulation of the enzyme aromatase in the granulosa cells. Aromatase converts DHEA and androstenedione into oestrogens inside granulosa cells. This LH-mediated expression of aromatase also causes a synthesis of oestrogens in the adipocytes. For most of the menstrual cycle, oestrogen provides negative feedback on LH secretion.

FSH promotes the development of the ovarian follicles. Inhibin is formed as a by-product of this process and provides negative feedback on FSH for most of the menstrual cycle.

Oogenesis

This is the production of a secondary ovum (fully mature) from a primordial germ cell (**Figure 6.23**). The process begins in utero,

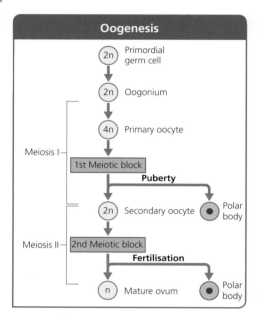

Figure 6.23 Oogenesis. The first meiotic block is held until puberty; the second meiotic block is ended by fertilisation.

when primordial germ cells proliferate to form a large number of cells called oogonia. The oogonia enter meiosis, are then termed primary oocytes, but meiosis halts at the crossing-over point of prophase I. This is known as the first meiotic block and the cells are held at this stage until puberty.

After puberty, meiosis is restarted in several primary oocytes each month in response to stimulation by FSH. At this point, they are known as secondary oocytes. However, although the second meiotic division now begins, it halts at metaphase II – the second meiotic block. This is not lifted until fusion of the sperm and egg, when the final polar body is produced (and a mature ovum remains). The polar bodies have no specific function and are degraded.

Folliculogenesis

Like oogenesis, folliculogenesis – the of development of a follicle – occurs in several stages (**Figure 6.24** and **Table 6.3**). The initial primordial follicle develops successively into a primary, secondary and tertiary (or Graafian) follicle under the influence of LH and FSH. The production of a mature (tertiary) follicle takes approximately 13 months. Each month, several follicles begin folliculogenesis, but usually only one ultimately undergoes ovulation.

A primordial follicle is composed of only a single layer of cells surrounding a primary oocyte. By the time the follicle has become a secondary follicle, the ovum is surrounded by a glycoprotein coat, the zona pellucida, which is important for its protection and for fertilisation. A number of granulosa cells, known as the corona radiata, surround the zona pellucida. The ooycte and corona radiata are suspended in follicular fluid, secreted from further granulosa

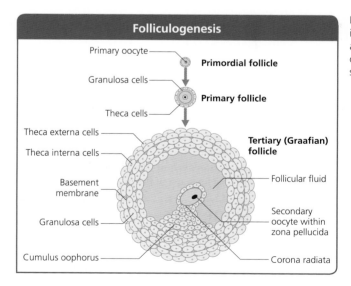

Figure 6.24 Folliculogenesis. An increasing number of granulosa and theca cells surrounds the ovum during development. The secondary follicle is not shown.

Stages of folliculogenesis and oogenesis		
Stage of folliculogenesis	Stages of oogenesis	
Primordial follicle	A single layer of granulosa cells covers the primary oocytes; they have not yet entered folliculogenesis	Oogonia pre-puberty Primary oocyte post-puberty
Primary follicle	The zona pellucida (a glycoprotein coat) develops around the oocyte; there are thickened granulosa cells with a basement membrane outside which theca cells grow to form the corona radiata	Primary oocyte
Secondary follicle	The theca cells separate into the theca interna and theca externa; there is thickening of the granulosa cells	Primary oocyte
Tertiary follicle	Follicular fluid is produced by the granulosa cells; a corona radiata surrounds the oocyte, attached by stalk of cumulus oophorus	Secondary oocyte

Table 6.3 Progression from a primordial follicle to a preovulatory tertiary follicle, which takes 13 cycles to complete

cells, by a stalk known as the cumulus oophorus. This connects the corona radiata to the other granulosa cells. The granulosa cells are surrounded by a basement membrane, outside which lie cells of the theca interna and externa.

At ovulation, the follicle that is most sensitive to LH becomes the dominant follicle. The resulting changes in hormone level (see the next section) stimulate an increase in the production of follicular fluid, causing a rise in pressure until the follicle ruptures. The ovum and its surrounding corona radiata are then released.

The remaining granulosa and theca cells together form the corpus luteum, which is important for hormone production in the luteal phase of the menstrual cycle (see page 186). Eventually, the corpus luteum involutes (dies and stops producing hormones) and is known as the corpus albicans (which is degraded).

Menstrual cycle

The menstrual cycle occurs approximately once a month during a woman's reproductive life (roughly from puberty to 50 years old) to produce an ovum and menses. During the cycle there are a series of hormonal changes (in oestrogen, progesterone, LH, and FSH), which cause specific effects on the ovaries and endometrium (inner lining of the uterus) (**Figure 6.25**). This underlies normal menstruation and fertility.

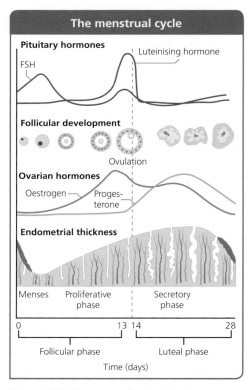

Figure 6.25 The menstrual cycle. The changes in luteinising hormone (LH), follicle-stimulating hormone (FSH), oestrogen and progesterone are shown, along with the gross histology of the endometrium and the stages of development of the follicle.

Follicular phase

The follicular phase lasts 6–16 days and begins on the first day of menses. During the early part of the phase, the rising level of oestrogen (in response to LH) initially provides negative feedback on the production of LH. Selection for a dominant follicle thus occurs in the setting of limited LH. The dominant follicle grows rapidly, synthesising oestrogen, and at this stage feedback on the pituitary switches so that oestrogen gives positive feedback on LH release. The resulting LH peak causes rupture of the dominant follicle and ovulation.

The high oestrogen also stimulates endometrial hyperplasia (proliferation of cells); this is the first step in establishing an endometrium – known as the endometrial decidua – that is receptive to the implantation of an embryo.

Luteal phase

The luteal phase always lasts 14 days. In this phase, the corpus luteum takes over hormone production (stimulated by LH and FSH), producing more progesterone than oestrogen. These, along with inhibin (also from the corpus luteum), provide negative feedback on LH and FSH.

Progesterone also increases the vascularity of the endometrium and causes dilatation of vessels, as well as increasing mucus secretions from endothelial glands.

Menses

If fertilisation does not occur, the corpus luteum involutes due to the falling levels of LH and FSH. This in turn causes a decrease in the synthesis of progesterone and oestrogen, which were maintaining the decidua. Consequently, the endometrial vessels vasoconstrict and epithelial proliferation ceases, resulting in a sloughing off of the dead endometrium that manifests as menses.

The low levels of progesterone, oestrogen and inhibin that are now present during this late luteal phase allow LH and FSH production to increase, which initiates another follicular phase and thus another cycle.

The placenta requires a huge blood supply, which is generated by remodelling the endometrial vasculature. Maternal cardiac output, blood volume, glomerular filtration rate and tidal ventilation all rise. The placenta produces hormones including human chorionic gonadotropin, which maintain the corpus luteum and keep it active. By week 10 of pregnancy, the placenta has taken over production of pregnancy hormones, and the corpus luteum begins to involute. High levels of progesterone maintain the dilated blood vessels in the uterus.

Fetal changes at birth

When air inflates the lungs during the baby's first breath after birth, the amniotic fluid that has filled the lungs is pushed out into the lung's interstitial space. The expansion of lungs facilitates an increase in pulmonary blood flow, due to drastically reduced pulmonary vascular resistance. In addition, clamping of the umbilical artery (in the umbilical cord) causes a rise in total peripheral resistance (see page 81).

The sequence of events leading to birth is initiated by a rise in fetal cortisol which can cross the placenta. This leads to a reduction in maternal progesterone and increases sensitivity of the maternal myometrium to oestrogen and oxytocin, which initiate labour.

Taken together, these changes cause the pressures in the left side of the heart to exceed those on the right. This results in a reversal of blood flow through the foramen ovale between the atria of the heart, and causes it to close. The ductus arteriosus constricts and eventually fibroses in response to the increased oxygen tensions. In addition, the ductus venosus fibroses as a result of the reduced blood flow after the umbilical vein has been clamped (see page 74).

These changes to the circulation start at birth but are not complete until the baby is

24 hours old. If the fetal circulation persists (e.g. there is a persistent ductus arteriosus), this causes left-to-right cardiac shunting and may result in heart failure.

Breasts

The breasts are specialised exocrine glands surrounded by fat and supported by fibrous septae. Their general structure is similar to that of other exocrine glands with milk being secreted by the alveolar epithelial cells into the acini. The milk is stored here until contraction of the myoepithelial cells surrounding the acini causes it to be expelled along the mammary ducts.

Lactogenesis

Breast milk is a unique fluid composed of water, solutes, proteins and lipids. Because of its specific nature, its production (lactogenesis) is more complicated than the exocrine secretion process for other glands. The process involves:

- **Exocytosis** – this is the packaging of proteins and large carbohydrates into secretory vesicles that are exported via the Golgi apparatus
- **Lipid synthesis and secretion** – triglycerides are formed in the smooth endoplasmic reticulum. Triglycerides then migrate towards the apical membrane and bud off, surrounded by a layer of phospholipid

- **Transcytosis** – immunoglobulin (especially IgA) moves through the alveolar cells, where it is modified to its secretory form. Some IgA may also move in a paracellular manner during pregnancy
- **Apical transporters** – these bring about the movement of monosaccharides and salts across the apical membrane
- **Paracellular movement** – salts and water move by diffusion through leaky occluding junctions between acinar cells

The main hormones involved in stimulating milk production are prolactin and human placental lactogen. Oxytocin, secreted in response to suckling, is responsible for myoepithelial contraction and milk expulsion.

> **Raised serum prolactin (hyperprolactinaemia)** is caused by prolactin-secreting pituitary tumours (prolactinomas), pharmacological dopamine blockade (e.g. haloperidol) or by disruption of dopaminergic inhibition of prolactin secretion by a large pituitary mass (macroadenoma).
>
> Because prolactin suppresses LH and FSH, hyperprolactinaemia causes amenorrhoea, loss of libido and infertility so serum prolactin should always be measured when investigating infertility. Hyperprolactinaemia also causes galactorrhoea, spontaneous excretion of breast milk not related to pregnancy and lactation.

Male reproductive system

The male reproductive system comprises anatomical components (e.g. testes, penis) and hormones (e.g. GnRH, LH, testosterone), which integrate to produce sperm. These all contribute to a man's fertility (i.e. the capacity to produce offspring).

Structure and function

The male reproductive system is much more straightforward as it does not undergo cyclical changes or show alterations in feedback. The majority of male sex steroids are produced in the testes and are required for the production of sperm as well as the development of secondary sexual characteristics.

The testes are composed largely of Leydig cells and Sertoli cells that lie within seminiferous tubules, the site of spermatogenesis (**Figure 6.26**). The Leydig and Sertoli cells interact to produce 5-dihydroxytestosterone in a mechanism akin to oestrogen synthesis

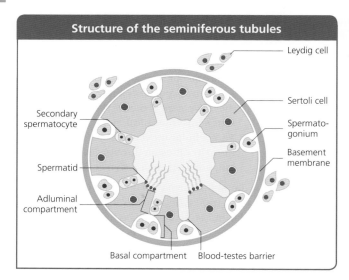

Figure 6.26 Structure of the seminiferous tubules. Spermatogenesis occurs within the tubules, supported by the Sertoli cells. The Leydig cells reside outside the tubule.

in the ovary (i.e. one cell produces a precursor, another cell produces the rate-limiting enzyme).

> **Testicular cancer is the most common malignancy in men aged 18–35 years.** It arises from any cell within the testes, usually from partially differentiated or undifferentiated germ cells. The most common tumours are seminomas or teratomas. The presentation is usually insidious, with a painless lump in one testicle. Testicular cancer has a high rate of metastasis but, as it also has a high response rate to chemotherapy even apparently advanced disease has a high cure rate.

Hypothalamic–pituitary–testicular axis

Pulsatile gonadotropin-releasing hormone (GnRH) released from the hypothalamus stimulates the secretion of LH and FSH from the anterior pituitary (**Figure 6.27**).

LH increases the rate of testosterone synthesis in the Leydig cells. Testosterone diffuses through the basement membrane of the seminiferous tubules and into the Sertoli cells, which express the enzyme 5α-reductase. Here, testosterone is converted into the more active form 5-dihydroxytestosterone. This is particularly important for the intrauterine development of the external genitalia, and for the development of the secondary sexual characteristics later in life.

FSH drives the development of mature spermatozoa. Inhibin is a by-product of this process and provides negative feedback on the pituitary to decrease FSH production.

Spermatogenesis

Spermatogenesis is the production of mature spermatozoa from spermatogonia (immature gametes that contain 2n genetic material).

During development of the testes, primordial germ cells populate the basal compartment of the seminiferous tubules. From puberty onwards, these are known as prospermatogonia and serve as a stem cell population. Each prospermatogonium divides to produce one type A spermatogonium and a new prospermatogonium.

The type A spermatogonia migrate into the adluminal compartment of the seminiferous tubules. Here they are separated from the stem cell population by the blood–testes barrier. The cells then undergo six rounds of cell division (mitosis), passing through a type B spermatogonium stage to become primary spermatocytes (**Figure 6.28**).

Each primary spermatocyte undergoes the first meiotic division, immediately followed by

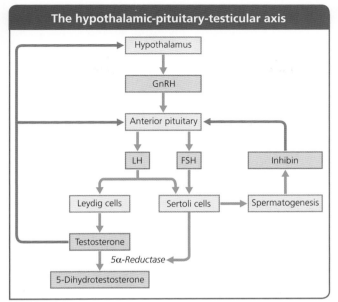

Figure 6.27 The hypothalamic-pituitary-testicular axis. Sertoli cell 5a-reductase is necessary to make active 5-dihydrotestosterone (5-DHT). FSH, follicle-stimulating hormone; GnRH, gonadotropin-releasing hormone; LH, luteinising hormone.

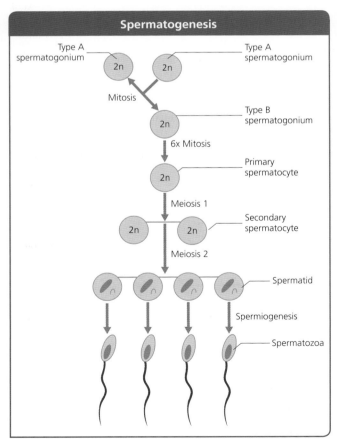

Figure 6.28 Spermatogenesis. Type A spermatogonia act as a stem cell population. Spermatids undergo spermiogenesis as a fused syncytium (n = 1 of each of the 23 chromosomes).

the second meiotic division, to generate four round spermatids that reside in the lumen of the seminiferous tubule, but are connected to Sertoli cells. The four spermatids remain connected via a cytoplasmic cord to facilitate the sharing of proteins needed for further development. This is necessary because, during meiosis, some spermatids lose their X chromosome, which contains genetic information necessary for the final differentiation stage in formation of the spermatozoa.

Spermiogenesis

The differentiation of the round spermatids into mature spermatozoa is known as spermiogenesis. It involves a number of structural and functional changes to the cells, as outlined in **Table 6.4**. Once this is complete, the connecting cytoplasmic cord breaks, and the spermatozoa are freed from Sertoli cells into the lumen of the tubule.

Sperm maturation and capacitation

Although the sperm leaving the seminiferous tubules are physically mature (**Figure 6.29**), they are not yet capable of swimming or of fertilising an ovum. The sperm mature

Spermiogenesis	
Component	Detail
Nucleus	Condensation with exchange of protamines (which are smaller) for histones
Acrosome	Formation of a modified Golgi apparatus containing hydrolytic enzymes to penetrate the zona pellucida
Flagellum	Centrioles migrate to beneath the nucleus and synthesise an axoneme that forms the tail (needed for motility)
Mitochondria	Assemble in a helical arrangement as a mid-piece for the spermatozoa's high energy demand
Cytoplasm	Excess cytoplasm is cleaved off as a cytoplasmic droplet (to make the spermatozoa as efficient as possible) and phagocytosed by the Sertoli cells

Table 6.4 Changes that occur during spermiogenesis in the formation of mature spermatozoa

further during their passage through the rete testis to the long, coiled epididymis. This passage takes several weeks. However, it is only when they are mixed with fluid from the seminal glands and prostate that they undergo capacitation and become motile.

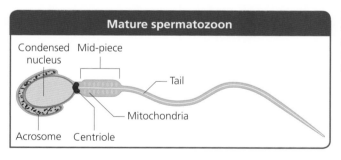

Figure 6.29 Mature spermatozoon with an acrosome covering a condensed nucleus, a mid-piece containing mitochondria and a motile tail formed by centrioles.

Answers to starter questions

1. Most endocrine glands are controlled by hormones secreted by the pituitary, e.g. TSH, LH, ACTH. The pituitary gland is also a key point for negative feedback and therefore regulates the majority of the body's hormonal axes. The pituitary is controlled in turn by the hypothalamus, which receives input from higher centres in the brain.

2. The four small parathyroid glands lie on the posterior aspect of the thyroid. During surgery to remove the thyroid (total thyroidectomy) preserving the parathyroids can be difficult. The parathyroids normally produce parathyroid hormone (PTH) that raises serum calcium levels. If the surgery cannot preserve enough of the parathyroids this can cause hypocalcaemia (low calcium levels).

3. Addison's disease (adrenal insufficiency) results in low cortisol levels. Cortisol normally inhibits ACTH production, which causes a rise in ACTH in Addison's disease. Every time ACTH is synthesised, melanocyte-stimulating hormone (MSH) is produced as a by-product. Raised MSH activates melanocytes to increase the rate of melanin production, which results in darkening of the skin (hyperpigmentation).

4. The menstrual cycle has two phases: the follicular phase and the luteal phase. The luteal phase equates to the lifespan of the corpus luteum and is therefore always 14 days long. The follicular phase varies from 6–16 days, because it is determined by a number of factors including the rate of follicular development, follicular competition for LH, and pituitary change from negative to positive feedback in response to oestrogen.

5. Unlike oogenesis in women, spermatogenesis occurs throughout life supported by the stem cell population of spermatogonia. Over 50 years there is a gradual decline in the activity of the male reproductive organs and sex steroid levels (the androgenopause) but there is no definitive cessation in reproductive capacity.

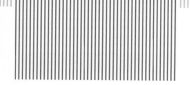

Chapter 7
Gastrointestinal system

Starter questions

Answers to the following questions are on page 237.

1. Why isn't the stomach's lining damaged by gastric acid?
2. How can antibiotics give patients diarrhoea?
3. Why does flatulence occur?
4. How does anxiety cause diarrhoea?
5. Why does prolonged fasting cause the blood to become more acidic?
6. What makes us vomit?

Introduction

The gastrointestinal (GI) tract is a muscular mucosal tube from the mouth to the anus. The GI system also includes the liver, pancreas and gallbladder.

The central function of the GI system is to transfer the nutrients in food from the external environment of the lumen to body tissues, via absorption and distribution in the blood. Food and water are moved through the tract and substances are absorbed at different stages into the blood. These functions are under local, hormonal and nervous control.

As the lumen is effectively outside the body, the GI system plays an important role in immunity by acting as a barrier to infection. The GI immune system also has a complex developmental symbiosis with a bacterial microbiome present in the colon.

Most GI disease is due to dysfunction of motility, absorption or immunity.

Case 7 Abdominal pain and weeks of diarrhoea

Presentation

Raphael is a 23-year-old man who visits his general practitioner after suffering several weeks of intermittently bloody diarrhoea. He also complains of lower abdominal pain, but has not been vomiting. He has just finished his degree and spent the summer in Brazil, including a trip to the Amazon. He has smoked 10 cigarettes a day since starting at university and, other than antimalarials, he is taking no regular medication.

Analysis

Abdominal pain and weeks of diarrhoea in an otherwise fit young man is suggestive of an inflammatory bowel disease (IBD), such as ulcerative colitis or Crohn's disease, or a chronic GI infection.

Compared to IBD, traveller's diarrhoea usually presents with a shorter history of more intense symptoms, often including nausea and vomiting. Bloody diarrhoea is rare in viral infections and food poisoning, but can occur in some bacterial infections, such as *Shigella* and *Campylobacter*. Colonic *Clostridium difficile (C. diff)* infection can present in this way, but usually occurs after antibacterial therapy in hospitalised patients with comorbidities.

Chronic diarrhoea can also occur in giardiasis – a protozoan infection – or *Tropherema whipplei* infection, also known as Whipple's disease.

Other possibilities include diverticulitis, which usually presents more acutely, or GI malignancy, which is rare in those under 50 years of age.

Further case

Raphael reports an episode in his mid-teens of diarrhoea, pain and tenderness

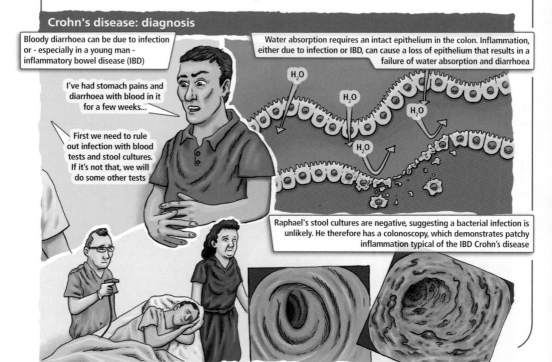

Crohn's disease: diagnosis

Bloody diarrhoea can be due to infection or - especially in a young man - inflammatory bowel disease (IBD)

I've had stomach pains and diarrhoea with blood in it for a few weeks...

First we need to rule out infection with blood tests and stool cultures. If it's not that, we will do some other tests

Water absorption requires an intact epithelium in the colon. Inflammation, either due to infection or IBD, can cause a loss of epithelium that results in a failure of water absorption and diarrhoea

H₂O

Raphael's stool cultures are negative, suggesting a bacterial infection is unlikely. He therefore has a colonoscopy, which demonstrates patchy inflammation typical of the IBD Crohn's disease in his right iliac fossa, which was thought to be appendicitis but was managed conservatively. He has been well whilst travelling. He has a low-grade fever (37.6°C) and mild abdominal tenderness without guarding. Rectal examination shows a couple of anal skin tags. Stool is positive for blood on testing. A stool sample is sent for microscopy and cultures for infectious agents, but none are found.

A colonoscopy is performed, which reveals discrete patches of very inflamed mucosa throughout the colon. Biopsies reveal transmural inflammation with granulomas. An abdominal X-ray using a barium contrast shows narrowing and scarring around the ileocaecal junction.

Further analysis

Raphael's previous history of a similar episode of abdominal pain; his low-grade fever, anal skin tags and the lack of infectious agent all suggest he has IBD rather than an infection. The colonoscopy, biopsy and imaging features of colonic inflammation also strongly support this.

Colonic inflammation in ulcerative colitis starts in the rectum and is a continuous lesion limited to the mucosa, and granulomas are not seen. Crohn's disease, on the other hand, can involve patches of inflammation anywhere along the GI tract. Lesions extend beyond the mucosal layer (i.e. are transmural), and are associated with granuloma and perineal skin tags. His previous 'appendicitis' was likely an early episode of Crohn's disease affecting the terminal ileum.

> **IBD is thought to be caused by a failure of the normal immune tolerance to the bacteria in the gut,** causing a T cell-mediated chronic inflammation. There is a substantial genetic component and changes in the gut flora appear to be involved, together with abnormal activation of T cells.

Crohn's disease is managed principally by use of steroids and/or immunomodulators. Surgery may be necessary in severe episodes, such as where an abscess or fistula has formed.

Overview of gastrointestinal anatomy

The GI tract is 9 metres long and consists of 15 sections, embryologically divided into upper, middle and lower tracts (**Figure 7.1** and **Table 7.1**). Clinically, it is divided into upper (mouth to ileum) and lower tracts, although sometimes – for example when differentiating a site of bleeding – this border is considered to be at the duodenojejunal junction of the small intestine.

The gastrointestinal wall

The gastrointestinal wall typically has four layers (**Figure 7.2**):

1. **Serosa** – a smooth membrane of two epithelial layers that secretes serous (i.e. clear) fluid, which lubricates the outside of the GI tract to allow movement and prevent adhesions
2. **Muscularis propria** – with longitudinal and circular smooth muscle. Longitudinal contraction shortens the GI tract while circular contraction constricts the lumen to propel food boluses
3. **Submucosa** – a connective tissue supporting the mucosa and the site of blood and lymphatic vessels and nerves

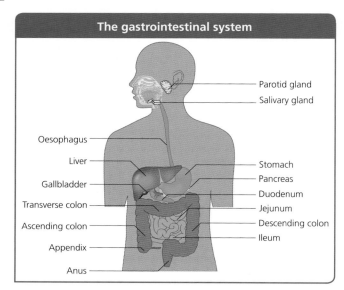

The gastrointestinal system

- Parotid gland
- Salivary gland
- Oesophagus
- Liver
- Gallbladder
- Transverse colon
- Ascending colon
- Appendix
- Anus
- Stomach
- Pancreas
- Duodenum
- Jejunum
- Descending colon
- Ileum

Figure 7.1 The gastrointestinal system consists of the GI tract and accessory organs: the liver, gallbladder and pancreas.

The gastrointestinal tract

Embryological division	Clinical division	Section		Length	Function
Upper tract (foregut)	Upper	Mouth			Mastication and enzymal digestion
		Oral cavity			
		Oropharynx			
		Oesophagus		25 cm	
		Stomach		25 cm	Acidic and enzymal digestion
Middle tract (midgut)	Lower	Small intestine or bowel	Duodenum	25 cm	Digestion and most nutrient absorption
			Jejunum	4–6 m	
			Ileum		
		Large intestine or bowel or colon	Caecum and appendix	6 cm	Water absorption, GI microbiota
			Ascending colon	20 cm	
			Transverse colon	30–60 cm	
			Descending colon	25 cm	
Lower tract (hindgut)			Sigmoid colon	40 cm	
			Rectum	10 cm	
		Anus			

Table 7.1 The embryological, clinical and sectional divisions of the gastrointestinal (GI) tract. Embryological divisions: upper is mouth to the duodenal papilla (i.e. where the bile duct enters); middle is from the papilla to the mid-transverse colon; and lower is from there to the anus. Their arterial blood supplies are the coeliac trunk, superior and inferior mesenteric arteries, respectively.

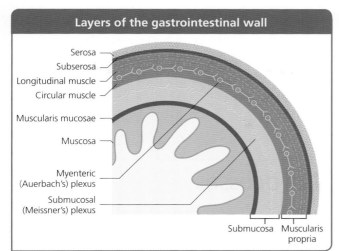

Figure 7.2 There are four main layers of the gastrointestinal wall: mucosa, submucosa, muscularis propria and serosa. The submucosal plexus lies in the submucosa and the myenteric plexus lies between the circular and longitudinal muscle layers.

4. **Mucosa** – with a glandular epithelium, the site of absorption and mucus production.

The stomach has an additional inner oblique layer of muscle inside the circular muscle, which creates the churning motion to break down food.

Blood supply to the gastrointestinal tract

The GI tract has a rich blood supply that reflects its role in absorption. It receives 20–25% of cardiac output in the unfed state, but this increases during active digestion. Almost the entire tract, from the bottom third of the oesophagus onwards, receives arterial blood from the aorta via three arteries: the coeliac, superior mesenteric and inferior mesenteric (**Table 7.2**).

> Like any arteries, mesenteric arteries can be blocked by the fatty inflammatory deposits of atheroma to cause mesenteric ischaemia and intestinal necrosis. Acute presentations are an emergency indicating surgical removal. Chronic ischaemia presents with 'abdominal angina': pain after eating in response to the increased blood flow.

Arteries of the gastrointestinal tract

Artery	Origin	Area supplied
Coeliac trunk	Foregut	Stomach and duodenum (to ampulla of Vater)
		Liver, spleen and pancreas
Superior mesenteric	Midgut	Duodenum (from ampulla of Vater distally) to 2/3rd transverse colon
		Pancreas
Inferior mesenteric	Hindgut	Distal 1/3rd transverse colon to dentate line in rectum

Table 7.2 The arteries supplying the gastrointestinal tract.

Postprandial hyperemia

Postprandial hyperemia is the large increase in intestinal blood flow that occurs after a meal. It is regulated by a complex mixture of neural, hormonal and local factors:

■ Enteric nervous system (ENS) and its reflexes
■ Hormones and peptides
■ Local vasoactive compounds
■ Direct affects of absorbed nutrients, particularly lipids, bile salts and glucose.

Blood flow is concentrated to each segment as it is distended and stimulated by contents.

Hepatic portal system

Nutrient-rich blood from the GI tract drains into the hepatic portal vein and into the liver. This is a portal system, as blood passes from one capillary bed, via a vein, into another. The hepatic portal system allows absorbed foodstuffs to be processed by the liver before entering the general circulation.

> The first-pass metabolism of the hepatic portal system means some drugs are inactivated by the liver and are therefore ineffective orally, while others are converted to active forms by the liver.

Gastrointestinal processes

Digestion involves five processes of the GI tract:

- Motility – the movement of GI lumenal contents
- Mechanical breakdown by muscular contractions
- Secretions of water, ions, digestive enzymes and hormones into the lumen
- Absorption of water, ions and nutrients into the blood
- Storage and expulsion of undigested waste.

Gastrointestinal motility

The GI tract controls the rate at which ingested material passes through each region so that effective digestion and absorption can occur. This motility is controlled by:

- Intrinsic properties of the tract's smooth muscle
- Sphincter muscles
- The ENS and its reflex pathways
- The autonomic nervous system (ANS)
- Circulating hormones.

Smooth muscle

Muscle contractions mix and move chyme (partially digested contents with a paste-like consistency) through the lumen, and periodic waves of contractions along the small intestine ensure undigested contents continue to move along the tract. Muscle activity:

- Mixes contents
- Moves contents by peristalsis
- Clears contents in interdigestive periods.

Electrophysiology of gastrointestinal muscle

The resting membrane potential of gastrointestinal smooth muscle is between -40mV and –80mV, however it is not constant and shows oscillations. These oscillations are a series of gradual depolarisations and hyperpolarisations, occurring 3–12 times per minute. This rhythm is termed the basal electric rhythm (BER, or slow waves) of gastrointestinal smooth muscle.

Slow waves are electrical changes (depolarisations), not mechanical contractions, because they are mediated by Na^+ entry rather than Ca^{2+} entry, which is required for contraction. BER is initiated by the interstitial cells of Cajal that lie between the circular and longitudinal layers of muscle. They act as pacemakers and then spread the slow waves across the GI smooth muscle through gap junctions.

At the peak of a slow wave, the threshold for activation of voltage-gated cation channels may be surpassed. If this occurs, one or more action potentials are initiated. Action potentials result in Ca^{2+} entry and forceful smooth muscle contraction.

The overall activity of GI smooth muscle is controlled by multiple neural and hormonal inputs that influence the amplitude of slow waves and therefore the frequency of action potentials.

Mixing contractions

As circular muscle of the GI wall is distended by chyme, reflexive contractions take place to mix ingredients. This occurs in a segmented manner, so that alternate sections of tract contract and relax, squeezing the gut contents back and forth, mixing and churning it. Haustrations are similar, but slower, mixing contractions of the colon.

Movement by peristalsis

Peristalsis moves material along the tract by sequential contractions of circular muscle behind the food bolus, coupled with longitudinal muscle contractions that shorten the gut over the bolus of contents. These waves normally move contents towards the anus, but reverse peristalsis occurs in vomiting.

Migrating motor complexes

Most peristaltic waves only persist for a short distance, but when the gut is almost empty, i.e. several hours after a meal, migrating motor complexes (MMC) occur in the small intestine. These inter-digestive contractions occur approximately every 100 minutes, start in the gastric antrum and pass along the intestine at 5 cm/min to the ileocaecal valve. This 'housekeeping' moves undigested material along and prevents reflux of colonic contents into the terminal ileum.

Motilin

The peptide hormone motilin, secreted from crypts in the duodenum and jejunum, is an important initiating factor for MMC.

Colonic migrating contractions

Colonic waves of contractions are similar to MMC (but are not necessarily synchronous) and occur a few times a day. These waves move material along a significant fraction of the colon and initiate defecation.

Sphincter muscles

The GI tract has five thickened muscular rings (sphincter muscles) that control the movement of substances from one region to another:

- **The upper oesophageal sphincter** (UOS) prevents air entry and reflux exiting
- **The lower oesophageal sphincter** (LOS) prevents the reflux of stomach contents into the oesophagus.

- **The pyloric sphincter** separates the stomach from the duodenum
- **The ileocaecal valve** separates the ileum and the bacteria-rich colon
- **The anus** controls the expulsion of faeces.

The UOS and LOS are physiological sphincters (unlike the others listed above which are anatomical), as they lack a distinct thickening of skeletal muscle, though the UOS has some.

Like security gates, sphincters are usually closed by default, and need parasympathetic stimulation to open.

Mechanical breakdown

Mechanical breakdown of food begins with chewing in the mouth. Large chunks of food are then broken down into smaller pieces through churning in the stomach. The three layers of smooth muscle (circular, longitudinal and oblique) interact to achieve this (see gastric motility below). Segmental contraction of small bowel smooth muscle helps to mix and break down any large food boluses that remain.

Gastrointestinal secretions

Seven of the 9 litres of fluid that pass through the GI tract each day are secreted by GI epithelial cells and GI glands (**Table 7.3**). Most of this fluid is water and electrolytes, including Na^+, H^+ and HCO_3^-, but exocrine glands of the oral cavity, stomach, small intestine and pancreas also secrete digestive enzymes. Other secretions into the lumen include:

- **Bile acids** from the liver, which allow absorption of lipids and fat-soluble vitamins
- **Mucus**, which protects the GI epithelia from digestive acid and enzymes, and lubricates chyme and faecal movement.

Water and ion secretion

Luminal epithelial cells and exocrine gland acinar cells secrete ions (e.g. Cl^-) across their apical membrane. Water follows the

Gastrointestinal secretions				
Location	Site	Secretion	Contents	Function
Oral cavity	Salivary glands	Saliva	Amylase	Lubrication, break down of carbohydrates
			Lipase	Triglyceride digestion
	Minor salivary glands	Mucus	Glycoproteins	Protects and lubricates
Stomach	Parietal cells	Gastric acid	Hydrochloric acid	Antimicrobial, activates pepsin
	Chief cells	Gastric pepsinogen	Pepsin	Protein breakdown
		Gastric lipase	Lipase	Triglyceride breakdown
	Foveoar cells	Mucus	Glycoproteins	Protects and lubricates
Small intestine	Enterocytes	Digestive enzymes	Peptidases, sucrase, maltase	Breakdown of polypeptides, polysaccharides and disaccharides
		Enterokinase		Activates proteases
	Goblet cells	Mucus	Glycoproteins	Protects and lubricates
Pancreas	Acinar cells	Pancreatic amylase	Amylase	Starch breakdown
		Pancreatic lipase	Lipase	Trigylceride breakdown
		Phospholipase	Phospholipase	Phospholipase breakdown
		Trypsinogen	Trypsin	Peptide breakdown
		Chemotrypsinogen	Chemotrypsin	Peptide breakdown
	Ductular cells	Mucus, water, mucus, HCO_3^-	Neutralise gastric acid	Activates enzymes
	Colon	Enterocytes	Mucus, water, HCO_3^-	Lubrication
Liver	Hepatocytes	Bile	Bile salts, HCO_3^-, toxins	Lipid digestion, waste excretion

Table 7.3 The secretions of the gastrointestinal (GI) tract epithelia and GI glands

movement of these ions in order to maintain osmolality and can pass transcellularly or paracellularly across the membrane (see page 18).

Gastrointestinal glands

Glands are structures that produce secretions. Exocrine glands secrete into ducts that lead to lumens (e.g. the pancreatic duct into the duodenal lumen), whereas endocrine glands secrete directly into the blood stream (e.g. the thyroid gland). In addition, the GI tract has a variety of glands that lie in the bowel mucosa.

Exocrine (complex, branching) glands

The pancreas, breast, salivary glands and prostate are all exocrine glands with a similar structure (**Figure 7.4**). They are formed of acini (small groups of epithelial cells, also called acinar cells or lobular cells) that secrete into an acinus; this is primary secretion.

The primary secretion then flows down ducts, lined by ductular cells. Ductular cells reabsorb and secrete substances that alter the composition of the primary secretion; this process is known as secondary modification.

Myoepithelial cells (contractile cells) lie outside the acini. When myoepithelial cells contract this causes stored fluid in the acini to be secreted. In addition, there are usually myoepithelial cells in the walls of ducts to help with expulsion, particularly in the breast.

Single cell mucus glands

These are also known as goblet cells and are found in the walls of many lumens (e.g. the respiratory tract, GI tract and female reproductive tract). They are single cells that sit in line with the rest of the epithelium. They secrete a highly viscous substance called mucin, which is a mixture of hydrated glycoproteins and proteoglycans.

Pit glands

These are short (10–20 cells deep), single lumen invaginations of the epithelial surface and are found in the stomach. They contain secretory cells (for enzymes and ions) at the base and down the walls of the lumen. There are often multiple different types of secretory cell present, including goblet cells.

Deep tubular glands

These are also single lumen glands that invaginate from an epithelial surface, but they are much deeper (around 40 cells deep). Secretory cells that produce enzymes lie at the base and cells that secrete ions and water line the walls nearer the surface. Deep tubular glands are found in the small bowel and stomach.

Control of secretion

Similar to most other secretions in the body, GI secretions are produced constitutively (constantly, irrespective of stimulus), but have the potential to increase production. Increases in secretion are mediated by circulating hormones that bind to epithelial cells or neurotransmitters released from enteric or autonomic nervous system neurones, in response to meals. Therefore, whilst fasting there is a continuous low rate of secretion but when eating, secretions greatly increase.

The enteric nervous system

The ENS is a largely autonomous system with 200–600 million neurones, significantly more than the spinal cord, and at least 40 different neurotransmitters (**Figure 7.3**). It has a large effect on:

- Local GI tract motility and patterns of movement
- Gastric acid secretion
- Fluid movement across the GI epithelium
- GI nutrient absorption and secretion
- Blood flow to the gut
- GI endocrine and immune responses.

The ENS is regulated by intrinsic neural pathways between different GI regions and extrinsic pathways to and from the ANS, which integrate GI activity within the body.

Major plexuses

The main components of the ENS are collections of parasympathetic nerves (i.e. plexuses) in the gut wall from the oesophagus to the anus (**Figure 7.2**):

- The **submucosal plexuses (Meissner's plexus)** sense the luminal environment, control mucosal secretory and absorptive processes and regulate blood flow
- The **myenteric plexuses (Auerbach's plexus),** between the circular and longitudinal muscle layers, coordinate muscular contractions in the gut wall.

Their numbers vary along the tract according to regional function; for example, there are few submucosal plexuses in the oesophagus.

> **Hirschsprung's disease is a congenital absence of myenteric plexus cells in the colon,** preventing the coordinated intestinal contraction. It presents with a failure of newborns to defecate within 24 hours of birth.

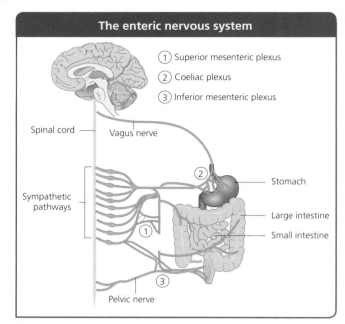

Figure 7.3 The enteric nervous system (ENS) is an autonomous collection of nerve bundles (i.e. plexuses) throughout the GI tract that controls secretion and smooth muscle contraction. The autonomic nervous system (ANS) moderates ENS function to the needs of the body and communicates satiety, hunger and nausea to the central nervous system (CNS).

Minor plexuses

There are also smaller neural plexuses in the mucosa, circular muscle and underneath the serosa, formed of three types of neurone:

- Motor neurones act on smooth muscle, secretory and endocrine cells
- Sensory neurones have receptors in muscle and mucosa that respond to chemical, heat, mechanical and osmotic stimuli
- Interneurones integrate sensory and motor neurones, plexuses, reflexes and the ANS.

Gastrointestinal reflexes

GI reflexes are neuronal circuits that begin and end in the GI tract and regulate motility and secretion of digestive substances and hormones (**Table 7.4**). They obey the same principles as neuronal reflexes (see Chapter 2).

Reflexes are categorised by how localised or broad their effects are, which is indicated by the location of the interneurones in the pathway:

- **A local reflex** has its interneurones within the ENS

- **Short-range reflex** interneurones are in local autonomic plexi
- **Long-range reflex** ANS interneurones are in the brainstem or spinal cord.

Local reflexes

Local GI reflexes have afferent neurones that connect to efferent neurones via enteric interneurones, so that a local GI stimulus results in a local GI motor or secretory effect. They are involved in the control of peristalsis, secretion, and mixing contractions.

Short-range reflexes

Short-range reflexes have sensory nerves to interneurones in local autonomic plexuses (i.e. the coeliac plexus and the superior and inferior mesenteric plexuses) and efferent nerves to regions of the GI tract. For example, presence of food in the stomach activates mechanoreceptors, which signal through the coeliac plexus to increase parasympathetic stimulation to the duodenum. This increases the duodenal secretions in preparation for more food.

Gastrointestinal reflexes			
Reflex	Stimulus	Outcome	Local/short/long reflex
Cephalogastric	Sight, smell and taste of food	Increased gastric acid Stomach muscle relaxation	Long
Gastrogastric	Peptides in the gastric lumen	Increased gastric acid Pepsinogen secretion	Local
Enterogastric reflex	Distension or irritation of the small intestine	Decrease in gastric motor and secretory activity	Short
Ileogastric	Acid in the duodenum Peptides in the intestinal lumen	Reduced gastric acid Increased pepsinogen Decreased emptying	Long
Ileopancreatic	Peptides, fats and sugars in the duodenal lumen	Increased pancreatic enzyme secretion	Short
Gastrocolic	Gastric distension	Increased colonic motility	Long

Table 7.4 Examples of gastrointestinal reflexes

Long–range reflexes

Long-range reflexes generally involve nerves of the ANS that enable a stimulus at one site to elicit a global GI response at distant sites by passing through the CNS. For example, tasting food in the mouth activates a number of areas in the brain, including the vagus nerve, which activates multiple areas in the GI tract (e.g. stomach, pancreas and duodenum). This causes an increase in their secretion and motor activity in preparation for reception of food.

The autonomic nervous system

As well as modulating long-range GI reflexes, the autonomic nervous system exerts control over the ENS to affect GI motility and secretion (**Figure 7.3**).

Input from the ANS coordinates GI activity with other activity, with sympathetic stimulation largely inhibiting GI secretory, and motor activity and parasympathetic activity stimulating it (**Table 7.5**). Sensory information from the GI tract is conveyed via the vagus nerve to

Autonomic control of GI plexuses		
Autonomic division	Submucosal plexus	Myenteric plexus
Parasympathetic (mainly via the vagus nerve)	Increases mucosal secretion	Increases activity in intermittent smooth muscle and relaxes sphincters
Sympathetic (via thoracic and lumbar splanchnic nerves)	Reduces or alters composition of mucosal secretion	Contracts sphincters and relaxes intermittent muscle

Table 7.5 The actions of the autonomic nervous system on the gastrointestinal (GI) system

brainstem nuclei in the CNS to affect behaviour and global homeostasis.

However, the ENS is largely autonomous and is referred to as a 'second brain'. For example, damage to the ANS does not inhibit ENS activity as pacemaker cells located within the plexuses are responsible for initiating peristalsis.

Gastrointestinal hormones

Gastrointestinal hormones (**Table 7.6**) are secreted by the GI tract (e.g. stomach and jejunum) and associated organs (e.g. pancreas) into the bloodstream. They have multiple and far-reaching affects on the gut, liver, adipose tissue and brain.

Gastrointestinal hormones			
Hormone	Secretion	Stimulant	Effects
Gastrin	G cells in pylorus and duodenum into blood	Peptides or distension in stomach	Stimulates gastric acid secretion by parietal cells
Cholecystokinin	I cells in duodenum	Fatty acids in duodenum	Decreases gastric acid secretion, stimulates pancreatic secretion, gallbladder contraction
Secretin	S cells in duodenum	Acid in duodenum	Reduces gastric acid
Somatostatin	Delta-cells of pancreas	Parasympathetic stimulation	Inhibits vasoactive intestinal peptide, gastrin and cholecystokinin
Motilin	M cells in stomach and small bowel	Unknown	Increases intestinal motility and the migrating motor complex
Glucagon-like peptide-1	L cells in small bowel	Luminal carbohydrate	Increased insulin secretion, reduced appetite
Vasoactive intestinal peptide	Enteric nervous system neurones	Unknown	Increased pancreatic and small bowel secretions, reduced gastric acid, smooth muscle relaxation
Pancreatic polypeptide	PP cells in pancreas	Fed state	Increases pancreatic secretions
Ghrelin	Ghrelin cells in stomach	Fasting state	Promotes hunger
Gastric inhibitory peptide	K cells in small bowel	Luminal carbohydrate	Reduced gastric acid and motility, increased insulin secretion, reduced appetite

Table 7.6 Gastrointestinal (peptide) hormones and their effects

The gastrointestinal immune system

All areas of the GI tract act as a barrier to prevent infection (**Table 7.7**). The barrier consists of epithelial cells, the tight junctions between them and mucus and acid that some sections of the tract secrete. This barrier is tightly controlled and varies along the tract according to a section's function.

Gastrointestinal-associated lymphoid tissue

Infection is also prevented by immune cells present in gastrointestinal-associated lymphoid tissue (GALT). These nodes and nodules are the site of B and T lymphocyte proliferation during the adaptive immune response.

Peyer's patches

Peyer's patches are small nodules scattered in the gut mucosa, especially in the distal ileum and colon. B lymphocytes in Peyer's patches secrete IgA, which can be transported across the epithelium into the lumen, to bind bacterial antigens and prevent infection.

Small intestine immune functions	
Component	Mechanism of action
Peyer's patches	Lymphoid aggregates in the submucosa of small intestine that act in a similar method to lymph nodes
Secretory IgA	B cells resident in the small intestine wall produce IgA that can cross the epithelium and enter the lumen. They bind viral attachment proteins to prevent adhesion
Epithelial barrier	Occluding junctions between epithelial cells prevent bacterial movement into the bloodstream

Table 7.7 The immune functions of the small intestine. IgA, immunoglobulin A

Peritoneal lymphoid tissue

There are also many lymph nodes in the greater omentum of the peritoneum, the membranous sheet anterior to the GI tract in the abdomen.

The mouth and oesophagus

The mouth consists of the vestibule and oral cavity, where the mechanical and chemical breakdown of food begins. The teeth, tongue and palate break up food, whilst saliva softens it and starts enzymatic digestion.

The cavity ends at the uvula, where it becomes continuous with the oropharynx, with the nasopharynx above and laryngopharynx below. The respiratory and digestive pathways diverge in the laryngopharynx, to form the larynx and oesophagus, respectively.

Starting and ending in two gate-keeping sphincters, the oesophagus is a GI tube that runs through the thorax connecting the pharynx to the stomach. Its peristaltic contractions end the swallowing reflex.

Mechanical breakdown

Chewing, or mastication, is needed to break up large items of food into smaller boluses. It is particularly important for breaking up hard foodstuffs that contain high amounts of cellulose, which is otherwise indigestible.

By breaking food up, chewing increases the surface area available for salivary and GI enzyme action, mixes it with saliva and softens food to facilitate swallowing.

Secretions in the mouth and oesophagus

The mucous membranes of the mouth and tongue contain three major, and many minor, salivary glands (**Table 7.8**).

Saliva

Saliva is a watery secretion containing mucus, digestive enzymes, electrolytes, glycoproteins

Salivary glands		
Gland	Fraction of total saliva	Content of secretions
Parotid	25%	Mainly serous Main source of salivary amylase
Submandibular	70%	Mixed serous and mucous Main source of lysozyme and lactoperoxidase
Sublingual	5%	Mainly mucous Main source of lingual lipase

Table 7.8 The three major salivary glands and their secretions

and antibacterial agents. Mucus lubricates the bolus of food and prevents epithelial damage as it passes along the GI tract.

It also contributes to oral hygiene and immunity, regulates acidity in the mouth and distributes food chemicals to taste receptors.

Salivary glands

Salivary glands are typical exocrine glands composed of acini, which produce a primary secretion similar in ionic composition to plasma, but also containing mucus, digestive enzymes and antimicrobial molecules. This is then modified as it passes along the ducts, with reabsorption of salt and the secretion of HCO_3^-, resulting in more alkaline saliva (**Figure 7.4**).

Salivary enzymes

There are four enzymes in saliva:

- **Amylase** hydrolyses about 30% of ingested starch, a polysaccharide, into di- and trisaccharides
- **Lipase** hydrolyses triglycerides into glycerides and fatty acids
- **Lysozyme** hydrolyses bacterial cell walls
- **Lactoperoxidase** generates bactericidal oxidised compounds.

> **Sialolithiasis is the formation of stones in the salivary glands.** They can block the duct and cause pain and swelling. Sour food is often more painful, as it stimulates more contraction of salivary myoepithelial cells over the stone. Stones can develop at almost any exocrine gland, as ions (e.g. Ca^{2+} and PO_4^{3-}) can precipitate out of solution in acini or ducts.

Antibacterial contents

As well as the antibacterial enzymes lysozyme and lactoperoxidase, saliva contains a glycoprotein, lactoferrin. Lactoferrin binds iron to immunoglobin A (IgA, the main antibody secreted in mucosal membranes) to reduce bacterial growth, which in turn clears antigens and bacteria, and blocks bacterial access to epithelial cells.

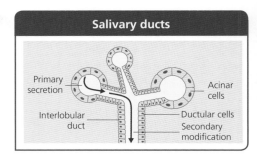

Figure 7.4 Acinar cells line the hemi-spherical lobules (i.e. acini) and produce the primary salivary secretion. These drain into interlobular ducts that unite to form interlobar ducts; ductular cells line both.

Autonomic control of salivary secretion

When we anticipate eating or there is food in the mouth, there is activation of the parasympathetic neurones supplying salivary glands, leading to increased secretion by acinar cells (**Figure 7.5**). The higher flow rate leaves less time for secondary modification, resulting in more watery and less alkaline saliva. Sympathetic stimulation also causes a small increase salivary secretion, but results in more mucus-rich saliva – hence the feeling of a dry mouth at times of anxiety.

Taste

Taste is a combination of sensorial input from taste receptors: mechanoreceptor input on texture and olfactory input on smell.

50–100 taste receptor cells are grouped within taste buds, which in turn are grouped on papillae, the thousands of raised cylinders of mucosa seen on the upper surface of the tongue.

Taste pathway

Ions and molecules are distributed by saliva and enter the pores of taste buds and activate receptors via ion channels or membrane receptor activation, such as G-protein linked receptors (see page 21). Afferent nerves carry signals via cranial nerves VII, IX and X from receptors in the tongue, soft palate and oesophagus to the gustatory nucleus of the medulla. The perception of taste is then

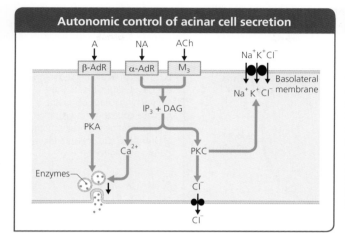

Figure 7.5 Parasympathetic stimulation by nerves secreting acetylcholine (ACh) and noradrenaline (NA) activate the PIP_2 pathway to raise intracellular Ca^{2+}. This activates the exocytosis of vesicles containing enzyme and Cl^- channel activation. Sympathetic β-adrenergic activation (A) increases vesicle exocytosis but not Cl^- movement. α-AdR, α-adrenoceptor; β-AdR, β-adrenoceptor; DAG, diacyl glycerol; IP_3, inositol trisphosphate; M_3, subtype 3 muscarinic receptor; PK A/C, protein kinase A/C.

processed in the gustatory cortex of the frontal lobe.

Motility in the mouth and oesophagus

Once partially broken down and mixed with saliva, food leaves the oral cavity via the swallowing reflex, which carries it through the pharynx and oesophagus and into the stomach.

Swallowing reflex

There are 3 phases to swallowing: oral, pharyngeal and oesophageal.

Oral phase

In the oral phase, the food bolus is moved towards the posterior third of the tongue and oropharyngeal wall, which activates vagal (CN X) and glossopharyngeal (CN IX) afferent nerves that signal to the medulla.

Pharyngeal phase

During the pharyngeal phase the soft palate is elevated to prevent nasal regurgitation of food. The epiglottis is pulled across to occlude the larynx and prevent inhalation and expose the UOS, which relaxes.

Oesophageal phase

Peristalsis propels the food bolus through the UOS and down the oesophagus, before the LOS relaxes to permit entry into the stomach. A second peristaltic wave follows to clear any remaining food and the LOS contracts to prevent reflux. Difficulty swallowing (dysphagia) can be caused by a lesion to any of the structures controlling this reflex, e.g. cranial nerve paralysis, oesophageal tumour or achalasia.

The lower oesophageal sphincter

The lower oesophageal sphincter is a 'physiological' sphincter; it is an area of tonically contracted smooth muscle. Several factors contribute its ability to remain closed (i.e. its competence), including gravity (**Figure 7.6**). Factors that increase intra-abdominal pressure, including obesity or chronic cough, or reduce lower oesophageal sphincter function, such as gastric herniation into the thorax (hiatus hernia), contribute to reflux.

> **A 41-year-old obese man, who smokes, develops intermittent burning retrosternal chest pain.** It is worse after eating spicy foods and often occurs when lying flat following a large meal.
>
> **Gastro-oesophageal reflux disease (GORD)** is a spectrum of clinical disease resulting from incompetence of the lower oesophageal sphincter, including: no symptoms, heartburn or severe oesophageal inflammation (oesophagitis). In chronic cases, the erosive effect causes ulcers or Barrett's oesophagus: a change in epithelial cell type (i.e. metaplasia) from squamous to intestinal-type columnar cells.

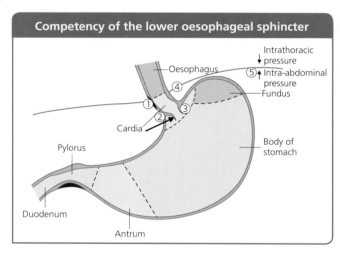

Competency of the lower oesophageal sphincter

Oesophagus
Intrathoracic ↓ pressure
⑤ ↑ Intra-abdominal pressure
Fundus
④
①
③
②
Cardia
Pylorus
Body of stomach
Duodenum
Antrum

Figure 7.6 The balance of pressures either side of the lower oesophageal sphincter (LOS) determines its competency. Factors involved are: ① The LOS; ② An acute angle where the oesophagus meets the stomach; ③ Flaps of gastric mucosa covering this entrance; ④ Diaphragmatic contraction; and ⑤ Intrathoracic pressure increase during exhalation.

The stomach

The stomach is a distended organ at the beginning of the abdominal GI tract, with five regions (**Figure 7.6** and **Table 7.9**).

Functions of the stomach

The stomach digests solid foodstuffs to form partially digested chyme, with a paste-like consistency, which passes into the duodenum. Protein digestion begins in the stomach; there is little fat or carbohydrate digestion. The stomach has six main functions:

- Storage of food – accommodation
- Motility
- Mechanical breakdown of food
- Secretion of pepsin and gastric acidic
- Stimulation of digestion via hormones and reflexes
- Antiseptic – largely due to gastric acid.

Its absorption and excretion functions are minimal; it absorbs alcohol quickly and small amounts of water and solutes.

Histology of the stomach

The gastric wall consists of the typical 4 layers of the GI tract (**Figure 7.2**) but with an extra inner oblique layer of muscle in the muscularis externa. Muscle is innervated by

Gastric regions		
Region	Location	Function
Fundus	Uppermost region, under the dome of the diaphragm	Highly distensible region, allowing stomach volume to expand from 50 mL to 1.5 L
Cardia	Immediately around the entrance of the oesophagus	Oblique muscle layer enhances mixing of food with gastric fluid to form chyme
Body	Remainder of the upper part of the stomach	
Pyloric antrum	Lower curve of the stomach	Muscular 'antral pump'
Pyloric sphincter	Ring of thickened smooth muscle	Controls passage of fine particles of chyme into duodenum. Muscle is relaxed by vagal nerve stimulation and contracted by duodenal hormone feedback

Table 7.9 The anatomical regions of the stomach and their function

efferent nerves originating in Auerbach plexuses in the muscularis externa.

Gastric mucosa

The deep pit glands of the stomach contain 6 different types of cells with different secretory function (**Table 7.10** and **Figure 7.7**). Their distribution in the mucosa varies between areas of the stomach, reflecting functions of the different areas. Cells that interact are often found close to each other, e.g. enterochromaffin-like-cells and parietal cells, which interact to increase gastric acid production.

The epithelial cells of the mucosa secrete mucus and HCO_3^- (bicarbonate ions), which form a protective layer against lumenal acid and microbes.

Accommodation of the stomach

The fundus of the stomach is highly distensible and acts as a store for food eaten during

Gastric mucosa cell types		
Cell type	Location	Function
Parietal cells	Fundus and corpus	Most numerous cell type. Secrete gastric acid and make intrinsic factor
Chief cells	Fundus and corpus	Secrete pepsin
APUD cells (amine precursor uptake decarboxylase cells)	Throughout stomach	Secrete somatostatin
G cells	Throughout, especially in antrum	Secrete gastrin
Mucus-secreting cells (foveoar cells)	Throughout stomach	Produce protective, alkaline mucus Surface cells make thicker mucus than deeper cells that make watery mucus
Enterochromaffin-like cells (ECL)	Corpus and fundus – near parietal cells	Secrete histamine, to stimulate parietal cells

Table 7.10 Cells of the gastric mucosa and their function

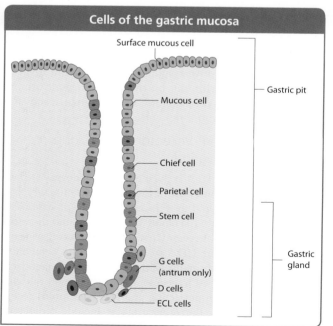

Cells of the gastric mucosa

Surface mucous cell
Mucous cell
Gastric pit
Chief cell
Parietal cell
Stem cell
G cells (antrum only)
D cells
ECL cells
Gastric gland

Figure 7.7 The gastric mucosa is arranged into pits; the deepest are gastric glands. Stem cells proliferate in the middle regions and migrate upwards as they divide to become mucous cells, or downwards to become specialised secretory cells. The gastric glands contain enteroendocrine cells, the hormone secreting cells of the gastrointestinal tract.

a meal. This gastric accommodation occurs when vagal nerve stimulation relaxes fundal smooth muscle via two reflexes:

- **Cephalogastric reflex** initiated by food in the mouth
- **Gastrogastric reflex** activated by distension of the stomach.

The mucosal layer is also expandable due to multiple folds called rugae that flatten as the stomach fills.

Motility and mechanical breakdown in the stomach

The muscular stomach churns food in waves of contractions to break it down and only passes it into the duodenum once it is in small particles.

The inner oblique muscle layer, which is particularly thick in the antrum, enables effective churning of contents. Contraction allows movement in all planes, like squashing a balloon from all angles.

Migrating motor complexes

Periodic MMC waves starting in the antrum remove undigested contents between digestive periods. These increase in intensity over a period of hours to cause 'hunger contractions' that can be felt.

Mixing peristaltic waves

During a digestive period, peristaltic waves start in the antrum to force chyme against the pyloric sphincter – this is termed propulsion. Large particles are unable to pass through and stimulate pyloric contraction that forces chyme back towards the antrum. Churning occurs as the antral pump moves contents downstream, and the pyloric contractions cause its retropulsion.

This breaks food down into increasingly smaller particles that can be easily digested and also regulates the rate at which chyme passes into the small intestine.

Gastric emptying

Chyme that has been broken down to a particle size of around $1mm^3$ or less is able to pass through the pyloric sphincter. Progressive waves of antral pumping empty around 5 mL of chyme at a time into the duodenum.

Vomiting

Vomiting – or emesis – is the forced expulsion of the contents of the upper GI tract. It can be induced by a range of GI, CNS or metabolic conditions, or by drugs.

Vomiting centre

Vomiting occurs due to activation of the vomiting centre, a nucleus in the medulla oblongata of the brainstem. The vomiting centre is activated by the chemoreceptor trigger zone (CTZ), the inner ear and parts of the cerebral cortex.

> **Haematemesis is the presence of blood in vomit and can be due to bleeding into the:**
>
> - Stomach
> - Duodenum
> - Oesophagus, such as from oesophageal varices, commonly a consequence of portal hypertension associated with chronic liver disease.

Activation of the vomiting centre

Vomiting occurs when stimulatory inputs reach a threshold (**Figure 7.8**). Some factors act directly on the vomiting centre (e.g. histaminergic neurones from the inner ear and cognitive responses to worrying or disgusting stimuli), but many emetogenic stimuli pass through the CTZ which in turn activates the vomiting centre.

Chemoreceptor trigger zone activation

The CTZ is located on the dorsal surface of the brain in the area postrema, which is unusual as this means it is not contained within the blood–brain barrier and therefore can be receptive to many circulating triggers.

The CTZ can be acti-vated by vagal afferents from the GI tract; these signal via muscarinic-ACh receptor or by systemically released serotonin acting at $5\text{-}HT_3$ (serotonin) receptors. The other triggers include circulating dopamine, serotonin and histamine.

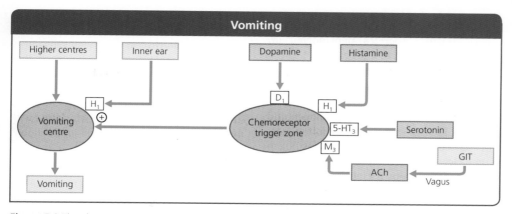

Figure 7.8 The chemoreceptor trigger zone (CTZ) receives many inputs, especially from the gastrointestinal system via the vagus nerve or 5-HT$_3$ (serotonin). The vomiting centre is stimulated by the CTZ, and gives the output that causes vomiting.

Process of vomiting

The physical process of vomiting can begin in the small intestine or stomach:

1. Changes occur in the normal peristaltic pattern of activity
2. Depending on the site of the stimulus, retrograde peristalsis starts in the stomach or small intestine
3. Forceful contractions in the gastric antrum run up towards the cardia, in combination with diaphragmatic contractions, to cause retching
4. Finally, the lower oesophageal sphincter relaxes whilst the abdominal wall musculature contracts to propel chyme out of the stomach, and retrograde peristalsis in the oesophagus carries the vomit out.

Nasal regurgitation is prevented by contraction of the soft palate and aspiration into the trachea is prevented by inhibition of respiration.

Secretions of the stomach

The stomach, as well as mechanically breaking food down, produces: mucus and HCO$_3^-$ to protect itself and for lubrication, and acid and enzymes for digestion.

Mucus

Gastric mucus consists of mucin (proteoglycans and glycoproteins), water, salts and bicarbonate. It forms a layer that sits on top of the epithelium and protects the underlying cells from damage by physically blocking gastric acid from penetrating down to the mucosa. If any acid does reach the mucosa, it is neutralised by HCO$_3^-$. Its secretion is matched to acid secretion as they are both stimulated by acetylcholine, which is released by parasympathetic neurones during vagal activation.

Prostaglandins

Prostaglandins (PGs), as well as their many other local hormone-like effects (see page 24), are central to gastric mucus and acid production. PGE$_2$, for example, is produced by many cells in the gastric mucosa both constitutively and in response to parasympathetic stimulation. PGE$_2$ increases mucus production and inhibits acid secretion via its G-protein coupled receptor on parietal cells.

> **The protective effect of prostaglandins (PGs) on the gastric mucosa is compromised by non-steroidal anti-inflammatory drugs (NSAIDs) such as aspirin,** leading to GI inflammation and ulcers. NSAIDs block the enzyme cyclooxygenase, which produces PGs, thereby decreasing protective gastric mucus and HCO$_3^-$ and increasing erosive gastric acid.

Enzyme secretion

Gastric mucosa secretes pepsinogen, an inactive precursor (i.e. a proenzyme) to the protease pepsin (**Table 7.10**).

Pepsinogen

Chief, or peptic, cells make pepsinogen and secrete it in response to acetylcholine, gastrin and secretin in the stomach. Pepsinogen is then cleaved to active pepsin in the lumen by gastric acid or pepsin itself. Pepsin is a protease that cleaves large proteins into shorter polypeptides and oligopeptides. This system means pepsin does not digest proteins of the mucosa itself.

Acid secretion

Parietal (oxyntic) cells secrete hydrochloric acid (H^+Cl^-) from their apical membrane. This maintains a lumenal pH of 2, which:

- Denatures proteins
- Helps enzyme function, e.g. it is the optimum pH for pepsin production and activity
- Aids iron absorption
- Creates a hostile environment for almost all pathogens.

Generation of hydrochloric acid

Parietal cells take CO_2, Cl^-, Na^+ and water from the blood, actively excrete HCl into the lumen, and in turn release HCO_3^- into the blood (**Figure 7.9**).

Carbonic anhydrase in parietal cell cytosol converts CO_2 and water to carbonic acid. Proton pumps (apical H^+/K^+-ATPase antiporters) actively move H^+ ions out of the cell and into the stomach lumen. Proton pumps are stored in vesicles within parietal cells, which fuse with the apical membrane when acid production is stimulated.

Alkaline tide

Apical H^+ secretion leaves HCO_3^- inside the cell, which diffuses across the basolateral membrane, into the bloodstream. The resulting 'alkaline tide' temporarily raises blood pH after meals. This is neutralised by pancreatic H^+ secretion into the circulation, as it secretes HCO_3^- into bile.

Control of acid secretion

Acid secretion is stimulated by the vagus nerve, gastrin and, most significantly, histamine. It is reduced by secretin and somatostatin (**Figure 7.10**).

Stimulation

The vagus nerve stimulates parietal cells directly via cholinergic (muscarinic) receptors and also indirectly, by stimulating G cells to release gastrin. Gastrin directly stimulates parietal acid secretion, and causes enterochromaffin cells to release histamine. Histamine acts via H_2 G-protein-linked receptors on parietal cells.

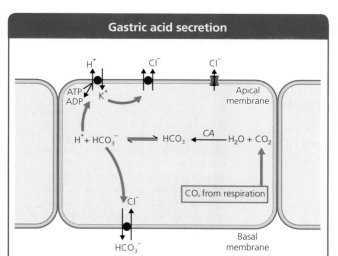

Gastric acid secretion

Figure 7.9 Parietal cells secrete HCl (hydrochloric acid) into the gastric lumen. Carbonic anhydrase (CA) acts on water to generate H^+ that are secreted into the lumen using the K^+/H^+ ATPase antiporter. HCO_3^- leaves via basolateral exchange for Cl^-, which passes through apical channels to the lumen.

Control of gastric acid secretion

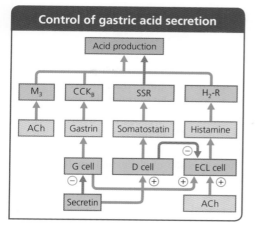

Figure 7.10 Activation of muscarinic, cholecystokinin (CCK) or histamine receptors on parietal cells promote acid production. Vesicles carrying the H+/K+ ATPase are inserted into the apical plasma membrane, greatly increasing its area. Somatostatin reduces HCl secretion. Secretin increases somatostatin production and reduces gastrin formation. Gastrin acts directly on CCK$_B$ receptor and by increasing histamine secretion thereby raising acid production. ACh, acetylcholine; CCK$_B$, cholecystokinin receptor subtype B; ECL cell, enterochromaffin-like cell; H$_2$-R, histamine receptor subtype 2; M$_3$, subtype 3 muscarinic receptor; SSR, somatostatin receptor.

Inhibition

Gastrin release is reduced by the action of secretin, a hormone released from S cells in response to acid in the duodenal lumen: a classical negative feedback system. Somatostatin from amine precursor uptake and decarboxylation (APUD) cells also reduces acid secretion, by inhibition of both parietal cell secretion and histamine release from ECL cells.

Excess gastric acid production erodes gastric mucosa to cause gastric or duodenal ulcers. These common conditions are life threatening if they bleed or perforate. The main drugs used to lower gastric acid secretion are:

■ Proton pump inhibitors, which inhibit apical H+/K+-ATPase antiporters
■ H$_2$ receptor antagonists, which block parietal histamine receptors.

Hormones and reflexes of the stomach

The stomach is involved in a number of GI reflexes (**Table 7.4**), as either the stimulus or the target organ. For example, the cephalo-gastric reflex is initiated when food is in the mouth which, via vagal stimulation, causes an increase in gastric activity.

The stomach also releases hormones (**Table 7.6**) that act locally (on the stomach mucosa) and on other sites in the GI tract. For example, gastrin stimulates production of gastric acid and also increases pancreatic secretions.

The small intestine

The small intestine begins at the pyloric sphincter, where the duodenum receives chyme from the stomach. After receiving pancreatic juice and hepatic bile from the biliary tract, it is the main site of the breakdown and absorption of food.

Structure of the small intestine

The small intestine is the longest section of the GI tract and takes a meandering course in the central abdomen. It has three regions:

■ **The duodenum** is 25 cm long and is where gastric chyme mixes with pancreatic and hepatic secretions
■ **The jejunum** is 4 m long and is the main site of absorption for most nutrients, including amino acids, lipids, carbohydrates, iron and Ca^{2+} (calcium ions)
■ **The ileum** is 2.5 m long and is also important for absorption, particularly of vitamin B12 and bile salts in the terminal ileum.

The ileum ends at the ileocaecal valve, through which chyme is passed into the caecum of the large intestine.

Functions of the small intestine

Functions of the small intestine include:

- Motility
- Mechanical breakdown of food
- Secretions, including bile from the biliary tract
- Absorption of nutrients
- Excretion
- Stimulation of digestion via hormones and reflexes
- Antimicrobial

Histology of the small intestine

The mucosa of the small intestine is structured to maximise the surface area for absorption at three levels:

- Gross circumferential folds called plicae circulares (valvulae conniventes) (**Figure 7.11**)

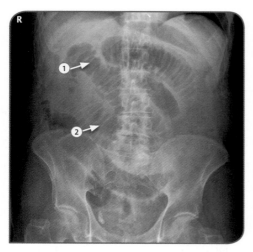

Figure 7.11 Abdominal X-ray showing a small bowel obstruction. There are multiple loops of distended bowel ①. The plicae circulares ② can be seen traversing the lumen of the bowel. There is no air visible in the rectum.

- Microscopically, there are finger-like projections of mucosa and submucosa called villi
- Cellularly, epithelial cells (or enterocytes) form a columnar epithelium with microvilli (**Figure 7.12**). These are responsible for nutrient absorption.

The duodenal mucosa has many enteroendocrine cells (**Table 7.11**), which regulate gastric, hepatic and pancreatic activity. These include cholecystokinin (CCK) from I-cells, in response to intraluminal lipid. CCK causes gallbladder contraction and increased production of hepatic bile. A further example is GLP-1 (glucagon-like peptide-1) from L-cells, in response to intraluminal carbohydrate. GLP-1 acts on the pancreas to increase insulin secretion (see page 177).

Crypts of Lieberkühn

The crypts of Lieberkühn are small glands at the base of small intestinal villi. These secrete a mucus- and HCO_3^- rich fluid that helps neutralise gastric acid. They also contain epithelial stem cells, which move up the villi progressively as they divide, so that those at the tip are the oldest, and are shed into the lumen after 4–6 days.

Motility and mechanical breakdown in the small intestine

Smooth muscle in the small intestine is predominantly used in motility; peristalsis causes movement of luminal contents distally. The migratory motor complex also passes through the small bowel, but there is relatively little mechanical breakdown (compared to in the stomach).

Patterns of motility

When there is chyme present, segmentation contractions churn and mix the intestinal chyme, and peristalsis moves it along (see page 199). Interdigestive MMC waves clear contents between meals.

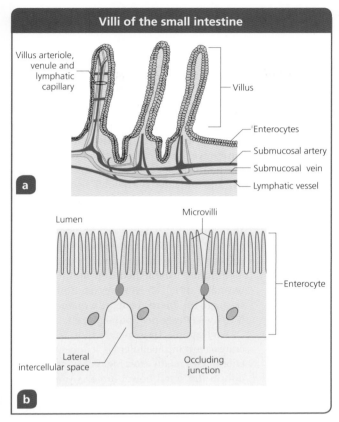

Villi of the small intestine

Villus arteriole, venule and lymphatic capillary

Villus

Enterocytes

Submucosal artery

Submucosal vein

Lymphatic vessel

a

Lumen

Microvilli

Enterocyte

Lateral intercellular space

Occluding junction

b

Figure 7.12 (a) Villi of the small intestine are composed of mucosal epithelium and a submucosal core containing blood vessels and lymphatics. At the base of each are the crypts of Lieberkühn. (b) The enterocytes that comprise the villus mucosa. Microvilli are projections of apical plasma membrane.

Duodenal mucosal cells

Type	Location	Function
Columnar epithelial cells	Throughout	Absorption
Goblet cells	Throughout	Mucus production
Brunner's glands	Throughout (submucosa)	Alkaline, mucous secretion
Enteroendocrine cells (e.g. I-cells, S-cells)	Multiple (e.g. cholecystokinin, secreti)	Various (see **Table 7.6**)

Table 7.11 Cells of the duodenal mucosa and their function

Control of motility

Motility is largely controlled by the ENS, as in most of the GI tract, with excitatory and inhibitory signals from the ANS. It is also affected by the following hormones:

- **Gastrin** produced by G-cells in the stomach – increases small bowel motility
- **Vasoactive intestinal peptide** (VIP) produced by enteric nerves – reduces small bowel motility
- **Motilin** produced by the stomach – promotes the migratory motor complex.

Secretion in the small intestine

The key digestive secretions added to chyme in the duodenum are hepatic bile (see page 228) and the pancreatic juice (see page 224).

The intestinal mucosa itself secrets a large volume of water into the lumen, and most is reabsorbed before the colon. Water enters the lumen due to an increased lumenal osmotic pressure generated by two factors:

- The breakdown of macromolecules

■ The transport of Cl⁻ into the lumen by cyclic AMP-dependent Cl⁻ channels.

Macromolecular digestion

Macromolecules (e.g. starch, polysaccharides, long-chain fatty acids and polypeptides) comprise multiple smaller units (e.g. glucose, amino acids). When macromolecules are broken down into their constituent parts by enzymatic cleavage, the number of osmotically active particles in the solution increases. For example when lactose is split into galactose and glucose, two osmotically active particles are present rather than one. This makes the lumen relatively hyperosmolar in comparison to enterocytes, therefore water moves by osmosis into the lumen.

Chloride ion secretion

Chloride moves across the apical membrane of enterocytes into the small bowel lumen via CFTR channels; water follows by osmosis. The movement is driven by the high enterocyte intracellular concentration of Cl⁻, which is established by basolateral uptake using the $Na^+/K^+/2Cl^-$ pump.

Basolateral uptake is a secondary active transport process. Basolateral uptake of Cl⁻ is coupled to Na^+, which has high concentration in the lateral intracellular space due to the action of the Na^+/K^+-ATPase pump. This is the main mechanism for chloride and water secretion in the salivary glands and pancreas.

Absorption in the small intestine

Most substances are absorbed in the small intestine, including macronutrients required in large amounts, mainly to generate energy, and micronutrients required in smaller amounts, to use as cofactors in metabolic reactions.

Macronutrients include carbohydrates, lipids and proteins, and also the inorganic ions (electrolytes) Ca^{2+}, Na^+, Cl^-, K^+ and Mg^{2+}. Micronutrients are only required in small amounts, and include other inorganic ions and trace elements and small organic compounds (i.e. vitamins).

Water can be considered a nutrient, though is better described as the solvent for all nutrients.

Principles of absorption

The small intestine is designed to have maximal surface area of absorption and all areas of the small bowel are able to absorb macronutrients and water. The duodenum and jejunum have similar absorptive functions, but the ileum is specialised to absorb vitamin B12 and bile salts (see below).

Source of energy

The source of energy for the absorption of most molecules and ions is the electrochemical Na^+ gradient across the epithelial membrane, established and maintained by basolateral Na^+/K^+-ATPases (sodium pumps; see page 19). There are approximately 150,000 Na^+/K^+-ATPases per epithelial cell.

For example, basolateral export of Na^+ generates a low intracellular Na^+ concentration in enterocytes relative to a higher Na^+ concentration in the small bowel lumen. Amino acids are absorbed through co-transporters with Na^+. Therefore, the concentration gradient of Na^+ drives the absorption of amino acids (**Figure 7.13**).

Routes of absorption

Lumenal compounds are absorbed into blood via two routes (**Figure 7.14**):

■ **The transcellular route**, through epithelial cells
■ **The paracellular route**, through occluding junctions between cells

Transcellular route

Substances absorbed transcellularly enter epithelial cells via the apical membrane, exit through the basolateral membrane into the interstitium, and finally cross the capillary endothelium to enter the blood.

The transcellular route allows for the possibility of active transport (see page 18) to enable efficient absorption from the gut. Most nutrients, such as glucose and amino acids, are absorbed across the apical plasma membrane via a secondary active transport process that exploits the Na⁺ gradient. Na⁺ entry across the apical membrane, following down its gradient, is coupled with the movement of other solutes (e.g. glucose) to carry them against their concentration gradient into the epithelial cell. These then leave the cells via passive transporters on the basolateral membrane because their concentration in the epithelial cell is higher than in the interstitium.

Paracellular route

Alternatively, some small molecules, including Cl⁻, K⁺ and H_2O, move by paracel-

lular transport through occluding junctions between epithelial cells (similar to Cl⁻ tubular reabsorption in the nephron, see page 14). This is always a passive process, so it will only be effective where plasma levels of the substance are significantly less that the concentration in the lumen. Occluding junction permeability varies depending on how closely the membranes of adjacent enterocytes are adhered to each other. If they are very firmly adhered, with dense proteins sealing the occluding junctions, then very little can pass via the paracellular route; these are called 'tight' occluding junctions and have low permeability. If adjacent membranes are loosely adhered to each other, with a low density of sealing proteins forming the junction, then they are termed 'leaky' occluding junctions and have high permeability (see page 25).

Water and electrolytes

Most of the water that we drink (approximately 2 litres a day), and that we secrete into the gut (approximately 6–7 litres), is (re)absorbed in the small intestine by paracellular transport, facilitated by 'leaky' tight junctions between epithelial cells. This is a passive process driven by the osmotic gradients established by the absorption of other solutes including Na⁺ and glucose.

80% of water is absorbed before the caecum. Water reabsorption in the colon is slower because the occluding junctions are less leaky.

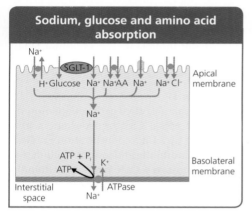

Figure 7.13 Na⁺, glucose and amino acid (AA) absorption in the small intestine. Most Na⁺ is absorbed via cotransport with glucose or amino acids, in addition to other channels, driven by the basolateral Na⁺/K⁺-ATPase antiporter pumps. Cotransported solutes such as glucose pass through passive transporters on the basolateral membrane.

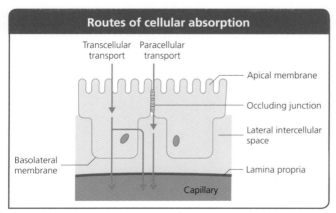

Figure 7.14 Transcellular absorption is the passage of substances across the apical membrane and into epithelial cell cytoplasm and then across the basolateral membrane. Paracellular movement occurs via the lateral intercellular spaces through epithelial tight junctions and is always passive.

Water absorption against its osmotic gradient

The absorption of other solutes (e.g. Na^+) generates an osmolar gradient for water reabsorption from the lumen (low osmolality) into enterocytes and intercellular space (higher osmolality). This is maintained by the Na^+/K^+-ATPase pump. However, the capillary blood is of lower osmolality than the lateral intercellular space, so water must move against its concentration gradient to enter the bloodstream. This is facilitated by a relatively high hydrostatic pressure in the lateral intercellular space, highly permeable capillary membrane and relatively high oncotic pressure in capillary blood. This balance of Starling's forces promotes uptake of water against its concentration gradient.

Electrolytes and dietary elements

Almost all ion absorption occurs in the small intestine, with some also occurring in the colon to drive water absorption (**Table 7.12**).

Dietary (or trace) elements are elements required in small amounts, often for use as enzyme cofactors, including iron), magnesium, copper, selenium and zinc. Most of these have Na^+-cotransporters to actively absorb them from the lumen in their ionic forms.

> **Oral rehydration solutions contain salt and sugar, which are cotransported by the mucosa of the small intestine providing a driving force for water reabsorption.** Their use has greatly reduced the mortality associated with infectious diarrhoea in the third world.

Hydrogen ions

H^+ is absorbed by cotransport with iron (Fe^{2+}) and dipeptides. These cotransporters utilise the H^+ ion gradient, generated by Na^+/H^+-exchange, and as a result H^+ ions are exported into the lumen. In the proximal small bowel a concentration gradient also exists due to the presence of gastric acid.

Calcium ions

Ca^{2+} is actively absorbed in the duodenum via specialised apical Ca^{2+} transporters; a process driven by a Ca^{2+} concentration gradient (high intraluminally and low intracellularly). Inside enterocytes Ca^{2+} binds to calbindin (a storage protein), which helps to maintain the concentration gradient for Ca^{2+} uptake.

Mechanisms of ion transport				
Ion	Transporters used in small intestine		Transporters used in colon	
	Apical transporters	Basolateral transporters	Apical transporters	Basolateral transporters
Na^+	Cotransporters and antiporters	Na^+/K^+-ATPase	Cotransporters and antiporters	Na^+/K^+-ATPase
Cl^-	Paracellular		Secretion via CFTR	Cotransporter
K^+	Paracellular		Secretion via K^+ channels or absorption via H^+/K^+ ATPase	Na^+/K^+-ATPase
Ca^{2+}	Duodenum: Ca^{2+} channels / Later paracellular	Ca^{2+} ATPase and Ca^{2+}/Na^+ antiporter	-	-
Fe^{2+}, Fe^{3+}	Reduced to Fe^{2+} by ferric reductase, then cotransport with H^+ on DMT1	Ferroportin / Transported in blood bound to transferrin	-	-

Table 7.12 Summary of ion transport and absorption. CFTR, cystic fibrosis transmembrane conductance regulator; DMT1, divalent metal transporter

The concentration gradient is established by active transport on the enterocyte basolateral membrane: Ca^{2+}-ATPase pumps Ca^{2+} out of enterocytes into the lateral intercellular space. There is also basolateral export of Ca^{2+} in exchange for Na^+ (Na^+/Ca^{2+}-exchange), driven by the Na^+ concentration gradient. This is regulated by vitamin D ($1,25$-$(OH)_2$-D_3), which increases synthesis of calbindin and increases Ca^{2+} transporter activity. There is further passive paracellular Ca^{2+} absorption in the rest of the small intestine.

Iron

Iron is ingested as Fe^{3+} or Fe^{2+}, though only the latter is absorbed, with the exception of iron contained in haem groups, which are endocytosed intact (**Figure 7.15**).

> **Coeliac disease is a lifelong sensitivity to gluten, a protein in wheat, barley and rye** in which the T cells attack a modified component of gluten. This causes mucosal inflammation of the small intestine, leading to flattened villi and decreased absorption. Symptoms can be mild and recurring or severe with weight loss, diarrhoea, abdominal pain, and bloating. There is increased risk of small intestine lymphoma due to chronic inflammation if gluten is not avoided.

Carbohydrate

The main carbohydrates consumed are the polysaccharides starch and cellulose, disaccharides lactose and sucrose, and monosaccharides glucose and fructose. The intestine can only absorb the monosaccharides glucose, galactose, and fructose, which are all hexoses (**Figure 7.16**).

Starch is a polysaccharide of α-glucose (OH group on C_1 extending down), and is ultimately broken down to glucose by amylase and hydrolase enzymes. Cellulose, on the other hand, is a polymer of β-glucose and is indigestible. However, it has a valuable contribution as fibre, which helps with the formation of stool. It is also known to reduce the risk of colorectal cancer and metabolic syndromes, such as obesity and type 2 diabetes.

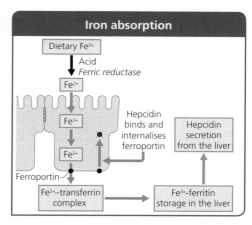

Figure 7.15 Ingested Fe^{3+} iron is reduced to Fe^{2+} by ferric reductase and gastric acid. This is absorbed into epithelial cells and exits into the circulation via the transporter ferroportin. Iron binds to transferrin in the blood and is stored in the liver bound to ferritin. High ferritin stores stimulate hepcidin secretion by the liver, which reduces the release of iron from epithelial cells.

Amylase and brush border hydrolases

Salivary and pancreatic amylase perform the first step in carbohydrate digestion by hydrolysing starch into the disaccharide maltose and glucose. Maltose is then broken down into glucose, galactose and fructose by a family of enzymes on the epithelial cell brush border, the microvilli-covered apical membrane of the mucosal epithelium:

- **Maltase** hydrolyses maltose into two glucose molecules
- **Lactase** hydrolyses lactose into glucose and galactose
- **Sucrase** hydrolyses sucrose into glucose and fructose.

Monosaccharide absorption

Glucose and galactose are absorbed into epithelial cells of the small intestine by cotransport with Na^+ through SGLUT-1 (sodium-glucose transporter) membrane transport proteins. Fructose is absorbed by facilitated diffusion via GLUT-5 protein channels.

All three monosaccharides then exit epithelial cells down their concentration gradient, through GLUT-2 hexose transporters on

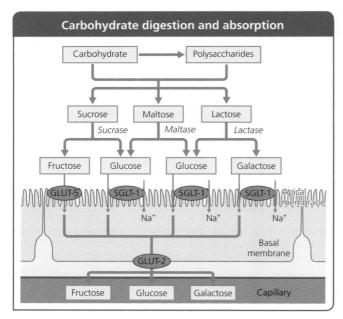

Carbohydrate digestion and absorption

Figure 7.16 Dietary polysaccharides are hydrolysed by salivary and pancreatic amylase. Disaccharides are split into their respective monosaccharides by brush border enzymes. Glucose and galactose are absorbed through SGLT-1 and fructose through GLUT-5. All exit via GLUT-2 basolaterally. GLUT-5, glucose transporter; SGLT, sodium-glucose linked transporter.

the basolateral membrane, and into the interstitium. Finally, they diffuse between endothelial cells and into capillary blood.

Protein

Proteins must be broken down by proteolytic enzymes to absorbable tri- and dipeptides or amino acids (**Figure 7.17**).

Pepsin and pancreatic proteases

Proteins are broken down by hydrolysis of their peptide bonds into short polypeptides. Gastric acid and pepsin start this process, which is taken further by proteases in pancreatic juice: trypsin, chymotrypsin and elastase. Peptidase enzymes, including aminopolypeptidase and multiple dipeptidases on the epithelial brush border, hydrolyse these chains further, to a combination of amino acids and di- and tri-peptides.

Amino acid and peptide absorption

Single amino acids are absorbed into epithelial cells by a family of sodium-linked cotransporters, with subtypes for acidic,

basic and neutral acids. They only bind amino acids once they have bound Na^+, and they then transport both into the epithelial cell.

> **Amino acid and monosaccharide absorption is dependent on the Na^+ electrochemical gradient across epithelial cell membranes**, and both, once in the interstitium, contribute to the osmotic gradient that drives the absorption of water.

Oligopeptides are transported by PepT1, a H^+-linked cotransporter. Within the cell, oligopeptides are broken down to single amino acids by cytosolic peptidases. Amino acids leave the cell via passive transporters on the basolateral membrane.

Fat

Most dietary fat is in the form of triglycerides, composed of three glycerol molecules, each with a fatty acid chain. The intestinal lumen also contains phospholipids and cholesterol from food and shed epithelial cells.

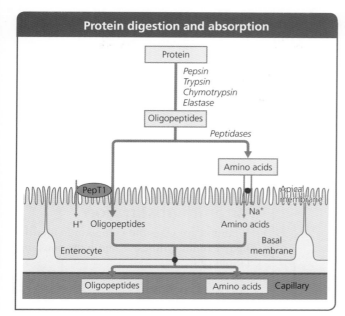

Protein digestion and absorption

Protein

Pepsin
Trypsin
Chymotrypsin
Elastase

Oligopeptides

Peptidases

Amino acids

PepT1

Apical
membrane

H^+ Oligopeptides

Na^+
Amino acids

Basal
membrane

Enterocyte

Oligopeptides

Amino acids Capillary

Figure 7.17 Pepsin and pancreatic proteases act on dietary protein to produce oligopeptides. Some are absorbed via PepT1 whilst some oligopeptides are broken down to amino acids by peptidases on the brush border before cotransport with Na^+.

Bile salt emulsification

Triglycerides are not very water-soluble and tend to form large globules with a relatively low surface area:volume ratio. The lipases that break down triglycerides are water-soluble, and can only act on the surface. Good digestion of fats thus depends on breaking the globules down into much smaller droplets, i.e. emulsification (**Figure 7.18**).

Emulsification is achieved by bile salts, cholesterol derivatives synthesised and conjugated with taurine or glycine by the liver, and secreted in bile. They are amphipathic, i.e. one end is lipophilic and will insert into the fat, whilst the other is hydrophilic and binds to water. Like a detergent, this results in fragmentation of the fat globules, into structures called micelles, and a huge increase in the surface area of exposed lipid. Micelles are small water-soluble spheres of lipids (internally) and bile acids (externally).

Pancreatic lipase hydrolysis

The increased surface area of the micelles allows pancreatic lipase to cleave the triglycerides into free fatty acids and monoglycerides.

Fat absorption

The monoglycerides (MG) and free fatty acids (FFA) form an unstirred layer close to the enterocytes. MG and FFA are small, lipophilic molecules and are therefore able to diffuse from this layer straight through the enterocyte apical cell membrane.

Chylomicrons

Triglycerides are re-formed in the endoplasmic reticulum of epithelial cells and combine with apolipoproteins to form chylomicrons. These are then exocytosed via the basolateral membrane into the interstitium, from where they enter lymphatic vessels associated with villi. After a fatty meal, these vessels are packed white with chylomicrons. Ultimately, these drain into systemic circulation and are distributed throughout the body.

Bile salt reabsorption

Most bile salts are reabsorbed in the distal part of the ileum or, after bacterial processing, in the colon. They then travel via the portal vein back to the liver where they are recycled (see page 228).

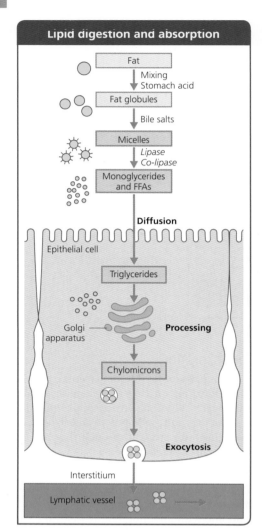

Lipid digestion and absorption

Figure 7.18 Dietary fat is partially emulsified by gastric acid and churning. Fat combines with bile to form micelles. Pancreatic lipase binds to micelles, releasing monoglycerides and free fatty acids (FFAs). These diffuse into epithelial cells where they are re-packaged as large chylomicrons, which pass into lymphatic capillaries.

Cholesterol absorption

Cholesterol is incorporated into micelles and then joins the unstirred layer of MG and FFA.

It is absorbed into enterocytes by diffusion, where they are also packaged into chylomicrons.

> The small intestine is relatively sterile compared to the colon but bacterial overgrowth can occur if there are changes in structure (e.g. due to surgery or radiotherapy) or metabolism (e.g. diabetes mellitus) that promote bacterial colonisation.

Vitamin absorption

Vitamins are essential compounds that the body cannot synthesise and must consume (**Table 7.13**).

Fat-soluble vitamins

Fat-soluble vitamins (A, D, E and K) are absorbed in a similar way to other fats, i.e. combined into chylomicrons. Most water-soluble vitamins, however, need specific Na^+-linked cotransporters for uptake; this occurs in the late jejunum and early ileum.

Vitamin B_{12}

Vitamin B_{12} is an essential cofactor required for DNA and protein methylation: a key mechanism of controlling gene and enzyme activity in cell metabolism, particularly for haematopoiesis and neural function.

Intrinsic factor (IF) is a peptide produced by parietal cells of the stomach that binds B_{12}. IF–B_{12} complexes travel to the terminal ileum and are endocytosed by epithelial cells with apical IF–B_{12} complex receptors.

> **Patients with pernicious anaemia** develop B_{12} deficiency due to reduced IF production, caused by autoimmune damage to parietal cells. Without IF, vitamin B_{12} cannot be absorbed.

Vitamins and their function		
Vitamin	Function	Disease of deficiency
Vitamin A (retinol)	Component of retinal, a visual pigment	Night-blindness
Vitamin B_1 (thiamine)	Cofactor in ketoacid decarboxylation; needed for normal central and peripheral nervous function, and cardiac function	Wernicke-Korsakoff syndrome; wet, and dry, beriberi
Vitamin B_3 (niacin)	Used in redox reactions (mitochondrial function for normal metabolism)	Pellagra (diarrhoea, dementia, dermatitis)
Vitamin B_6 (pyridoxine)	Cofactor for transamination, (synthesis of amino acids), haem synthesis, and decarboxylation	Neuropathy
Vitamin B_{12} (cobalamin)	Cofactor for DNA and protein methylation and in formation of succinyl-CoA	Pernicious anaemia, peripheral and central neuropathy
Vitamin C (ascorbic acid)	Cofactor for breakdown of dopamine, needed for collagen synthesis, helps iron absorption	Scurvy (bruising, gingivitis)
Vitamin D (cholecalciferol)	Absorption of Ca^{2+} and PO_4^{3-} (phosphate ion)	Rickets (children), osteomalacia (adults)
Vitamin E	Antioxidant in red blood cells	Haemolysis and neuropathy
Vitamin K	Synthesis of proteins for clotting cascade	Bleeding
Folic acid	Coenzyme for DNA methylation – regulation of gene expression and synthesis of DNA and RNA	Megaloblastic anaemia

Table 7.13. The main vitamins, their physiological function, and the consequence of their deficiency

The pancreas

The pancreas is both an endocrine and exocrine organ located behind the stomach. It produces and secretes the hormones insulin, glucagon, and somatostatin into the blood, which have a large effect on regulating body metabolism.

Its alkaline secretions into the duodenum neutralise acidic chyme and contain digestive enzymes, which are essential to the breakdown of lumen contents started by saliva and gastric secretions.

Structure of the pancreas

The pancreas is a 12–15 cm long, 2.5 cm wide retroperitoneal gland, which lies posterior to the stomach. It has a head, body and a tail, with the head attached to the duodenum (**Figure 7.19**).

Functions of the pancreas

The pancreas has endocrine and exocrine functions, the former including the production of insulin and glucagon, the key hormones of carbohydrate metabolism (see page 174). Its exocrine function is the production of pancreatic juice that is secreted into the duodenum via the sphincter of Oddi. Pancreatic juice is responsible for protein, carbohydrate, lipid and nucleic acid digestion in the small intestine.

Histology of the pancreas

Endocrine function (i.e. hormone production) is performed by the islets of Langerhans (see page 174), which make up 1–2% of the mass of the pancreas.

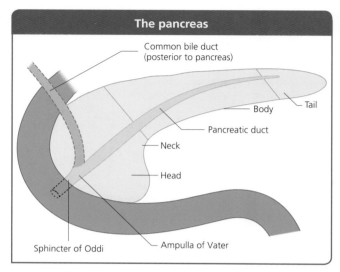

The pancreas

Common bile duct
(posterior to pancreas)

Body

Tail

Pancreatic duct

Neck

Head

Sphincter of Oddi

Ampulla of Vater

Figure 7.19 The pancreas is a retroperitoneal organ with a tail that projects towards the splenic hilum. The main pancreatic duct joins with the common bile duct at the ampulla of Vater. These open into the second part of the duodenum at the sphincter of Oddi.

The rest are exocrine acinar cells arranged in lobules, similar to those of the salivary glands. Acinar cells secrete a range of inactive digestive enzymes (**Table 7.14**) into a duct system that drains into the duodenum at the sphincter of Oddi.

The cystic fibrosis transmembrane conductance regulator (CTFR) is a Cl⁻ channel involved in fluid secretion in the exocrine pancreas. CFTR is absent in cystic fibrosis, resulting in inadequate Cl⁻ (and water) secretion in pancreatic fluid and bronchial mucus, but excess Cl⁻ in sweat. This causes viscous secretions that block pancreatic ducts, causing chronic pancreatitis. Patients need dietary supplements with pancreatic enzymes, as well as physiotherapy to clear mucus from the lungs.

Pancreatic juice		
Origin	Function	Ingredient
Acinar cells	Starch digestion	Pancreatic amylase
	Protein digestion (proteases)	Trypsin, chymotrypsin, carboxypeptidase, elastase
	Fat digestion	Pancreatic lipase
	RNA and DNA digestion	Ribonuclease, deoxyribonuclease
	Solvent	Water
Ductal epithelial cells	Fluid volume, membrane gradients and transport	Salts
	Buffers gastric acid	Sodium bicarbonate

Table 7.14 Pancreatic fluid contents and their function. 1.2–1.5 litres of this clear liquid is produced a day

Pancreatic juice

The pancreatic acinar cells produces 1–1.5 litres of pancreatic juice a day, a clear liquid with a pH of 7.1–8.2 containing:

- Water
- NaHCO$_3$
- Electrolytes
- Proenzymes for protein digestion: trypsinogen, chymotrypsinogen, procarboxypolypeptidase

- Enzymes for carbohydrate digestion: pancreatic amylase
- Enzymes for lipid digestion: pancreatic lipase, cholesterol esterase and phospholipase.

Trypsinogen is activated by enterokinase in the duodenum to form the protease trypsin, which in turn activates all three proteases. This prevents pancreatic autodigestion.

Acinar cell secretion

Secretion from pancreatic acinar cells is extremely similar to the primary secretion mechanism in salivary acinar cells (see page 207). Cl^- is secreted across the apical membrane down its concentration gradient through the CFTR channel. The concentration gradient is established by basolateral uptake through $Na^+/K^+/2Cl^-$ cotransporters. Water and Na^+ follow Cl^- movement through paracellular transport.

Pancreatic enzymes are stored in secretory vesicles prior to release. An increase in intracellular calcium (e.g. triggered by acetylcholine binding to muscarinic receptors) causes secretory vesicles to fuse with the apical membrane of acinar cells.

Water and bicarbonate ions

Water and HCO_3^- are mainly added to the pancreatic juice by epithelial cells of the pancreatic and biliary ducts, not the acinar cells. This secondary modification is very similar to the mechanism in salivary gland ductular cells (see page 207). There is secondary active reabsorption of Na^+ into ductular cells through the apical ENaC channel, driven by basolateral Na^+/K^+-ATPase. Water cannot follow due to the presence of relatively tight occluding junctions; therefore water is concentrated in ductular fluid. There is secretion of HCO_3^- using the HCO_3^-/Cl^- exchange channel on the apical membrane of ductular cells. This is driven by the high intraluminal concentration of Cl^-.

HCO_3^- is necessary to neutralise the acidic chyme from the stomach.

Regulation of secretion

Pancreatic secretion is regulated by neural and hormonal signals. The three main stimulants are:

■ **ACh** released by vagal and enteric nerve endings

■ **CCK** hormone secreted by duodenal epithelial cells when stimulated by food
■ **Secretin** hormone secreted by duodenal epithelial cells when stimulated by acidic food.

Neural control

Activation of the vagus nerve causes an increase in acinar cell secretion. Long-range enteric and autonomic reflexes control the phases of pancreatic secretion:

■ The **cephalopancreatic reflex** is activated by the anticipation of food and its taste
■ The **gastropancreatic reflex** is stimulated by peptides in the stomach's lumen
■ The **enteropancreatic reflex** contributes 60% of the pancreas' stimulation.

Low duodenal pH causes secretin release from S-cells, which acts on ductular cells to increase HCO_3^- secretion. Duodenal I-cells release CCK in response to lipid, which stimulates acinar cell secretion.

> **Acute pancreatitis is acute inflammation of the pancreas** that often presents with severe epigastric pain and vomiting. A common cause is gallstones blocking the flow of pancreatic juice and bile. If some pancreatic enzymes spontaneously cleave to their active form, a positive feedback loop of activation occurs. Proteases and lipases digest pancreatic tissue and stimulate a systemic inflammatory response that results in respiratory failure, hypotension and renal failure.

Hormonal control

APUD cells in the small intestine (and stomach) sense nutrients in the gut lumen and release hormones into the bloodstream, including cholecystokinin-pancreozymin (CCK, or CCK-PZ) and secretin. CCK stimulates pancreatic acinar secretion and gallbladder contraction, while secretin increases the secretion of fluid and HCO_3^-, in the pancreatic ducts and the biliary tree.

The liver and biliary system

The liver is the largest internal organ, with a large blood supply from both the heart and GI tract. It has roles in digestion, excretion, immunity and fluid balance. It is a synthesising factory, a processing and recycling plant, a detoxifier and a filter.

Structure of the liver

Grossly, the liver has a large right lobe and a smaller left lobe. Its vascular supply branches to supply eight segments. The hepatic artery and portal vein enter through the porta hepatis and the bile duct leaves through here too.

Functions of the liver

The liver's functions include:

- Synthesis of most plasma proteins
- Production of bile for fat digestion, and bilirubin and cholesterol excretion
- Metabolism of carbohydrates, proteins and lipids
- Regulation of carbohydrate, protein and lipid metabolism
- Processing of waste substances and toxins for excretion
- Regulation of body fluid volume by interacting with the cardiovascular, renal and respiratory systems
- Phagocytosing bacteria and regulating immune tolerance towards gut-derived antigens.

Histology of the liver

The liver consists of:

- **Hepatocytes**: the predominate functional cells of the liver
- **Sinusoids**: specialised, highly permeable capillaries
- **Bile canaliculi**: small canals that run between hepatocytes.

The networks of hepatocytes are arranged to receive a constant supply of arterial and portal vein blood via the sinusoids. Their products are then secreted into the blood and bile.

Cell types

The functional cells of the liver are the hepatocytes, sinusoidal endothelial cells, stellate cells and reticuloendothelial cells **(Figure 7.20)**.

Hepatocytes

Hepatocytes are specialised epithelial cells that perform the metabolic, secretory and endocrine functions of the liver. Like endothelial cells, they are capable of cell division despite being differentiated cells.

Hepatocytes form three-dimensional, one-cell thick laminae (plates) that line the vascular sinusoids. The lateral membrane of each two adjacent hepatocytes forms the wall of a bile canaliculus, which drains into a nearby bile duct.

Endothelial cells

The sinusoids are lined with endothelial cells that regulate the transport into hepatocytes and act as a barrier between the blood and hepatocytes. They are separated from hepatocytes by a small gap called the space of Disse.

Stellate cells

Stellate cells (Ito cells) are connective tissue cells within the space of Disse. They store vitamin A and have myofibroblastic activity that is increased in liver fibrosis.

Kupffer cells

Kupffer (or reticuloendothelial) cells are macrophage-like cells within the sinusoids that clean the blood. They phagocytose bacteria as a part of innate immunity, as well as old erythrocytes, lymphocytes and other large particles. Like most phagocytes, they also present antigens of phagocytosed contents to lymphocytes in the lymph nodes in order to initiate the adaptive immune response (see page 99).

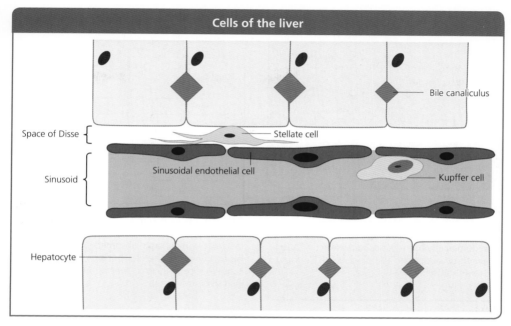

Cells of the liver

Space of Disse

Sinusoid

Hepatocyte

Bile canaliculus

Stellate cell

Sinusoidal endothelial cell

Kupffer cell

Figure 7.20 Hepatocytes are arranged in plates between sinusoids, lined by fenestrated endothelial cells (HSEC). The area between HSEC and hepatocytes is known as the space of Disse, containing stellate cells. Kupffer cells lie in the sinusoids.

Organisation

The liver can be organised either structurally (into lobules) or functionally (as acini) (**Figure 7.21**).

Classical lobules

Classical lobules are hexagonal and centred on a central vein. In each corner are portal triads, which contain branches of the hepatic artery and portal vein, together with a bile duct. A mixture of arterial and portal blood flows through the sinusoids, to drain into the central vein of the lobule. Portal lobules are triangular, centred on a portal triad, with the three adjacent central veins at each apex (**Figure 7.22**).

Acini

Acini of the liver and their zones are defined functionally, representing an area supplied with oxygen by one set of blood vessels:

■ Zone 1 hepatocytes, the closest to portal tracts, have access to the most oxygen and

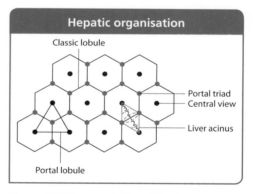

Hepatic organisation

Classic lobule

Portal triad
Central view

Liver acinus

Portal lobule

Figure 7.21 The organisation of the liver. Peripheral portal triads and a central vein define a hepatic lobule. A liver acinus is formed from hepatic veins at the edge and a portal triad in the middle. Hepatocyte zones describe decreasing oxygen concentration moving away from portal triads.

perform highly aerobic tasks including amino acid synthesis and β-oxidation of fat
■ Zone 2 cells are intermediate in function
■ Zone 3 are relatively oxygen-deficient and perform drug metabolism and glycolysis.

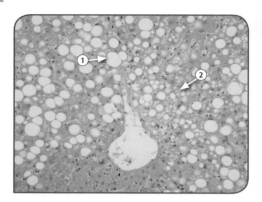

Figure 7.22 A section from a liver biopsy showing non-alcoholic fatty liver disease. Centrilobular hepatocytes show fatty change with a predominantly macrovesicular pattern ①. A few smaller fat vacuoles are also present ②. Courtesy of Stefan Hübscher.

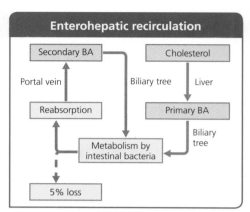

Figure 7.23 The enterohepatic recirculation of bile acids (BA). Primary BAs are exported into the biliary system, but most are reabsorbed in the terminal ileum. In addition, colonic bacteria metabolise some to secondary BAs. They return via the portal vein to be resecreted.

Bile

Bile is a green-brown hepatic secretion that consists of water, bile salts, cholesterol, lecithin (a phospholipid), bile pigments and electrolytes. Its functions are to supply bile acids to facilitate fat digestion and absorption in the small intestine, and to excrete bilirubin (a waste product of haem breakdown) and excess cholesterol.

Bile acids

Primary bile acids are synthesised de novo in hepatocytes from cholesterol, which is converted to cholic acid and chenodeoxycholic acid. These are conjugated (in hepatocytes) with glycine or taurine, which generate the hydrophilic and hydrophobic properties important in the breakdown and absorption of fats (see page 222). When bile acids bind to K^+ or Na^+ ions they are known as bile salts.

Reabsorption

Conjugated bile salts are reabsorbed actively in the distal ileum, but intestinal bacteria deconjugate and hydrolyse primary bile acids in the small intestine and colon to form secondary bile acids. These are absorbed passively in the colon and returned in the portal circulation to the liver for re conjugation.

This process is termed enterohepatic recirculation (**Figure 7.23**). This makes the process highly energy-efficient. 95% of all secreted bile acids undergo this process, while 5% are lost in the faeces.

Bile production

Bile production is driven by the secretion of electrolytes, bile acids and cholesterol across the canalicular membrane of hepatocytes and into the canaliculi. This generates an osmotic gradient for water movement. The cells making up the bile ducts secrete HCO_3^-, resulting in an alkaline fluid. The secretion mechanism of HCO_3^-, Na^+, Cl^- and water is similar to the mechanism of pancreatic electrolyte secretion (see page 225). Secretion is continuous, but increases during eating. 600–1000 mL is produced daily.

The biliary system

Bile travels through the canaliculi to the terminal bile ducts, which join to form the hepatic duct. This joins the cystic duct to form the common bile duct, which joins with the pancreatic duct to form the ampulla of Vater. This drains through the sphincter of Oddi muscle, into the duodenum at the duodenal papilla (**Figure 7.24**).

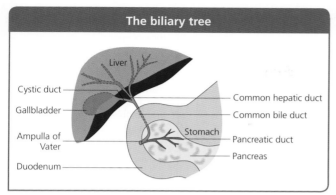

The biliary tree

Liver
Cystic duct
Gallbladder
Ampulla of Vater
Duodenum
Common hepatic duct
Common bile duct
Stomach
Pancreatic duct
Pancreas

Figure 7.24 The biliary system transports bile from the liver in the hepatic duct and stores and concentrates it in the gallbladder. When stimulated, bile is excreted into the common bile duct, where it joins pancreatic juice and is secreted through the sphincter of Oddi into the 2nd part of the duodenum.

Between meals, the sphincter of Oddi is closed so bile is stored and concentrated in the gallbladder over a period of minutes.

The gallbladder

Bile salts are concentrated in the gallbladder by reabsorption of NaCl and water. This is driven by active basolateral Na^+ reabsorption via Na^+-K^+-ATPase. Micelles containing cholesterol and bile salts form, reducing their osmotic effect and allowing more water to leave the gallbladder lumen.

Release of bile

The release of bile from the gallbladder is controlled by the hormone cholecystokinin (CCK). When fat or protein is detected in the lumen of the duodenum, I cells release CCK, which acts on gallbladder smooth muscle to cause contraction. It also causes relaxation of the sphincter of Oddi and increases pancreatic secretions.

Secondary ductal secretions

Biliary ductal epithelial cells (cholangiocytes) produce an alkaline secretion of HCO_3^- and Na^+ similar to pancreatic ductal cells. In contrast, gallbladder cells acidify the bile, which helps to reduce stone formation.

Bilirubin

Bilirubin is an organic compound called porphyrin formed from the breakdown of haemoglobin and other haem-containing proteins, such as cytochromes. It travels in the blood bound to albumin (**Figure 7.25**).

Hepatocytes conjugate bilirubin with glucuronate: this makes bilirubin water-soluble, allowing its excretion via bile.

A 38-year-old woman presents to the emergency department with upper right quadrant abdominal pain shortly after eating fish and chips. An ultrasound scan shows multiple gallstones within the gallbladder.

Gallstones (cholelithiasis) often present with biliary colic pain after eating fatty foods, as this stimulates release of cholecystokinin (CCK) from the duodenum, which causes gallbladder and biliary contraction. Gallstones are associated with high cholesterol levels in the bile, although there is no direct association with high serum cholesterol.

Stones can pass into the intestines without harm or they may lodge in the biliary system, obstructing the flow of bile or pancreatic fluid causing obstructive jaundice and/or pancreatitis.

Colonic conversion

Conjugated bilirubin secreted into the small intestine is converted into urobilinogen and then stercobilinogen by colonic bacteria and is excreted in faeces. Stercobilinogen is brown, which gives stool its brown colour. 20% of urobilinogen is not converted and is reabsorbed, some of which passes into the urine as urobilinogen is water-soluble. The remaining urobilinogen is recycled in the liver and excreted in the bile once more.

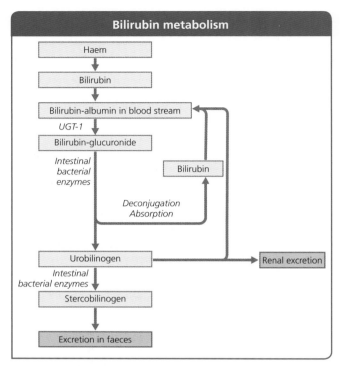

Figure 7.25 The liver conjugates bilirubin with glucuronide using the enzyme UGT-1. Bilirubin glucuronide, is then exported into the bile. Bacterial enzymes may deconjugate bilirubin allowing reabsorption. Other bacterial enzymes cause metabolism into urobilinogen (some passes into the urine) and stercobilinogen.

Other colonic bacteria deconjugate bilirubin before it is converted into urobilinogen, which is then be absorbed and recycled like bile salts.

A 45-year-old man presents to emergency department with yellow eyes and skin, a fever and vomiting a few days after returning from a holiday to Africa. He says he did not take all the recommended vaccinations before travelling.

Jaundice is the presence of raised bilirubin in the blood, and is caused by pre-, intra- or post-hepatic factors preventing its excretion:

- Pre-hepatic jaundice is due to increased erythrocyte breakdown (haemolysis) or reduced hepatocyte conjugation (e.g. Gilbert's syndrome)

- Hepatocyte damage (e.g. from viral hepatitis, the most likely cause here) causes intrahepatic jaundice

- Obstruction to bile flow, e.g. with gallstones, causes post-hepatic jaundice.

High bilirubin levels cause deposits in tissues giving them a yellow colour most easily seen in the sclerae.

Synthetic functions of the liver

Hepatocytes synthesise most plasma proteins, including albumin, clotting factors, globulins and fibrinogen.

Albumin

Albumin is a plasma protein with two main roles: exerting an oncotic force that retains water in blood vessels and binding and transporting other molecules in blood.

Albumin can bind ions (e.g. about 50% of circulating Ca^{2+} is bound to albumin), lipid-based molecules to make them more water-soluble (e.g. bilirubin), hormones and many drugs.

Hypoalbuminaemia (low plasma albumin concentration) is usually caused by decreased synthesis of albumin in liver disease or chronic illness, or loss in the urine due to renal disease. Reduced vascular oncotic pressure leads to tissue oedema and ascites as water escapes the vascular compartment into surrounding tissues.

Clotting factors

These are a group of over 15 proteins that interact to cause coagulation (see page 96). Like albumin, clotting factors are only synthesised in the liver, but they have a half-life of a day or less. Vitamin K is a fat-soluble cofactor for the synthesis of factors II, VII, IX and X.

Metabolic functions of the liver

The liver has a central role in the metabolism of absorbed and circulating carbohydrates, proteins and lipids, and in coordinating their availability to other tissues. This is tightly regulated by the effects of the pancreatic hormones insulin and glucagon (see page 174). Their role is modulated by a number of other hormones, including:

■ Thyroid hormone
■ Growth hormone
■ Stress hormones, such as glucocorticoids and adrenaline
■ Hormones involved in fat regulation and appetite, e.g. leptin, ghrelin and adiponectin.

These endocrine systems interact to synchronise liver metabolism with the availability of nutrients and the needs of the body.

Carbohydrate metabolism

Hepatocytes take up glucose from the blood when levels are relatively high and convert it into glycogen stores. When glucose levels fall, hepatocytes break down glycogen to release glucose into the blood, and also generate new glucose via gluconeogenesis. As hepatocytes possess the enzyme glucose-6-phosphatase, unlike all other human cells, they are able to dephosphorylate the glucose-6-phosphate created by these pathways and release it into the blood.

Protein metabolism

Amino acids arrive in the portal circulation from the small intestine or are generated by the peripheral breakdown of protein during fasting. The liver uses them to synthesise plasma proteins or deaminates them by removing an NH_2 group and uses the carbon chain for gluconeogenesis. The amino groups are converted to urea, which is excreted in urine.

Lipid metabolism

Fed state

Chylomicrons absorbed from the small intestine during a meal pass into the circulation. Lipoprotein lipase (LPL) on vascular endothelial cells releases free fatty acids (FFA) and monoglycerides (MG) from triglycerides in chylomicrons. This leaves chylomicron remnants, which travel back to the liver where they are taken up by hepatocytes for storage and processing (**Figure 7.26**). The FFA and MG diffuse through endothelial cells into the underlying tissues and provide an energy source.

$$\text{Triglyceride (TG)} \xrightarrow{LPL} \text{Free fatty-acids (FFA)} + \text{monoglycerides (MG)}$$

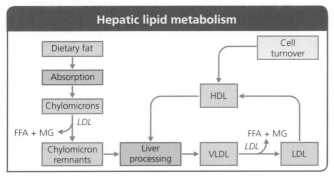

Figure 7.26 The liver's role in lipid metabolism. Lipoprotein lipase (LPL) on endothelial cells acts on chylomicrons, giving chylomicron remnants, which are then converted to very-low-density lipoproteins (VLDL) in the liver. VLDL are released during fasting, forming low-density lipoproteins (LDL) after further LPL metabolism. LDL binds high-density lipoproteins (HDL) for recycling back to the liver.

Fasting state

During fasting, hepatocytes release particles containing triglycerides, cholesterol and apolipoproteins called very-low-density lipoprotein (VLDL). These are broken down by LPL, releasing FFA and MG, which can be used as an energy source by most cells. The removal of triglycerides from VLDL, coupled with changes in apolipoproteins, causes VLDL to gradually become low-density lipoproteins (LDL). They are termed LDL once the cholesterol content of the particle exceeds the triglyceride content.

High-density lipoproteins (HDL) are formed as small apolipoprotein-rich particles by the liver. Their primary function is to take up cholesterol (generated in normal cell turnover) from tissues and transport it back to the liver. HDL exchanges apolipoproteins with VLDL and LDL; it also takes cholesterol from LDL. The exchange of apolipoproteins helps to promote binding of LDL to LDL-receptors on hepatocyte membranes. LDL (and its contained cholesterol) and HDL are then recycled in the hepatocytes.

Processing of waste substances and toxins for excretion

The liver is the main site for detoxification and metabolism of organic compounds, especially those that are lipid-soluble. These include endogenous compounds (e.g. bilirubin, cholesterol and steroid hormones) and exogenous compounds (e.g. drugs, pesticides and alcohol). Detoxification is generally performed in two phases:

- **Phase 1:** hydroxylation and oxidation reactions performed by the cytochrome P450 (CYP450) enzymes (CYP450) facilitate conjugation (phase 2)
- **Phase 2:** conjugation with water-soluble molecules (e.g. glutathione, sulphate and glucuronate) by conjugation enzymes makes the substance water-soluble

The phase 1 reactions may generate toxic intermediates between phase 1 oxidation and phase 2 conjugation; therefore, adequate stores of conjugation molecules are required for safe drug excretion. The water-soluble (conjugated) products can then be excreted in the bile or pass back into the blood to be excreted in urine.

There are multiple different CYP450 enzymes, each acting on specific molecular sequences on drugs, e.g. CYP2E1 metabolises ethanol (alcohol) and CYP2C9 metabolises warfarin. The activity of the CYP450 enzymes increases or decreases in response to availability of their substrate (e.g. CYP2E1, which metabolises alcohol, is increased with chronic alcohol ingestion) or drugs (e.g. the antibiotic rifampicin increases activity in all CYP enzymes).

Regulation of body fluid volume

The liver interacts with the renal, cardiovascular and pulmonary systems to maintain homeostasis in body fluids. It is best understood when considering the consequences of liver failure.

The liver is the site of albumin production, which is needed for normal plasma oncotic pressure. Reduction in albumin synthesis (causing hypoalbuminaemia) causes a loss of fluid into the tissue spaces (oedema) and activation of the renin–angiotensin–aldosterone system (RAAS).

The liver breaks down nitric oxide (NO), a key vasodilator. Loss of this function causes increased NO and systemic vasodilation, again activating the RAAS. Therefore, liver disease causes a hyperdynamic circulation.

Immune function of the liver

The liver promotes tolerance (i.e. lack of an immune response) to harmless antigens and helps to clear harmful bacteria that pass through the gut wall. Antigens from food (absorbed in the gut) travel to the liver where Kupffer cells promote tolerance towards them, despite them being foreign material. By contrast, bacteria passing through the gut wall and entering the liver via the portal vein are removed by Kupffer cells before they reach the systemic circulation. This is why patients with chronic liver disease are at increased risk of infections.

Metabolic states

Nutrients absorbed in the GI tract are subject to three states of metabolism, depending on the nutritional status of the body. These states are regulated by the balance of anabolic hormones (insulin) and catabolic hormones (e.g. glucagon and adrenaline) (**Table 7.15**).

Post-prandial state

In the post-prandial state the body enters a period of anabolism, during which large molecules are synthesised from foodstuffs. These include energy storage molecules like glycogen and triglycerides, and proteins and RNA for the maintenance and growth of cells. This leads to a positive nitrogen balance, as nitrogen in amino acids and nucleic acids are incorporated into the body.

Catabolic state

Once the energy in foodstuffs has been used, the body enters a state where storage molecules are broken down to release small molecules, that can be used as an energy source, for example glucose. This process is called catabolism. Since this includes the breakdown of protein and the use of amino acids for gluconeogenesis, this results in a negative nitrogen balance.

Starvation state

In more prolonged starvation, the body acts to protect muscle and protein by using fat to generate energy. Rapid lipolysis leads to the production of excess acetyl-CoA, which is then converted by the hepatocytes to the ketone bodies acetone and β-hydroxybutyrate. The brain adapts over a few days to use these as its major energy source, reducing the need for glucose.

Diabetic ketoacidosis is a state of starvation with high concentrations of ketone bodies in the blood due to a lack of insulin. Ketoacidosis also occurs in anorexia nervosa. The volatile ketone compounds cause a characteristic pear-drop smell on patients' breath.

Prandial and post-prandial states				
State	Plasma hormones	Liver	Muscle	Fat
Post-prandial	Insulin	Increased glycogenesis, Inhibited glycogenolysis, Inhibited gluconeogenesis	Increased proteogenesis, Inhibited proteolysis	Increased lipogenesis, Inhibited lipolysis
Fasting	Glucagon, Adrenaline, Growth hormone, Cortisol	Increased glycogenolysis, Increased gluconeogenesis, Increased ketone body formation, Increased deamination of amino acids, Inhibited glycogenesis	Increased glycogenolysis, Increased proteolysis, Inhibited proteogenesis	Increased lipolysis, Inhibited lipogenesis

Table 7.15 Summary of the post-prandial, i.e. anabolic, and fasting-catabolic states

The large intestine

The large intestine begins at the ileocaecal valve, extends clockwise for 150 cm around the edge of the abdominal cavity and finally connects with the anus medially. It is the major site for water absorption, storage of faecal matter and controls the expulsion of faeces during defecation.

Structure of the large intestine

The large intestine consists of six sections (**Figure 7.27**):

- Caecum (and appendix)
- Ascending, transverse, descending and sigmoid regions of the colon
- Rectum.

Functions of the large intestine

Approximately 1.5–2 litres of chyme pass into the caecum each day. The large intestine absorbs almost all of the water and electrolytes from this to produce about 100–200 mL of faeces. The large intestine does this by its:

- Motility
- Secretion

- Absorption
- Colonic flora.

These processes produce semi-solid faeces, consisting of 75% water and a solid component of dead bacteria, fibre, sloughed mucosal epithelia and inorganic ions. Little digestion occurs in the large intestine apart from that carried out by bacteria.

Histology of the large intestine

In contrast to the rest of the GI tract, the longitudinal muscle layer in the colon is not a continuous layer over the gut, but is gathered into 3 longitudinal bands: the taeniae coli. The tension of these, together with slow contractions of the circular muscle, forms the colon into a series of 'pockets' called haustra.

The mucosa of the large intestine is not arranged in villi, but is relatively flat. Deep pit glands secrete mucus to facilitate the movement of the increasingly solid faecal material.

Motility in the large intestine

Motility in the large intestine is slower than in the small intestine because it focuses on

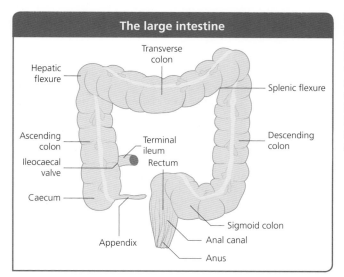

The large intestine

Transverse colon

Hepatic flexure

Splenic flexure

Ascending colon

Terminal ileum

Descending colon

Ileocaecal valve

Rectum

Caecum

Appendix

Sigmoid colon

Anal canal

Anus

Figure 7.27 The colon begins at the ileocaecal junction in the right iliac fossa. The caecum lies inferior to this, from which the appendix protrudes. The ascending and descending colon are retroperitoneal and are linked by the transverse colon, which lies in the omentum. The sigmoid colon connects the descending colon to the rectum.

mixing and churning, rather than propulsion. This gives the maximum time for water and electrolyte reabsorption.

Haustrations

Haustrations are slow contractions of the circular muscle similar to segmentation. They mix and compress gut contents without moving it aborally (away from the mouth).

Mass movements

Mass movements are the equivalent of the peristaltic waves in the small intestine. These occur a few times a day and move material substantial distances along the colon.

Reflexes

Like most GI movements large intestine activity is largely autonomous, but several reflexes can precipitate mass movements, including the:

- **Gastrocolic reflex**: associated with food in the stomach
- **Orthocolic reflex**: associated with gaining an upright posture in the morning.

When material moves into the rectum, the defecation reflex is triggered.

Defecation

Defecation is the passage of faeces out of the rectum and anus. It occurs via a four-stage reflex:

Colonic distension

Mass peristalsis moves colonic contents to fill the rectum, causing distension. Squatting or sitting facilitates this movement of contents.

Parasympathetic reflex

Distension activates a local parasympathetic reflex at spinal nerve roots S2–4 to stimulate contraction of the rectum and relaxation of the internal anal sphincter, which consists of smooth muscle.

Reinforcement

Movement of stool through the rectum and internal anal sphincter reinforces the reflex to increase rectal smooth muscle contraction.

Sphincter relaxation

Finally, there is relaxation of the external anal sphincter, which consists of striated muscle under voluntary control. The parasympathetic reflex causes an urge to relax the external sphincter, but it can be consciously overcome. When this happens, retrograde peristalsis moves the faecal material back up into the rectum, temporarily relieving the urge to defaecate. This is used clinically in the administration of suppositories.

Secretion in the large intestine

Colonic secretions contain large amounts of mucin, produced by goblet cells, and HCO_3^-. HCO_3^- is secreted using an apical Cl^-/HCO_3^- exchange, which also facilitates the uptake of Cl^-. Both these secretory processes are activated by parasympathetic stimulation and mechanical distension of the bowel caused by luminal contents.

Absorption in the large intestine

The core function of the large intestine is the absorption of water, of which it can absorb a maximum of 6 litres a day. Most of this occurs in the first half of the large intestine.

> **Diarrhoea is an increase in volume or frequency of stool.** It is caused by increased intestinal motility, reduction in absorption or increased secretion of ions and water in the large intestine. Crypt cells and the epithelium secrete fluid into the lumen in a similar method to salivary gland acinar cells. This can be increased by vasoactive intestinal peptide (VIP) or bacterial toxins, such as cholera, to cause a life-threatening degree of fluid loss.

Water and salt

Because water can move in both directions across the GI mucosa, absorption of water is dependent on the controlled absorption of electrolytes.

The colonic mucosa has a large number of Na$^+$/K$^+$-ATPases on its basolateral membrane that drive the absorption of Na$^+$ from the lumen into the epithelium, interstitium and blood. This mechanism is identical to Na$^+$ absorption in small bowel enterocytes.

The occluding junctions of the large intestine are 'tighter' than in the small intestine, preventing paracellular 'back-flow' of water and ions. This enables absorption of Na$^+$ against a higher gradient than in the small intestine.

> **Bacterial toxins** (e.g. *Clostridium difficile* toxins A and B) can cause life-threatening net solute and water secretion and severe diarrhoea.

Bacteria in the large intestine

The large intestine contains a microbiota (or 'gut flora') of over 500 species of bacteria. These have important roles in immunity and metabolism, including:

- Fermentation of undigested carbohydrates to short chain fatty acids
- Production of vitamins B and K
- Recycling of bile salts needed for lipid absorption and transport
- Preventing the growth of pathogenic bacteria
- A mutually-dependent relationship with the immune system.

Their importance is emphasised by their number, around 100,000,000,000, which is approximately ten-times the number of body cells. Similarly, dead bacteria constitute nearly a third of the solid matter in faeces.

Breakdown of nutrients

Certain colonic bacteria (e.g. *Bacteroides*) contain hydrolytic enzymes that break down lumen contents, including the fermentation of carbohydrates into short-chain fatty acids that are absorbed by passive diffusion. In addition, some bacteria (e.g. *Escherichia* species) produce vitamin K and B vitamins that are absorbed in the colon and process any bile salts not absorbed in the ileum, allowing them to be reabsorbed.

Immune development and tolerance

Colonic flora represent a potentially vast array of foreign antigens that must be tolerated by the immune system. This complex and dynamic relationship between the microbiota and the development and regulation of the GI and systemic immune systems is thought to be involved in many aspects of immune regulation. For example, they influence systemic immune tolerance to antigens that would otherwise provoke a strong immune response – a central feature of autoimmune disease and allergy.

Flatulence

Bacteria produce about 1 litre of nitrogen, hydrogen and CO$_2$ each day as a by-product of the fermentation process, which leaves the body as flatus. Depending on what foodstuffs reach them, methane, ammonia and hydrogen sulphide will also be produced causing the flatus to smell.

> **Alteration of intestinal microbiota may result in serious illness.** Antibiotics used to treat other infections (e.g. respiratory) also kill normal colonic bacteria. An absence of flora allows the proliferation of potentially pathogenic bacteria (e.g. *Clostridium difficile*) causing diarrhoea or invasive infection.

Answers to starter questions

1. The stomach produces hydrochloric acid with a pH of 2. However, the sensitive gastric epithelium is not damaged because of the presence of mucus. Goblet cells in the stomach lining secrete alkaline, viscous mucus in response to prostaglandin E. The acid is unable to penetrate the mucus which protects the epithelial cells. Mucus and acid production are linked; so when levels of acid rise, mucus secretion does too.

2. There are more bacteria within the colon than cells in the body. These bacteria form the microbiota, or 'flora', of the intestine, which is needed for normal processing of food and gut secretions, formation of stool and to prevent growth of pathogenic bacteria. Antibiotic therapy may kill these normal bacteria, allowing harmful bacteria that cause diarrhoea (or invasive infection) to multiply.

3. Flatulence can be due to either physiological or pathological causes (e.g. inflammatory bowel disease or gluten intolerance). Normal flatulence is due to the fermentation of carbohydrates in the colon, which produce a mixture of oxygen, carbon dioxide and hydrogen gas. Enzymes in the colon's bacterial flora catalyse this fermentation.

4. Diarrhoea is caused either by a change in luminal contents or by an increase in intestinal motility. Anxiety and fear increase parasympathetic innervation of the intestine resulting in increased motility. This decreases the time for absorbing water, resulting in diarrhoea.

5. During prolonged fasting the body's fat stores are broken down, producing an excess of acetyl-CoA. Acetyl-CoA is converted to ketone bodies which, when dissolved, form keto-acids. These can be used as an energy source for the brain but also reduce blood pH.

6. Being sick (vomiting) or feeling sick (nausea) occurs when there is activation of the vomiting centre in the medulla. The vomiting centre can be activated by strong emotions, sight or smells, disturbances in the inner ear or by the chemoreceptor trigger zone (CTZ). The CTZ responds to circulating drugs and hormones, which is why we feel sick with certain medications (e.g. opiates) or if there is damage to, or irritation of, the stomach or small intestine.

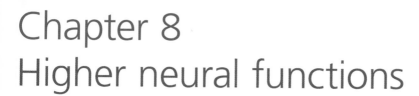

Chapter 8
Higher neural functions

Starter questions

Answers to the following questions are on page 268.

1. Why do some stimuli cause sharp pains and some cause burning pains?
2. Why can we not see in colour in low light?
3. How are memories stored?
4. What makes us dizzy after we spin around?
5. How is anger controlled?

Introduction

The central nervous system, which comprises the brain and the spinal cord, is the most complex part of the body. It is responsible for the automatic functions essential for life, such as breathing and digestion. It also controls the higher neural functions, i.e. those that enable people to sense their bodies and their environment and to interpret and respond to their experiences.

This chapter starts with an overview of perception, followed by descriptions of the sensory systems responsible for sight, hearing, balance, taste and smell. The perception of pain by the somatosensory system is then discussed; this warrants particular attention because of its importance in clinical care. Next, the roles of the main parts of the brain associated with higher neural functions are described. Consciousness is discussed separately, because it is an elusive phenomenon arising from several areas of the brain and is altered in clinical care (e.g. in anaesthesia)

Case 8 Seizure

Presentation

Alan, aged 27 years, is found unconscious on the floor by his mother. When she arrives, his arms and legs appear stiff and are making jerking movements. Alan's face looks blue and he has been urine incontinent.

After 3–4 min, the twitching stops but Alan is very drowsy. He is only semi-conscious for the next few hours; he does not remember being in the ambulance and is unable to recognise his mother.

Analysis

Alan's mother has provided a classic description of a tonic–clonic seizure followed by a post-ictal state. This type of seizure starts with the tonic phase: the muscles stiffen and consciousness is lost, typically causing the patient to fall to the ground, and they may become cyanosed. The tonic phase is followed by the clonic phase: all four limbs make rapid, symmetrical flexion–extension movements, usually over 1–3 min.

As the patient's movements stop, bladder or bowel control may be lost as their muscles relax. The seizure is immediately followed by a period of diminished or altered consciousness lasting up to 2–6 hours.

A seizure is the clinical manifestation of abnormal, excessive cortical depolarisation. Consciousness is lost because of widespread dysfunction in the cerebral cortex, and often also in the relay of information from the thalamus to the cortex (the thalamocortical relay). Seizures can be precipitated by certain factors (e.g. low levels of sodium), or they may be unprovoked.

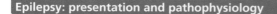

Epilepsy: presentation and pathophysiology

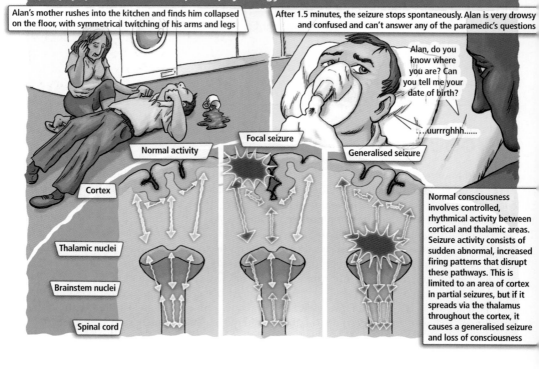

Alan's mother rushes into the kitchen and finds him collapsed on the floor, with symmetrical twitching of his arms and legs

After 1.5 minutes, the seizure stops spontaneously. Alan is very drowsy and confused and can't answer any of the paramedic's questions

Alan, do you know where you are? Can you tell me your date of birth?

....uurrrghhh......

Focal seizure

Generalised seizure

Normal activity

Cortex

Thalamic nuclei

Brainstem nuclei

Spinal cord

Normal consciousness involves controlled, rhythmical activity between cortical and thalamic areas. Seizure activity consists of sudden abnormal, increased firing patterns that disrupt these pathways. This is limited to an area of cortex in partial seizures, but if it spreads via the thalamus throughout the cortex, it causes a generalised seizure and loss of consciousness

Most seizures self-terminate, as in this case. However, if they continue for > 10 min, a rapidly acting depressant of the central nervous system (e.g. lorazepam) is given. This is the standard first-line treatment for status epilepticus. A prolonged tonic–clonic seizure (convulsive status epilepticus) can reduce oxygen supply to the brain and thus cause brain damage or death.

Further case

The results of blood tests and a computerised tomography scan of Alan's head are all normal. He is discharged from hospital and advised not to drive for 6 months. This requirement is highly inconvenient because he is a journalist.

The next week, Alan has a similar attack while at work after staying up late the previous night to finish a report. He is advised to avoid sleep deprivation, as well as the consumption of excessive amounts of alcohol.

Further analysis

Epilepsy is a tendency towards recurrent, stereotyped (similar), unprovoked seizures. Alan has had two seizures without a clear cause, so it is now reasonable to prescribe antiepileptic medication.

Antiepileptic agents are use-dependent neuronal blockers (the most active channels are inhibited first); most such drugs (e.g. valproate) block fast voltage-gated sodium channels to inhibit the propagation of action potentials. Patients are warned that sleep deprivation and alcohol withdrawal may provoke seizures. It is essential that patients at risk of further seizures do not drive, because driving would imperil not only their lives but also those of other people.

Perception: an overview

Perception can be defined as the ability to become aware of something through the senses. The body's sensory systems convert internal and external information into electrical signals that are sent to the brain. The brain then interprets the information and coordinates a response.

This chapter focuses on the sensory systems responsible for the sensations of sight, hearing, balance, taste and smell:

- The visual system is responsible for sight
- The auditory and vestibular systems, which are closely related, enable hearing and the maintenance of balance, respectively
- The gustatory and olfactory systems, again closely related, are responsible for taste and smell, respectively

Information on all stimuli, other than those detected by these five sensory systems, is transmitted to the brain through the somatosensory system. Receptors for somatosensory stimuli are distributed throughout the body, and different types of somatosensory receptor respond to a wide range of stimuli, including touch, pressure, temperature, proprioception and pain. In this chapter, special attention is paid to the perception of pain by the somatosensory system.

Each of the body's sensory systems has the following elements:

- **sensory receptors** to detect an internal or external stimulus and transduce it, i.e. turn the stimulus into an electrical signal that may or may not be propagated
- **neural pathways** to convey the signal through afferent neurones (usually two or three) to the brain
- **specific parts of the brain responsible for processing** the sensory information and coordinating the body's response

Sensory receptors

Sensory receptors are almost always specific for a particular stimulus. However, some are polymodal and may be activated by a few different stimuli.

Transduction occurs when activation of a sensory receptor causes a localised increase in its membrane potential, termed the receptor potential. The magnitude of this change depends on the intensity of the stimulus: the greater the stimulus, the greater the change in membrane potential. Receptor potentials can summate (spatially or temporally) or decay over time. If the increase in membrane potential reaches the threshold for triggering an action potential (see page 42), this electrical signal is propagated along the primary afferent neurone.

■ The **intensity** of a stimulus is coded by the frequency of action potentials in the afferent neurone; this is known as the 'frequency code'.
■ The **modality** of the sensation (e.g. pain or light touch) is coded by the afferent neurone; this is the 'line code' (each afferent neurone only ever conveys one modality, which allows the brain to recognise the sensation)

Receptors adapt slowly or rapidly depending on whether they are able to detect changes in the intensity, duration or rate of change of a stimulus (**Figure 8.1**).

■ **Rapidly adapting receptors** are activated by a change in the stimulus; however, they stop responding to a continuously applied stimulus and have minimal ability to determine stimulus intensity
■ **Slowly adapting receptors** do not respond as quickly as rapidly adapting receptors, but they code intensity well and remain activated for the duration of the stimulus

The skin contains several highly specialised sensory receptors (**Table 8.1**).

Neural pathways

The key somatosensory neural pathways are:

■ the spinothalamic pathway
■ the dorsal column pathway
■ the spinocerebellar pathway

Cutaneous receptors in the skin		
Receptor	Adaptation rate	Modality or modalities
Pacinian corpuscle	Rapid	Vibration and pressure
Meissner's corpuscle	Rapid	Vibration and pressure
Merkel's disc	Slow	Pressure and vibration (low frequency)
Ruffini's endings	Slow	Pressure (fingertips)
Free nerve endings	Rapid or slow	Pain and temperature

Table 8.1 The five main sensory receptors in the skin, their modalities and their rate of adaptation

Figure 8.1 Slowly adapting receptors show a graded response relative to stimulus intensity, whereas rapidly adapting receptors show a marked response to a change in the stimulus but do not continue to fire if the stimulus is maintained.

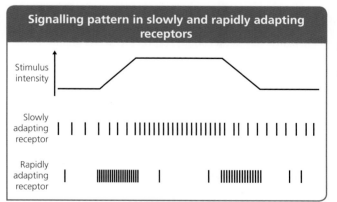

The spinothalamic pathway

This is a somatic sensory pathway that conveys fine touch (i.e. touch in a small area, e.g. 1–2 mm) pain and temperature. It is the only pathway for pain (and temperature); there is overlap with the dorsal column pathway for touch.

In the spinothalamic pathway, signals travel along three neurones (**Figure 8.2a**). The cell body of the primary afferent neurone is in the dorsal root ganglion; its axon runs from the peripheral receptor into the dorsal horn of the spinal cord. Before the primary afferent enters the dorsal horn, it ascends or descends a couple of spinal segments in the tract of Lissauer, which lies just peripheral to the dorsal horn (**Figure 8.3**).

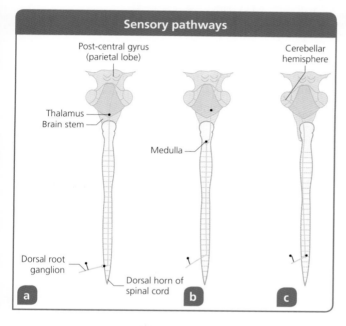

Sensory pathways

Post-central gyrus (parietal lobe)

Cerebellar hemisphere

Thalamus
Brain stem

Medulla

Dorsal root ganglion

Dorsal horn of spinal cord

a   b   c

Figure 8.2 The key somatosensory pathways. (a) Spinothalamic pathway. (b) Dorsal column pathway. (c) Spinocerebellar pathway.

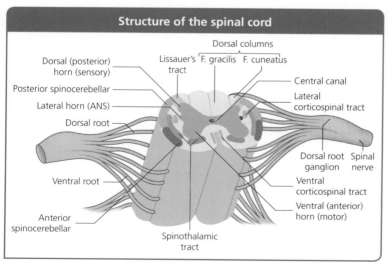

Structure of the spinal cord

Dorsal columns

Dorsal (posterior) horn (sensory)

Lissauer's tract   F. gracilis   F. cuneatus

Posterior spinocerebellar

Lateral horn (ANS)

Dorsal root

Central canal

Lateral corticospinal tract

Dorsal root ganglion   Spinal nerve

Ventral root

Ventral corticospinal tract

Ventral (anterior) horn (motor)

Anterior spinocerebellar

Spinothalamic tract

Figure 8.3 General structure of the spinal cord, with the major sensory tracts on the left and motor tracts on the right (both are present bilaterally).

The primary afferent synapses on to a second-order neurone, whose cell body is in the dorsal horn. The axon of this neurone crosses (decussates) to the contralateral side of the spinal cord through the white commissure; it then ascends to the thalamus, where it synapses. The third-order neurone runs from the thalamus to the post-central gyrus of the parietal lobe, the primary sensory cortex.

> **Dissociative sensory loss is the marked loss of some modalities with the preservation of others.** For example, in syringomyelia, expansion of the central canal in the brain stem and spinal cord compresses the spinothalamic pathway more than the dorsal columns. Patients lose their perception of pain and temperature but remain able to sense vibration and position and movement of their body.

The dorsal column pathway

This somatic pathway conveys information related to proprioception, vibration and two-point discrimination (the ability to distinguish between two stimuli that are close to each other), as well as some information on touch.

As in the spinothalamic pathway, signals travel along the dorsal column pathway across three neurones (**Figure 8.2b**), and the cell body of the first-order neurone is in the dorsal root ganglion. However, the primary afferent neurone ascends ipsilaterally (on the same side of the CNS) in the dorsal columns up to the medulla before synapsing with the second-order neurone The dorsal columns consist of the medial fasciculus gracilis and the lateral fasciculus cuneatus, which convey sensory information from the lower limbs and the upper half of the body, respectively.

The second-order neurone decussates at the level of the pons before ascending to the thalamus, where is synapses. The third-order neurone projects to the post-central gyrus.

The spinocerebellar pathway

This pathway mediates proprioception that is predominantly subconscious. It is involved in axial positioning and truncal stability. In contrast, the proprioception mediated by the dorsal columns is for fine movement of the limbs and digits.

The spinocerebellar pathway also differs from the dorsal column and spinothalamic pathway in that it comprises two neurones, and these remain ipsilateral (**Figure 8.2c**). The cell body of the primary afferent neurone is in the dorsal root ganglion; it synapses in Clarke's column in the dorsal horn. The second-order neurone ascends, without decussation, up to the cerebellum.

> **Damage to part of the spinal cord affects certain functions more than others, because of the distribution of tracts.** For example, injury of the posterior part of the spinal cord affects the dorsal columns, so patients experience a loss of vibration, proprioception and two-point discrimination below the level of the lesion.

The visual system

The sensory system responsible for vision enables a person's brain to form a mental representation of the world around them. An understanding of vision is vital to comprehension of the many pathologies that affect it, especially as loss of vision is highly debilitating.

Structure of the eye

The eye is a spheroid structure filled with aqueous humour anterior to the lens, and vitreous humour posterior to it (**Figure 8.4**). The aqueous humour is secreted into the posterior chamber (the space between the

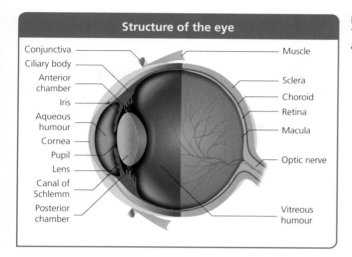

Structure of the eye

Conjunctiva
Ciliary body
Anterior chamber
Iris
Aqueous humour
Cornea
Pupil
Lens
Canal of Schlemm
Posterior chamber

Muscle
Sclera
Choroid
Retina
Macula
Optic nerve
Vitreous humour

Figure 8.4 Structure of the eye. The lens divides the eye into anterior and posterior chambers.

lens and the pupil) by the epithelium of the ciliary body. It passes through the pupil into the anterior chamber, and is then absorbed by passing into the canal of Schlemm. Once absorbed, it is able to enter the venous circulation.

The continuous production of aqueous humour maintains the pressure within the eye. However, if the drainage system becomes blocked, this intraocular pressure increases, which causes glaucoma.

Glaucoma is caused by increased intraocular pressure in the anterior chamber. The condition results from increased production and reduced drainage of aqueous humour. The increased pressure progressively damages the head of the optic nerve; the peripheral retinal fibres are affected first. The visual fields are greatly restricted before the patient becomes aware of any loss of vision. Eye drops are used to reduce aqueous production and increase outflow, and laser surgery is used to promote drainage in severe cases. Untreated glaucoma can lead to irreversible blindness.

Iris

The iris is an extension of the ciliary body. It contains muscle fibres arranged circularly and radially.

Sclera, cornea and conjunctiva

The external covering of the eye is the sclera, an opaque layer of connective tissue. At the front of the eye is the cornea, the specialised transparent region over the iris and pupil; this is covered by the conjunctiva, a thin layer of epithelium. There are no blood vessels carrying nutrients to this region, so it relies on diffusion of material carried in the aqueous humour and the tear film.

Lens

The lens is formed from multiple layers of clear epithelial cells, which synthesise proteins (crystallin) that help increase the density and transparency of the lens. It is surrounded by a suspensory ligament, which connects it to the ciliary muscles.

Retina

The retina consists of layers (**Figure 8.5**). A vascular supportive layer (the choroid) lies just inside the sclera. Above the choroid are the photoreceptors (rods and cones); these two classic types of photosensitive cell differ both structurally and functionally (**Table 8.2**).

The distribution of photoreceptors varies from the periphery of the retina to its centre (**Figure 8.6**).

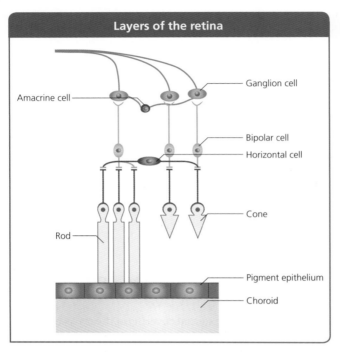

Figure 8.5 Layers of the retina. Photoreceptors lie deep to the ganglion cells and bipolar cells.

Photoreceptors		
Characteristic	Rods	Cones
Types	One type	Red, green and blue
Distribution	Peripheral retina	Macula and fovea
Connection with ganglion cells	Many rods to one ganglion cell	One cone to one ganglion cell
Photopigment	Rhodopsin (one type) at high density on intracellular discs	Photopsin (three types for colour) at lower density on membrane invaginations
Acuity	Low	High
Sensitivity	High	Low

Table 8.2 Comparison of the two kinds of photoreceptor: rods and cones.

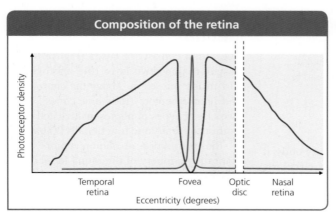

Figure 8.6 Composition of the retina. The periphery of the retina is formed of rods, which decrease in number towards the macula. At the fovea, there are only cones.

- **The periphery** is composed predominantly of rods
- **The macula** (the central retina) consists mainly of cones
- **The fovea** (the central macula) contains only cones

Above the photoreceptors are the layers of ganglion cells and amacrine cells. Ganglion cells are the only neurones in the retina.

The optic disc is the point where the optic nerve (cranial nerve II) is formed from the axons of ganglion cells as they pass through the retina. This is the blind spot, because it is devoid of photoreceptors.

Mechanism of vision

Refraction, the deflection of light as it passes through a medium or into another medium, occurs as light passes into and through the eye. At the front of the eye, light is refracted at the interface between the air in the environment and the tears (essentially water) on the corneal surface. Further refraction occurs as it passes through the lens.

This refraction helps focus light on to the retina, which contains the photoreceptors. Contraction of the ciliary muscles alters the shape of the lens so that the light rays converge on the macula.

Photoreception

At the retina, light passes through the layer of ganglion and amacrine cells to reach the photoreceptors.

All photoreceptors have the following elements, which enable them to transduce particles of light (photons) into an electrical signal (**Figure 8.7**):

- **an outer segment** containing membrane-bound photopigment (pigments that undergo a chemical change when they absorb light)
- **an inner segment** containing the nucleus and densely packed with mitochondria
- **a synaptic terminal** for communication with bipolar cells

Photoreceptors are able to depolarise or hyperpolarise, and to release neurotransmit-

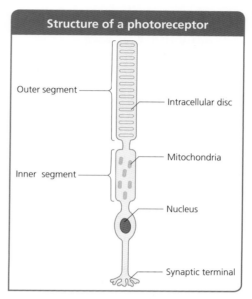

Structure of a photoreceptor

Outer segment

Intracellular disc

Inner segment

Mitochondria

Nucleus

Synaptic terminal

Figure 8.7 General structure of a photoreceptor. The outer segment contains membrane-bound photopigment. The photoreceptor has a high density of mitochondria because of its high energy requirement.

ter (usually glutamate) in response, but they cannot fire an action potential.

Rods

These are highly sensitive photoreceptors that transduce even at low light intensity. Rods contain a large amount of rhodopsin (their photopigment) packed into intracellular membrane discs.

Rods provide limited acuity; multiple rods converge on a single bipolar cell (see **Figure 8.5**), so the ganglion cell supplied by this bipolar cell receives information from a large area of retina. In compensation, rods produce a signal even in very low light. A single photon may be enough to produce a signal from a rod, and fewer than 10 photons are needed to sense light.

All rods respond identically to different wavelengths of light, therefore they simply differentiate between light and dark. This property manifests as black-and-white vision at low levels of light, for example at night. In daytime, much of the colour in our peripheral vision is a projection of the brain.

Retinitis pigmentosa is a group of conditions characterised by progressive loss of vision from a young age. Retinitis pigmentosa causes photoreceptor (particularly rod) degeneration and optic nerve damage. Visual impairment classically begins with night blindness from the loss of rods progressing to profound impairment, with a pigmented, damaged retina in advanced stages.

Cones

Cones contain less photopigment than rods, and they have a one-to-one relationship with bipolar cells. Therefore a higher light intensity is required to facilitate signalling. However, cones are high-acuity photoreceptors, because they transduce light from a small area of retina.

The three types of cone contain different variants of rhodopsin, which respond preferentially to light of different wavelengths in the approximate red, green and blue ranges. The brain integrates information from the cones to enable the perception of colour.

Phototransduction

Photoreceptors are unusual in that they are depolarised and release neurotransmitter in the absence of a signal (i.e. light). This is because open cyclic guanosine monophosphate (cGMP)-gated cation channels in the outer segment permit the entry of sodium ions (Na^+) (**Figure 8.8**). Na^+ entry increases the membrane potential to about -40 mV and enables the release of neurotransmitter from the synaptic terminal. A low cytosolic Na^+ concentration is maintained by Na^+/K^+ ATPase, mainly in the inner segment; this turnover leads to the 'dark current' (depolarising influx of Na^+ when in the dark) flowing through these cells.

Activation by light of photopigment in the photoreceptors triggers a secondary messenger cascade through the G-protein transducin. This increases the activity of a phosphodiesterase, which catalyses the breakdown of cGMP to 5'-GMP. The consequent decrease in cGMP concentration closes the cGMP-gated channels and thus hyperpolarises the cell. This, in turn, reduces neurotransmitter release from the photoreceptor.

Retinal processing

All photoreceptors, but not all bipolar cells and ganglion cells, hyperpolarise in response to light. Bipolar and ganglion cells are termed ON cells if they depolarise in the light, and OFF cells if they hyperpolarise in the light. ON bipolar cells from synapses with ON ganglion cells and OFF bipolar cells synapse with OFF ganglion cells. Whether bipolar and ganglion cells are ON or OFF cells is mediated by differences at the photoreceptor–bipolar cell synapse.

Almost all photoreceptors release glutamate. In response, OFF bipolar cells normally depolarise, and ON bipolar cells hyperpolarise.

The two types of cell help differentiate areas of light and dark (**Figure 8.9**).

- **ON** ganglion cells fire most rapidly when they are in light and the surrounding area is dark
- **OFF** ganglion cells have a high action potential frequency when they are in the dark and the surrounding area is light

These differences are mediated by different subtypes of receptor and different neurotransmitters. Further integration and processing occur in the retina, mediated by amacrine and horizontal cells.

Visual fields

The visual field is divided into two areas:

- **a central area** (the nasal field) of binocular vision
- **a peripheral area** (the temporal field), which is monocular because only one eye receives input from it

The image formed on the retina is reversed and inverted as it passes through the lens. Consequently, the temporal visual field is supplied by the nasal retina, and the nasal field is supplied by the temporal retina (**Figure 8.10**).

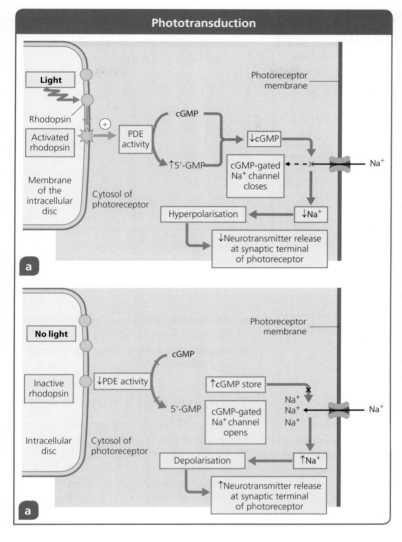

Phototransduction

Light

Photoreceptor membrane

Rhodopsin

Activated rhodopsin

PDE activity

cGMP

↑5'-GMP

↓cGMP

cGMP-gated Na⁺ channel closes

Na⁺

Membrane of the intracellular disc

Cytosol of photoreceptor

Hyperpolarisation

↓Na⁺

↓Neurotransmitter release at synaptic terminal of photoreceptor

a

No light

Photoreceptor membrane

Inactive rhodopsin

↓PDE activity

cGMP

↑cGMP store

5'-GMP

cGMP-gated Na⁺ channel opens

Na⁺
Na⁺
Na⁺

Na⁺

Intracellular disc

Cytosol of photoreceptor

Depolarisation

↑Na⁺

↑Neurotransmitter release at synaptic terminal of photoreceptor

a

Figure 8.8
Phototransduction is mediated by closure of cyclic guanosine monophosphate (cGMP)-gated sodium and calcium channels in response to light, which hyperpolarises photoreceptors. (a) In the presence of light, PDE is activated causing a fall in the levels of cGMP and closure of cation channels. The resulting hyperpolarisation reduces neurotransmitter release. (b) In the dark, high intracellular cGMP allows cation channels to remain open. The membrane is depolarised and neurotransmitter is released. PDE, phosphodiesterase.

A visual field defect is the loss of sight from damage to any part of the visual system. Lesions before the optic chiasm cause uniocular defects, and lesions after the optic chiasm cause contralateral field loss. A lesion of the optic chiasm itself damages the decussating fibres from the nasal retina, resulting in bilateral loss of the temporal visual fields. This is usually the result of compression of the superior chiasm by benign pituitary tumours (adenomas).

The central visual pathway

The centrally projecting axons of ganglion cells form the optic nerves. The optic nerves have a purely sensory role, relaying visual information from the retina to the brain. The left and right optic nerves communicate at the optic chiasm, just anterior and superior to the pituitary gland. Here, the fibres from the nasal retina decussate, bringing together information from both eyes for each part of the visual field.

From the optic chiasm, fibres pass to the lateral geniculate nucleus (of the thalamus) as

Retinal processing by bipolar and ganglion cells

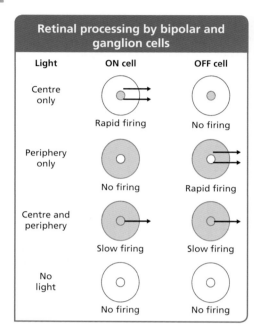

Figure 8.9 Retinal processing by ON and OFF bipolar and ganglion cells (which function together). Firing frequency is determined by whether light is at the centre or the periphery of the ganglion cell.

Visual fields and the central visual pathway

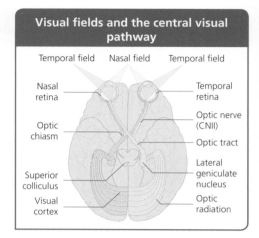

Figure 8.10 The visual fields and central visual pathway. There is monocular vision to the temporal visual fields from the nasal retina, and fibres from here cross at the optic chiasm.

the optic tract. Branches of these optic tract fibres send signals to the hypothalamus for the regulation of circadian rhythm, the changes in biological processes that occur over roughly 24-h periods correlating with the natural cycle of light and dark.

Fibres in the lateral geniculate nucleus pass to the primary visual cortex in the occipital lobe; this arrangement is called the optic radiation. The left visual cortex receives information from both eyes about the right visual field, and vice versa.

Branches from the lateral geniculate nucleus also run to two structures in the midbrain:

- **the superior colliculus** (their signals are used for the control of head movement)
- **the pretectal nucleus** (for the pupillary light reflex)

Conjugate eye movements

Movement of the eye is controlled by interactions between cranial nerves III, IV and VI, which innervate the extraocular muscles (Table 8.3).

Control of these nerves depends on the type of eye movement, i.e. saccades, smooth pursuit, vergence or vestibulo-ocular. Bilateral connections enable conjugate eye movements, so that the eyes move together while keeping an image fixed on both retinas.

Looking right requires activation of cranial nerve VI (supplying lateral rectus) for the right eye, and activation of cranial nerve III

Cranial nerves controlling extraocular muscles		
Nerve	Muscles innervated	Eye movement(s)
III (oculomotor)	Medial rectus, inferior rectus, superior rectus, inferior oblique and levator palpebrae superioris	Adduction, up-gaze, down-gaze and up-gaze when abducted and opening of the eyelid
IV (trochlear)	Superior oblique	Down-gaze when abducted
VI (abducens)	Lateral rectus	Abduction

Table 8.3 The three cranial nerves that interact to control the muscles of eye movement

activation (supplying medial rectus) on the left. Conversely, looking left requires activation of cranial nerve III for the right eye and activation of cranial nerve VI for the left eye. A key structure facilitating such movements is the median longitudinal fasciculus, which runs through the brain stem and connects the ocular muscle nuclei.

> **A 57-year-old man presents to the emergency department with sudden right-sided weakness, loss of the visual field on his right side and difficulty speaking.** A computerised tomography scan shows a large infarction in the territory of his left middle cerebral artery.
>
> Stroke is characterised by sudden loss of neurological function as a consequence of a vascular event. Most strokes are ischaemic, caused by thrombosis in situ or embolisation of a thrombus; however, they may also be haemorrhagic. Clinical features correlate with the region of brain affected. In this case, this patient has lost function of the area of cerebral cortex supplied by the left middle cerebral artery, including Broca's area and the optic tract. Loss of function in these areas produces aphasia and homonymous hemianopia, respectively.

Ocular reflexes

A reflex is an automatic reaction of a body in response to a stimulus. For normal sight, there are four key reflexes involved, as described below. These all abide by the principles of reflexes described in Chapter 2.

Pupillary light and accommodation reflexes

The amount of light entering the eye is regulated by changes to the diameter of the pupil. This process is mediated by contraction and relaxation of two muscles in the iris:

- **constrictor pupillae** (supplied by parasympathetic fibres in cranial nerve III)
- **dilator pupillae** (supplied by sympathetic fibres in the ophthalmic division of cranial nerve V)

Constriction of the pupil in response to an increase in light intensity is mediated by an increase in parasympathetic activity and a reduction in sympathetic activity. Conversely, dilation in response to low light intensity is mediated by a decrease in parasympathetic activity and an increase in sympathetic activity.

The afferent limb of the pupillary light reflex is the optic nerve, and the efferent limb is a bilateral response through cranial nerve III (the oculomotor nerve). Consequently, when light is shone in the right eye, for example, the pupils of both the right eye and the left eye constrict (as a result of the direct reflex and the consensual reflex, respectively).

The accommodation reflex is ciliary muscle contraction and bilateral pupil constriction that occur during convergence (focusing on a near object). The reflex is initiated by signals from afferent fibre in the optic nerve, which pass to the occipital cortex. These signals cause cranial nerve III and Edinger–Westphal nuclei (the centre for parasympathetic supply to the eye) to activate medial rectus and constrictor pupillae.

The light and accommodation reflexes can become separated in cases of serious central nervous system damage or disease. In such cases, patients may have what is termed an Argyll Robertson pupil, which responds to accommodation but not to light.

> **Relative afferent pupillary defects occur in patients with unilateral optic nerve damage.** When a light is shone into the unaffected eye, the consensual light reflex causes the affected eye to constrict. If the light is quickly moved to the affected eye, the affected eye continues to dilate because the afferent optic nerve is damaged (e.g. from optic neuritis). The absence of light from the opposite eye (the consensual reflex) is detected as a stronger stimulus than the direct light reflex of the affected eye.

Corneal reflex

In this reflex, stimulation of the cornea causes the eyelid to close. This reflex arc has an afferent limb through cranial nerve V (the ophthalmic branch), with a unilateral cranial nerve VII (facial nerve) efferent branch to supply orbicularis oculi.

Vestibulo-ocular reflex

This reflex allows gaze to be fixed on an object while the head turns, without the object blurring or the image being displaced from the retina. The head movement is transduced by the semicircular canals (in the vestibular system), which signal to the vestibular nuclei in the brain stem (see page 255). Bilateral connections to the nuclei for cranial nerves III and VI ensure that turning the head to the left, for example, results in left eye medial rectus activation and right eye lateral rectus activation.

The auditory and vestibular systems

Hearing and the ability to maintain balance warrant detailed discussion because they are affected by a variety of pathologies throughout life, for example as a result of infection or as adverse effects of certain drugs. Damage causes significant functional impairment.

Structure of the ear

The ear is divided into outer, middle and inner segments (**Figure 8.11**).

Outer ear

The outer ear is formed from the elastic cartilage auricle. It is connected to the middle ear by the external acoustic meatus (the ear canal). Like the auricle, the first part of the external acoustic meatus also consists of cartilage, but it soon becomes part of the temporal bone at the side of the skull. The external acoustic meatus ends at the tympanic membrane (eardrum), which marks the start of the middle ear.

Middle ear

The middle ear is an air-filled bony chamber that contains the three ossicle bones:

- **the malleus,** which sits on the tympanic membrane
- **the incus,** connecting the malleus and the stapes
- **the stapes,** which is attached to the oval window (the entrance to the cochlea)

The muscles tensor tympani (supplied by cranial nerve V) and stapedius (supplied by cranial nerve VII) insert on to the ossicles.

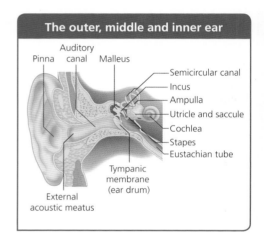

The outer, middle and inner ear

Pinna — Auditory canal — Malleus — Semicircular canal — Incus — Ampulla — Utricle and saccule — Cochlea — Stapes — Eustachian tube — Tympanic membrane (ear drum) — External acoustic meatus

Figure 8.11 Anatomy of the outer, middle and inner ear.

The middle ear is kept at atmospheric pressure through its communication with the nasopharynx, i.e. the pharyngotympanic tubule (Eustachian tube).

Otosclerosis is an autosomal dominant condition with incomplete penetrance in which conductive hearing loss develops from fusion of the ossicle bones. In particular, the foot of the stapes becomes fused to the oval window; this prevents the normal amplification of sounds through the middle ear and limits movement of the oval window. Hearing aid implants provide some benefit to patients with otosclerosis.

The inner ear

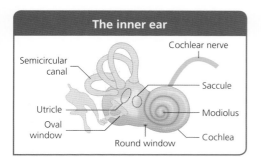

Figure 8.12 Anatomy of the inner ear.

Inner ear

The inner ear is a fluid-filled bony chamber with several compartments (**Figure 8.12**). It contains the cochlea, a helical bony canal consisting of three fluid-filled channels separated by membranes:

- the scala media
- the scala tympani
- the scala vestibuli

Figure 8.13 shows a cross-section through an 'unwound' cochlea. The scala vestibuli and scala tympani both contain perilymph, a fluid similar to tissue fluid, and communicate with each other at the cochlea's apex through the helicotrema. In contrast, the scala media contains endolymph, a fluid with an extremely high concentration of potassium (about 150 mmol/L) and secreted by the stria vascularis (capillaries in the wall of the scala media)

On the basilar membrane, which separates the scala tympani and the scala media, sits the organ of Corti. This contains highly specialised hair cells. The hair cells have stereocilia that project upwards and into the tectorial membrane, a relatively fixed structure in the scala vestibuli.

The vestibule contains the utricle and saccule, i.e. the otolith organs, which are surrounded by fluid. The three semicircular canals communicate with the vestibule.

The cochlear nerve enters at the modiolus, which lies at the centre of the cochlea.

Semicircular canals

These are three bony canals filled with endolymph that sit at right angles to each other. Each has an area of dilation, the ampulla, which contains a group of hair cells; these hair cells lie on a ridge termed the crista (**Figure 8.14**). The hair cells have stereocilia covered in a gelatinous projection called the cupula.

Otolith organs

The utricle and saccule are specialised regions of hair cells in the vestibule of the inner ear. They are innervated by the vestibular nerve.

The otolith organs are composed of hair cells with stereocilia, similar to those in the organ of Corti (**Figure 8.15**). However, the stereocilia in the utricle and saccule are encased in a gelatinous cap topped with otoliths (calcium crystals).

Cochlea: cross-section

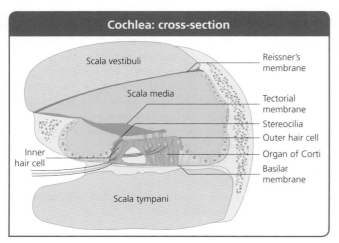

Figure 8.13 Cross-section through (an unwound) cochlea, showing the three fluid-filled channels and the organ of Corti (the site of sound transduction), which sits on the basilar membrane.

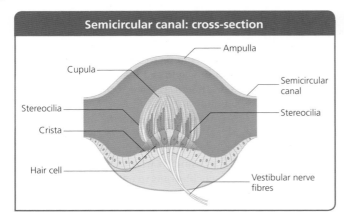

Semicircular canal: cross-section

- Ampulla
- Cupula
- Semicircular canal
- Stereocilia
- Stereocilia
- Crista
- Hair cell
- Vestibular nerve fibres

Figure 8.14 Cross-section through part of a semicircular canal, showing the site of transduction of rotation. The cupula moves in response to endolymph flow through the canal, which activates vestibular nerve afferents.

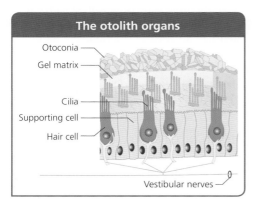

The otolith organs

- Otoconia
- Gel matrix
- Cilia
- Supporting cell
- Hair cell
- Vestibular nerves

Figure 8.15 Microanatomy of the otolith organs (the utricle and saccule).

Mechanism of hearing

First, the elastic cartilage auricle of the outer ear funnels sound (as vibrations of the air) into the external acoustic meatus. The sound then travels along the auditory canal, and the tympanic membrane vibrates in response.

The function of the ossicles is to amplify and focus vibrations of the larger tympanic membrane, which responds to movement of the air, on to the smaller oval window, which is backed by fluid. The malleus moves when the tympanic membrane moves, thus transmitting vibrations through the incus to the stapes. Movement of the stapes on the oval window causes vibrations of the fluid in the scala vestibuli of the cochlea. These are transmitted to the scala tympani at the helicotrema, which communicates with the round window. The round window has no direct external contacts, but it facilitates movement in the scala tympani.

The volume of sound is regulated by tensor tympani and stapedius. Contraction of these muscles reduces ossicle vibration and therefore lowers the volume.

Vibrations in the scala vestibuli and scala tympani are transmitted to the scala media through Reissner's membrane and the basilar membrane. This causes the specialised hair cells in the organ of Corti to move in response to the transmitted vibrations. The tips of the stereocilia are fixed in position at the tectorial membrane, which results in bending between the stereocilia and the hair cells as the structures move.

Transduction occurs when mechanically gated potassium channels on the stereocilia open with their movement. Because of the high potassium concentration in endolymph, potassium ions (K^+) enter the hair cells along the electrochemical gradient. The resulting depolarisation causes the release of glutamate from the basal end of the hair cells. The released glutamate then stimulates afferent fibres in the cochlear nerve.

There are two kinds of hair cell: inner and outer.

- The single row of inner hair cells transduces sound
- The three rows of outer hair cells help amplify sound

Pitch is coded by the resistance of the basilar membrane. At the apex, it is wide and flexible, enabling maximum vibration at low-frequency sounds; the converse is true for the base.

The central auditory pathway

Auditory stimuli are processed bilaterally. Primary afferent neurones in the cochlear nerve synapse in the cochlear nuclei in the medulla (**Figure 8.16**). Most fibres then cross to the contralateral inferior colliculus, where the fibres synapse. However, some fibres remain ipsilateral.

The inferior colliculus projects to the medial geniculate nucleus of the thalamus. It then passes to the primary auditory cortex, present bilaterally on the superior temporal lobe. This bilateral input is used to localise sound by comparing signals from the left and right ear.

Mechanism of balance

When the position of the head changes, the otoliths and the gelatinous cap that encases them move with gravity, pulling the stereocilia of the inner ear with them. The otolith organs are also surrounded by high K^+ concentration endolymph, so they depolarise in response to K^+ entry, thus activating the vestibular nerve.

In response to rotation, endolymph moves in the semicircular canals and displaces the cupula. This moves the stereocilia of the hair cells, thereby opening mechanically gated potassium channels and depolarising these cells.

Central processing of balance

The vestibular nerve synapses on the ipsilateral vestibular nuclei in the brain stem. The brain stem then communicates with other regions:

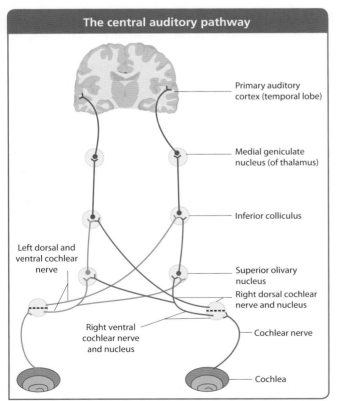

The central auditory pathway

- Primary auditory cortex (temporal lobe)
- Medial geniculate nucleus (of thalamus)
- Inferior colliculus
- Left dorsal and ventral cochlear nerve
- Superior olivary nucleus
- Right dorsal cochlear nerve and nucleus
- Right ventral cochlear nerve and nucleus
- Cochlear nerve
- Cochlea

Figure 8.16 The central auditory pathway. The ventral cochlear nerve provides bilateral connections at the superior olivary nucleus.

- oculomotor (cranial nerve III) and abducens (cranial nerve VI) nuclei, through the medial longitudinal fasciculus, for the vestibulo-ocular reflex, which allows the eyes to track an object as the head moves
- the cerebellum, for integration with ascending proprioceptive signals
- the upper cervical spinal cord, to control head movement in response to gravity

> **Benign positional paroxysmal vertigo is a common and potentially disabling condition characterised by short-lived periods of severe vertigo with nausea.** These episodes are often precipitated by head movement, such as when rolling over in bed. Benign positional paroxysmal vertigo occurs when calcium carbonate crystals (otoliths) in the semicircular canals cause continued and excessive cupula movement with small changes in head position.

The gustatory and olfactory systems

Differentiation of flavours is made possible by the gustatory and olfactory systems. Loss of these senses is less debilitating than failure of the visual or auditory systems. However, as well as being distressing for patients, gustatory and olfactory loss can contribute to reduced appetite and therefore affect nutritional status, as occurs in many elderly patients for example.

Taste

Taste buds are located on the lateral wall of fungiform papillae on the tongue and parts of the oropharynx (the part of the throat just behind the mouth) (**Figure 8.17**). Each taste bud contains several types of taste cell, and each cell may have more than one kind of taste receptor, although one predominates.

Mechanism of transduction of taste

There is a different receptor for each of the five main tastes: salt, sour, sweet, bitter and umami (a savoury taste). Each type of receptor uses a different mechanism to transduce taste stimuli (**Table 8.4**):

- Na^+ entry for salt
- H^+ entry for acid
- activation of G-protein-coupled receptors for sweet, bitter and umami

Activation of each type of receptor depolarises taste cells, which activates voltage-gated calcium channels. Calcium ions (Ca^{2+}) enter the cell, which stimulates neurotransmitter release (ATP and 5-HT) and thereby activates afferent gustatory nerves. Taste receptors adapt rapidly, so intensity of taste diminishes with continued stimulation.

Central processing of taste

Afferents in cranial nerve VII (from the anterior two thirds of the tongue) and cranial nerve IX (from the posterior third of the tongue) pass to the gustatory nucleus in the brain stem. The brain stem signals to the primary gustatory cortex (in the temporal lobe) through the thalamus. The gustatory nucleus also communicates with the medulla to activate the swallow or gag reflexes, and with the hypothalamus for communicate palatability and satiety.

Smell

Olfaction is the only sense in which the transducing cells are neurones. Primary afferents from the olfactory bulb project through the cribriform plate, an area in the ethmoid bone, into the nasal cavity.

Mechanism of transduction of smell

Only one kind of receptor is present on each olfactory neurone. However, it is possible to distinguish thousands of different smells

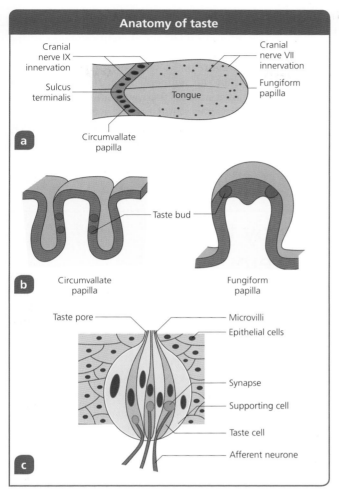

Anatomy of taste

a
Cranial nerve IX innervation
Sulcus terminalis
Circumvallate papilla
Tongue
Cranial nerve VII innervation
Fungiform papilla

b
Taste bud
Circumvallate papilla
Fungiform papilla

c
Taste pore
Microvilli
Epithelial cells
Synapse
Supporting cell
Taste cell
Afferent neurone

Figure 8.17 The anatomy of taste buds. (a) Location and innervation of papillae on the tongue. (b) The main forms of papillae. (c) Microanatomy of a taste bud.

Transduction of taste

Taste	Mechanism of transduction*
Salt	Na$^+$ entry through non-gated channels → depolarisation → voltage-gated Ca^{2+} entry
Sour	H$^+$ blockage of K$^+$ efflux channels → reduced K$^+$ efflux → depolarisation → voltage-gated Ca^{2+} entry
Sweet	Saccharide binds type 1 taste receptors (G-protein-coupled receptors) → activation of phospholipase C → Ca^{2+} release
Bitter	Substances bind type 2 taste receptors (G-protein-coupled receptors) → activation of phospholipase C → Ca^{2+} release
Umami	Amino acids bind to G-protein-coupled receptors → activation of phospholipase C → Ca^{2+} release

*Each of these mechanisms increases intracellular Ca^{2+} to release neurotransmitters.

Table 8.4 The five tastes and their mechanism of transduction

because each receptor is able to bind many different odorants, and there are hundreds of kinds of receptor.

Olfactory receptors are G-protein–coupled receptors that, when they bind their odorant, cause sodium and calcium channels to open. This causes Na^+ and Ca^{2+} to enter the taste cell, thereby increasing its membrane potential. If the threshold for an action potential is reached, the olfactory neurones fire. Like taste receptors, olfactory receptors adapt rapidly.

Central processing of smell

Primary olfactory afferents synapse in the olfactory bulb and then connect to a few different regions. The primary olfactory cortex is in the temporal lobe; the second-order afferents pass there without synapsing in the thalamus (unlike sight, hearing and taste). Some second-order neurones communicate with the orbitofrontal cortex (through the thalamus) for recognition; others pass to the limbic system for further association.

Perception of pain by the somatosensory system

Clinicians require an understanding of what pain is, and how the body senses it, to be able to treat its diverse manifestations.

Pain is subjective. The perception of pain varies between individuals; the same painful stimulus can be experienced differently by different people. Furthermore, many people report pain in the absence of such a stimulus, so pain is considered a psychological state with or without a physical cause. These characteristics of pain are summarised by its International Association for the Study of Pain definition: 'an unpleasant sensory and emotional experience associated with actual or potential tissue damage, or described in terms of such damage'.

Gate control theory of pain

The gate control theory helps explain the subjective nature of pain perception, and why it is not simply a product of the intensity of a painful stimulus and the degree of damage to affected tissue.

This theory postulates that whether or not pain is experienced is determined by a 'gate' at the level of the spinal cord, which is influenced by ascending stimulatory and descending inhibitory inputs.

Peripheral transduction

The ascending pain signal is carried by spinothalamic afferents that innervate nociceptors, which transduce the physical component of pain.

There are two types of nociceptor.

- **Mechanical nociceptors** are specialised mechanoreceptors that are activated only by a strong physical force (i.e. force that is potentially damaging to tissues); they are innervated by Aγ afferent fibres
- **Polymodal nociceptors** respond to various painful stimuli (e.g. heat, toxins, inflammatory mediators and physical force); they are innervated by C fibres

Spinal cord 'gate'

The gate is located in lamina II (the substantia gelatinosa) or lamina V of the dorsal horn. It is concerned with controlling activity in the output neurone, which projects the pain signal centrally (**Figure 8.18**). The output neurone is subject to both tonic and phasic inhibition; spinal cord interneurones and descending signals provide the tonic inhibition.

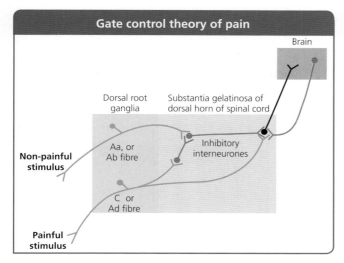

Figure 8.18 The gate control theory of pain. Pain is experienced when the output neurone is activated. There are descending and ascending inhibitory fibres (red) and ascending activating fibres (green).

A transient increase in inhibition occurs when Aβ afferent fibres are stimulated; stimulation of these fibres is the basis for certain forms of pain relief therapy. To experience pain, this inhibition must be removed and the output neurone stimulated; C fibres have this role.

Exaggerated pain

In certain situations, people experience a higher level of pain than would normally be felt. This occurs in cases of hyperalgesia, allodynia or both.

- **Hyperalgesia** is an increase in the intensity of a normally painful stimulus
- **Allodynia** is a painful sensation in response to a normally non-painful stimulus

These conditions are caused by changes in both the periphery and the spinal cord.

Peripheral hyperalgesia

Tissue damage results in an inflammatory response, with consequent:

- acidic environment
- K^+ release
- increased levels of prostaglandins or histamine

These factors act on polymodal nociceptors to reduce their threshold for activation. As a result, signalling along C fibres increases, eliciting greater pain.

Central hyperalgesia

Persistence of pain over a long period changes transmission between the neurones in the periphery and those in the spinal cord; this effect is called synaptic plasticity. Consequently, signalling from the output neurone becomes disproportionate to the intensity of the incoming stimulus (**Figure 8.19**). This phenomenon, known as 'wind-up', is mediated by an increase in the sensitivity of the post-synaptic membrane (**Figure 8.20**).

Normally, the primary afferent neurone releases glutamate, which binds to α-amino 3-hydroxy 5-methyl 4-isoxazolepropionic acid (AMPA) receptors (one of several types of glutamate receptor) on the post-synaptic terminal. Activation of the AMPA receptor

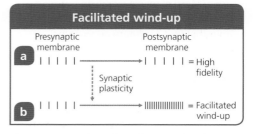

Figure 8.19 Facilitated wind-up, mediated by synaptic plasticity, transforms a synaptic connection from a high-fidelity response (a) to disproportionate hyperactivation (b). Each vertical line represents an action potential.

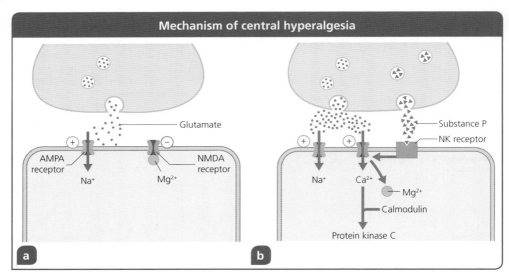

Figure 8.20 (a) In physiological situations, glutamate binds to AMPA receptors and NMDA receptors are blocked. (b) Central hyperalgesia (and long-term potentiation of memory) is mediated by sensitisation of the post-synaptic membrane. With chronic or high-level stimulation, substance P signalling removes the blockade of post-synaptic N-methyl D-aspartic acid (NMDA) channels by Mg^{2+}, which allows Ca^{2+} entry and thereby increases the likelihood of an excitatory post-synaptic potential being triggered. AMPA, α-amino 3-hydroxy-5-methyl-4-isoxazolepropionic acid; Glu, glutamate.

causes Na^+ to enter the output neurone, which triggers an excitatory post-synaptic potential.

Chronic or high-level stimulation sensitises the output neurone to further stimulation as follows.

1. With this type of stimulation, the afferent neurone releases substance P as well as glutamate
2. Substance P binds to post-synaptic neurokinin (NK) receptors
3. Activation of these receptors removes the blockade by intracellular magnesium ions (Mg^{2+}) of post-synaptic membrane N-methyl D-aspartic acid (NMDA) receptors (another type of glutamate receptor)
4. Removal of the Mg^{2+} block enables the glutamate released by the afferent neurone to bind to NMDA receptors as well as AMPA receptors
5. Activation of the NMDA receptors allows Ca^{2+} to enter the cell, which further increases the membrane potential, thereby making an excitatory post-synaptic potential more likely

Analgesic drugs target specific pathways. Non-steroidal anti-inflammatory drugs (i.e. cyclo-oxygenase inhibitors) reduce the synthesis of prostaglandins, which are key mediators in the stimulation and sensitisation of polymodal nociceptors (receptors responding to multiple painful stimuli). Opioids such as morphine act at μ, κ and λ receptors, thus promoting inhibition of neural output signalling pain in the spinal cord and increasing activation of euphoria-inducing reward pathways in the limbic system.

Functions of the basal ganglia

The basal ganglia are a collection of deep cerebral and midbrain nuclei (**Figure 8.21**). Together, they predominantly regulate motor activity (see page 48) and motor learning.

- **Most input** enters the putamen and caudate nucleus, which are known as the striatum because of their striped appearance; much of this input comes from the cerebral cortex, but additional input is supplied by a wide range of other sources (e.g. the spinal cord and cerebellum)
- **Most output** passes from parts of the globus pallidus and substantia nigra, through the thalamus, to the region of the cortex controlling voluntary movement (the motor cortex); the thalamus receives much sensory information, which through thalamocortical relay is relayed to the cortex

Connections both within the basal ganglia and with other structures are complex and remain poorly understood. Overall, their role appears to be to help coordinate learned movements and to suppress unnecessary ones. Many of the neurones in the basal ganglia are inhibitory (GABA-ergic), but inhibition of an inhibitory centre increases activity.

Disorders of the basal ganglia can lead to both hypokinetic disorders such as Parkinson's disease and hyperkinetic ones such as Huntington's disease, a condition in which unintended and uncontrolled movements occur spontaneously.

> **Parkinson's disease is characterised by difficulty in initiating movement, slowed movement (bradykinesia), rigidity and postural instability.** The condition arises from the loss of nigrostriatal dopaminergic neurones. Treatment focuses on dopamine replacement using the neurotransmitter's precursor, levodopa.

Motor control by direct and indirect pathways

The striatum (the main site of input to the basal ganglia) communicates with the substantia

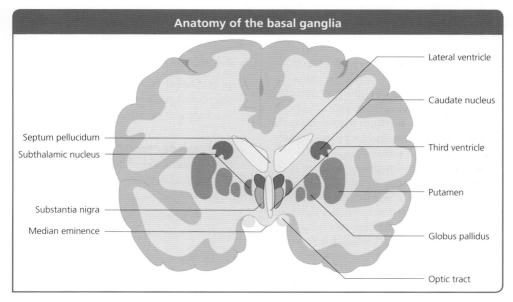

Anatomy of the basal ganglia

Lateral ventricle

Caudate nucleus

Septum pellucidum

Subthalamic nucleus

Third ventricle

Putamen

Substantia nigra

Median eminence

Globus pallidus

Optic tract

Figure 8.21 Coronal section of the brain, showing the anatomy of the basal ganglia.

nigra pars reticulata and globus pallidus interna in two ways: through a direct pathway and an indirect pathway (**Figure 8.22**).

- **The direct pathway** helps to facilitate movement by inhibiting output from the substantia nigra pars reticulata and globus pallidus interna
- **The indirect pathway** signals through the globus pallidus externa and subthalamic nuclei to activate the substantia nigra pars reticulata and external globus pallidus; consequently, the indirect pathway reduces motor activity by augmenting inhibition of the thalamocortical relay

The role of dopamine

Dopaminergic neurones originate in the substantia nigra pars compacta and synapse on neurones of the striatum. Dopamine facilitates movement by:

- activating D_1 receptors on direct pathway neurones, which increases their activity
- activating D_2 receptors on indirect pathway neurones, which reduces their activity

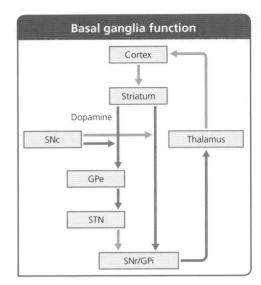

Figure 8.22 Input to the basal ganglia is through a direct pathway (which promotes movement) or an indirect pathway (which reduces or slows movement). Dopamine from the substantia nigra pars reticulata promotes movement by activating the direct pathway and inhibiting the indirect pathway. Activating signals are in green; inhibitory signals are in red. GPe, globus pallidus externa; GPi, globus pallidus interna; SNC, substantia nigra pars compacta; SNr, substantia nigra pars reticularis; STN, subthalamic nucleus.

Functions of the cerebellum

The cerebellum is part of the hindbrain in the posterior fossa, and is separated from the occipital lobes of the cortex by the tentorium cerebelli. The cerebellar cortex comprises two hemispheres lying either side of a central vermis. Tucked underneath the vermis is the flocculonodular lobe, and four pairs of nuclei lie deep within the vermis.

The cerebellum integrates sensory information about the body's position and movements, and uses this information to fine-tune motor activity. Therefore cerebellar functions are essential for the maintenance of balance and posture and for the smooth performance of voluntary movements.

The cerebellum connects with the rest of the brain through the cerebellar peduncles

(**Table 8.5**). It receives a wide range of sensory and motor input, including:

- **proprioceptive input** (information about the relative positions of different parts of the body and the effort used to move them)

Cerebellar peduncles	
Peduncle	Signals conveyed
Superior	Output to ipsilateral midbrain
Middle	Input from contralateral cerebral cortex
Inferior	Input from ascending spinal cord afferents

Table 8.5 The cerebellar peduncles: the nerve tracts conveying signals in and out of the cerebellum

- **vestibular input** (information relating to balance)

Output passes from the cerebellar cortex to the cerebellar nuclei. From these structures, it travels to either the thalamus (for transmission to the cerebral cortex) or the red nucleus (in the midbrain, for passage to the spinal cord).

Functional components of the cerebellum

The cerebellum is divided into three main functional components:

- the vestibulocerebellum
- the spinocerebellum
- the cerebropontocerebellum

Vestibulocerebellum

This structure is in the flocculonodular lobe and is evolutionarily the oldest part of the cerebellum. It uses information from the vestibular system to coordinate posture, balance and eye movements. Cross-communication between the spinocerebellar pathway and the vestibular system enables balance to be maintained.

Spinocerebellum

The vermis receives proprioceptive information through the spinocerebellar pathway and vestibular nucleus.

- The spinocerebellar pathway provides gross proprioception, which is important for movements of the trunk and axial skeleton and for larger actions of the limbs
- Dorsal column proprioception concerns fine movements of the distal extremities

Cerebropontocerebellum

The cerebellar hemispheres are predominantly responsible for motor learning and control of the timing, distance and speed of voluntary movements. The cerebropontocerebellum is part of a feedback loop that compares intended movement with actual movement input and provides an 'error' signal (**Figure 8.23**).

> **Ataxia is caused by damage to the cerebellum, for example by stroke.** Ataxia describes a group of neurological disorders in which movements are jerky and difficult to control, and balance is difficult to maintain. Spinocerebellar or vestibulocerebellar damage causes truncal ataxia in which patients struggle to maintain balance even when sitting on the edge of a bed. Vision partially compensates for this problem, but the effect is negated when the patient closes their eyes (Romberg's sign).

Motor control by the cerebellum

The cerebropontocerebellar loop highlights the central role of the cerebellum

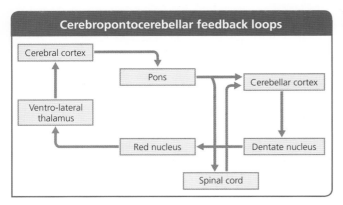

Cerebropontocerebellar feedback loops

Cerebral cortex

Pons

Cerebellar cortex

Ventro-lateral thalamus

Red nucleus

Dentate nucleus

Spinal cord

Figure 8.23
Cerebropontocerebellar feedback loops allow the cerebellum to compare descending 'intended' and ascending 'actual' inputs.

in integrating descending (cortical) and ascending (spinal cord) signals. Collaterals from cortical motor neurones pass through the pons to the cerebellum. As an action is performed, proprioceptive and other sensory information feeds back to the cerebellar cortex. Descending 'intended' and ascending 'actual' signals are then integrated, with an 'error' signal generated in cases of discrepancy. The dentate nucleus passes the error signal through the thalamus to the cortex to allow movements to be fine-tuned.

To learn a complex series of actions, such as those used to drive a car, the patterned cortical output is changed from the non-learned state to a finely tuned final product; this process is partly mediated by changes in the cerebellar cortex. Synaptic plasticity (changes in synaptic communication) in the cerebellar cortex allows the error signal to be incorporated into the motor output.

Functions of the limbic system

The limbic system includes the amygdala, hippocampus, hypothalamus, olfactory cortex and prefrontal cortex. The hypothalamus is an evolutionarily ancient part of the brain that sits just beneath the third ventricle, above the pituitary gland.

The limbic system has roles in the perception of smell and consciousness. The hypothalamus connects with various parts of the central nervous system to carry out its functions, which include the regulation of appetite and emotion (**Table 8.6**). The endocrine roles of the hypothalamus are covered in Chapters 5 and 6.

and the central nervous system. Appetite is controlled by the hypothalamus, which integrates signals from various hormones (**Table 8.7**), as well as sensory input from the gut and cerebral cortex.

Emotional control by the limbic system

The key structures in the control of emotion are shown in the Papez circuit (**Figure 8.24**), which forms the limbic system. It is not known precisely how integration occurs to

Appetite control by the limbic system

The balance between satiety and hunger is a complex interplay between the gut

Hypothalamic functions	
Type	Function
Autonomic	Initiation and control of autonomic activity, with output to the medulla
Circadian rhythm	Optic nerve input and regulation by clock protein determine natural daily rhythm
Appetite	See Table 8.7
Emotion	Interaction with the limbic system (including the amygdala, hippocampus and prefrontal cortex)
Endocrine	As the master endocrine gland, controls pituitary function (see page 166)

Table 8.6 The main functions of the hypothalamus

Control of appetite	
Factor	Mechanism
Leptin	Released by adipocytes in direct proportion to amount of stored fat
	Reduces appetite
Adiponectin	Released by adipocytes
	Inversely proportional to amount of stored fat
	Promotes hunger
Glucagon-like peptide-1	Released by small bowel enterocytes in response to consumed carbohydrate
	Reduces appetite
Ghrelin	Released by cells in the gut
	Promotes hunger
Neuropeptide Y	Key signalling molecule in the hypothalamus
	Increases with hunger

Table 8.7 Key factors in the neuroendocrine control of appetite

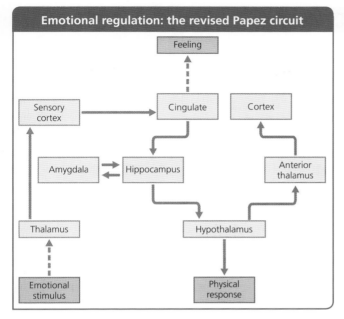

Figure 8.24 The Papez circuit connects the key parts of the central nervous system that regulate emotion.

produce emotion, but certain components are thought to have specific roles.

- **The amygdala** particularly controls anger and aggression
- **The hippocampus** is responsible for emotional memory
- **The hypothalamus** provides the physical (autonomic) output associated with emotion
- **The frontal cortex** integrates other cortical functions and associations
- **Cortisol** has an important role in mounting the physiological response to chronic stress

Anxiety and depression are the two most common disorders related to emotional dysfunction. Moderate and severe depression includes symptoms of low mood, anhedonia (the inability to experience enjoyment) and physical disturbances, including poor sleep and appetite. Antidepressant agents target monoamine synapses (noradrenaline and serotonin), which are implicated in the aetiology of depression.

Functions of the cerebral cortex

The cerebral cortex is the outermost layer of the cerebrum. It is divided into the left and right hemispheres bridged by the corpus callosum. Each cerebral hemisphere is divided into four lobes (**Figure 8.25**), which together are responsible for many higher neural functions.

- **The frontal lobe** governs movement, motor control of speech, personality, planning and social interaction

- **The temporal lobe** contains centres of taste, smell, hearing, understanding speech, and emotion
- **The parietal lobe** is responsible for sensation, awareness and linking experiences to sensory input
- **The occipital lobe** is primarily concerned with vision

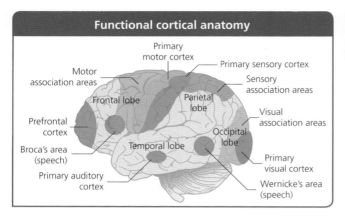

Functional cortical anatomy

Primary motor cortex
Primary sensory cortex
Motor association areas
Sensory association areas
Frontal lobe
Parietal lobe
Visual association areas
Prefrontal cortex
Occipital lobe
Broca's area (speech)
Temporal lobe
Primary visual cortex
Primary auditory cortex
Wernicke's area (speech)

Figure 8.25 Functional cortical anatomy: the main areas of the cerebral cortex responsible for higher neural functions.

Speech and the cerebral cortex

The two main regions of the central nervous system responsible for speech are Broca's area and Wernicke's area (see **Figure 8.25**), which are connected by the arcuate fasciculus.

- **Broca's area**, in the frontal lobe, is expressive, i.e. it controls motor production of speech
- **Wernicke's area**, in the temporal lobe, is receptive, i.e. it allows the comprehension of speech

These are located in the dominant cerebral hemisphere, which is usually the left hemisphere. However, to produce normal speech an intact arcuate fasciculus, as well as all the normal elements of motor control, are required.

Broca's area

Located on at the inferolateral aspect of the frontal lobe, Broca's area mediates formation of speech. It is termed the 'expressive' area, because it allows a thought to be turned into the motor co-ordination required for vocalisation of the sentence. Therefore its output is to the primary motor cortex, which controls the muscles required for speech. However, more recent evidence has suggested that Broca's area also has a role in comprehension.

Wernicke's area

Understanding of the spoken word is mediated by Wernicke's area, which lies on the posterior part of the superior temporal gyrus. It receives input from the auditory centres, as well as from visual and other sensory areas.

Wernicke's area is described as the 'receptive' area, because it facilitates comprehension of sentences and confers the ability to follow complex tasks and engage in conversation. Wernicke's area is also important for the production of meaningful speech.

Aphasia (or dysphasia) is caused by damage to Broca's area or Wernicke's area.

Damage to Broca's area leads to expressive aphasia: patients are unable to express their thoughts verbally, cannot find the correct words and their speech is halting.

Damage to Wernicke's area leads to receptive aphasia: patients lack understanding of language and cannot comprehend complex instructions; their speech is superficially fluent, but nonsensical.

Memory and the cerebral cortex

Memory, the ability to recall experiences and information, is crucial for learning.

Types of memory

Memory can be divided into short-term or long-term. Short-term memory, or 'working' memory, lasts only about 30 seconds and is mediated by the prefrontal cortex. The average person is able to store only seven or eight different items in their working memory at any one time, and the memories decay unless repeated.

Long-term memory can be split into declarative and non-declarative memory.

- Procedures, behaviours and skills (e.g. driving a car) make up non-declarative memory; these are controlled by the basal ganglia, cerebellum and supplementary motor areas of the frontal lobe
- Declarative memories are those that can be described or explained, such as what you had for lunch yesterday or the height of the Eiffel Tower

Declarative memories are subdivided into episodic memories, context-dependent personal life memories and semantic memories (facts independent of context). The hippocampus appears to be crucial in laying down new long-term memories. However, the actual location at which they are stored is unclear; indeed, it may not be a single location for any given memory.

Long-term potentiation

Storage of memories in the hippocampus requires a change in the communication between CA3 and CA1 neurones. This synaptic plasticity occurs through a similar mechanism to that for central hyperalgesia (see **Figure 8.20**); it is induced by brief, tetanic firing of the presynaptic neurone. How this synaptic plasticity results in storage of episodic memory that we can access and internally visualise is not understood.

Consciousness

Consciousness is difficult to define. However, it can be considered a person's awareness of their mind and their surroundings.

Unlike the higher neural functions of speech and memory, consciousness does not emanate from a single area in the brain. Instead, multiple bilateral areas of the cortex are involved in consciousness, particularly the sensory association areas and the cingulate gyrus. Therefore it is uncommon for a unilateral, focal insult (e.g. an ischaemic stroke) to cause loss of consciousness.

Activity in all of these areas depends on the thalamocortical relay and the ascending reticular activating system. The basal ganglia and limbic system also play a role, though the precise details are unclear.

Ascending reticular activating system

The reticular formation is a collection of nuclei and tracts that run through the brain stem, into the midbrain and up to the thalamus. It also helps produce motor activity (particularly walking) as the pontine and medullary reticulospinal tracts.

One part of the reticular formation is the ascending reticular activating system, which provides tonic activity to the thalamocortical relay. Interruption to this supply causes widespread reduced cortical activity, with resultant loss of consciousness.

Dementia is a chronic, progressive, life-limiting condition characterised by loss of cognitive function. The condition has several forms, depending on the underlying pathology. The most common type is Alzheimer's disease; patients have early progressive loss of memory and word-finding abilities. People with severe cerebrovascular disease develop vascular dementia, with a step-wise decline as further intracerebral ischaemic events occur (**Figure 8.26**). The common factor is cortical atrophy, with shrinkage of the brain, opening of the sulci and sometimes enlargement of the ventricles.

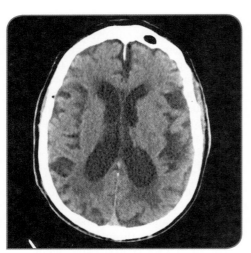

Figure 8.26 Computerised tomography scan of the head, showing significant loss of cortical volume, with ventricular enlargement; these changes result from cerebrovascular disease. This patient had advanced vascular dementia.

Answers to starter questions

1. Different sensations of pain are caused by the activation of different types of pain receptors and nerve fibres. Sharp pain is mediated by high-threshold mechanoreceptors and innervated by Aδ afferent fibres; it is often felt very quickly after a painful physical stimulus. Burning pain is mediated by polymodal nociceptors and innervated by slower C fibres; it is felt later after a painful physical stimulus or with other toxic damage, such as inflammation.

2. Vision in low light is mediated by rods, the most sensitive photoreceptors. However, there is only one kind of rod, which has one kind of photopigment that responds only to either the presence or absence of light; hence why we can only see in black and white in low light.

3. Memories come in several different forms. Those that we commonly refer to as 'memories' (e.g. where I went last summer holiday) are known as episodic declarative memories. The hippocampus is particularly important for storage of these memories using a mechanism known as long-term potentiation. How exactly this generates memories that we can recall is not clear. It is intimately linked to emotion, which is why strongly emotional events are often more clearly remembered.

4. Spinning around causes endolymph (fluid) in the semicircular canals of the inner ear to move. This displaces the cupula and activates the hair cells that transduce head rotation (to cause the sensation of dizziness). The endolymph continues to move after you stop spinning, causing continued activation of the hair cells and the sensation of vertigo (dizziness).

5. Most emotions are controlled by the limbic system, which includes the amygdala, hippocampus, hypothalamus and prefrontal cortex. The amygdala is particularly important in the control of anger, though it is not clear exactly how. The physical manifestations (i.e. the surge of adrenaline) come from the hypothalamus, which activates the ventral medulla to stimulate the sympathetic nervous system.

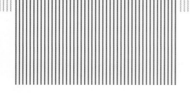

Chapter 9
Applied physiology

Starter questions

Answers to the following questions are on page 281.

1. Why is urine volume reduced and its concentration increased after a haemorrhage?
2. Why does intense exercise cause muscle pain?
3. Why is infection associated with a fever?
4. Why does a gradual ascent up a mountain reduce altitude sickness?
5. Why does chronic stress cause weight loss?

Introduction

It is common practice to learn physiology in terms of the functions of individual systems in isolation. However, the human body works through the interaction of multiple systems. Therefore the examples described in this chapter illustrate the need to consider various different systems when trying to identify the cause of pathological changes.

Several of the descriptions of physiological processes relate to extreme situations, such as thermoregulation in subzero temperatures. However, the same processes are also responsible for homeostasis in normal conditions.

Case 9 Massive blood loss

Presentation

Four hours ago, and 2 weeks past term, 33-year-old Emma gave birth to a healthy baby boy. However, she has suddenly developed profuse vaginal bleeding requiring urgent assessment and treatment by the obstetric team.

Emma is immediately given intravenous fluid, and cross-matched blood is ordered. By the time the haemorrhage has stopped, she is estimated to have lost > 5 L of blood. She receives a transfusion of 10 units of packed red cells.

Analysis

Postpartum haemorrhage is a terrifying and potentially life-threatening complication of childbirth. An enormous amount of blood may be lost before the bleeding can be stopped. However, if intravenous access is adequate, blood and other fluids can be administered to compensate for this loss.

Further case

Emma's condition stabilises. However, once a catheter is inserted, only 15 mL of urine is drained.

Repeat blood tests show mildly increased plasma urea concentration (10.2 mM; normal range, 2.5–6.7mM), low platelet concentration (75×10^9/L; normal range, 150–400 $\times$ 10^9/L) and prolonged prothrombin clotting times (28 seconds; normal range 10–14 seconds). Emma's temperature has decreased to 34.3°C, and she is having a little difficulty breathing.

Plasma cryoprecipitate (containing clotting factors) and platelets are administered intravenously. Diuretic agents are administered orally. Active warming, for example using warm air through a bear

Postpartum haemorrhage: fluid overload

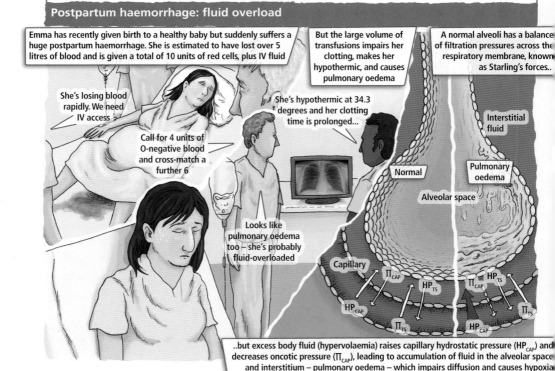

Emma has recently given birth to a healthy baby but suddenly suffers a huge postpartum haemorrhage. She is estimated to have lost over 5 litres of blood and is given a total of 10 units of red cells, plus IV fluid

But the large volume of transfusions impairs her clotting, makes her hypothermic, and causes pulmonary oedema

A normal alveoli has a balance of filtration pressures across the respiratory membrane, known as Starling's forces..

She's losing blood rapidly. We need IV access

Call for 4 units of O-negative blood and cross-match a further 6

She's hypothermic at 34.3 degrees and her clotting time is prolonged...

Interstitial fluid

Normal

Pulmonary oedema

Alveolar space

Looks like pulmonary oedema too – she's probably fluid-overloaded

Capillary

Π_{CAP} HP_{TS} Π_{CAP} HP_{TS}

HP_{CAP} Π_{TS} Π_{TS}

Π_{TS} HP_{CAP}

..but excess body fluid (hypervolaemia) raises capillary hydrostatic pressure (HP_{CAP}) and decreases oncotic pressure (Π_{CAP}), leading to accumulation of fluid in the alveolar space and interstitium – pulmonary oedema – which impairs diffusion and causes hypoxia

hugger is also used. Over the next two days Emma's renal function and other tests return to normal, and she is able to go home with her son.

Further analysis

Emma's low urine output is a consequence of reduced renal perfusion in response to the loss of effective circulating volume as well as activation of the sympathetic nervous system and renin–angiotensin–aldosterone system. Compare this situation with that of case 4 (see page 132), where two different methods of injury have both lead to reduction in circulating volume.

Packed red cells are required for oxygen delivery but do not contain platelets or clotting factors, so these must be administered in addition. The citrate with which red cells are stored impairs coagulation. Red cells are stored at 4°C, so massive transfusion (replacement of over half the total vascular volume in < 24) is associated with hypothermia.

Excessive volume replacement is not uncommon in the struggle to maintain adequate blood pressure. The excess fluid further decreases the concentration of plasma proteins, which are already depleted by the bleeding; oncotic pressure is reduced in consequence. This shift in the Starling forces (see page 86) causes fluid to accumulate in the tissue, including the lungs (pulmonary oedema). Management of these complications includes encouraging the patient to maintain an upright posture, oxygen therapy and the administration of diuretics.

Exercise

Exercise is the term for the multitude of activities requiring physical effort, to which the body produces a coordinated response, including chronic adaptation.

Types of exercise

Exercise can be broadly divided into static and dynamic.

- In static exercise, muscles contract to work against a resistance, so their length does not change and the joint does not move (isometric contraction); an example of such exercise is holding shopping bags.
- In dynamic exercise, muscles alternately contract and relax changing in length, hence moving the joint; examples include walking or running.

Intensity of exercise is expressed in several ways. For static exercise, the percentage of maximum voluntary contraction is used. This is a measurement of the intensity of exercise relative to the patient's perceived maximal effort.

Dynamic exercise is usually graded by oxygen consumption (V_{O_2}) or carbon dioxide production (V_{CO_2}). For a patient with a normal diet and fully aerobic metabolism, the respiratory quotient (V_{O_2}/V_{CO_2}) is about 0.8, because some oxygen is used to convert hydrogen to water. Therefore in theory either V_{O_2} or V_{CO_2} could be used, but in practice the former is more common.

Central control of exercise

Central responses to exercise are coordinated by hypothalamic and medullary centres. These receive input from the cerebral cortex, which is responsible for planning movements; this information enables the body to anticipate the demands placed on it.

Transduction

The hypothalamic centres also receive feedback from the periphery. Through the process of transduction, the conversion of sensory stimuli into neural signals, muscles and joints send information from various metaboreceptors and proprioceptors.

- **Metaboreceptors** in skeletal muscle are stimulated by products of metabolic activity, such as hydrogen ions, potassium ions, phosphate and adenosine, which accumulate in the interstitial space before being carried away in the bloodstream
- **Proprioceptors** sense the position, length and movement of muscles and joints, thus enabling the body to assess the intensity of exercise as it is happening and to anticipate the need for increased cardiorespiratory and metabolic activity

Baroreceptors and chemoreceptors monitoring blood pressure and composition, also send information to the hypothalamus (see page 92).

Neural output

Afferent fibres bring information to the area of the hypothalamus that coordinates exercise. The hypothalamus then generates the appropriate patterned response, coordinating changes in heart rate and breathing with the planned exercise. These changes are driven by the corresponding medullary centres (**Figure 9.1**).

Generally, exercise activates the sympathetic nervous system and inhibits the parasympathetic nervous system. The consequences are increased cardiac output and peripheral vasoconstriction. The hypothalamus also activates the medullary inspiratory centre to increase the rate and depth of ventilation.

Neurally mediated vasoconstriction occurs mostly in the skin, gut, kidneys and inactive skeletal muscle. However, activation of metaboreceptors in exercising muscle causes vasodilation, which results in metabolic hyperaemia (increased blood flow). This effect, combined with vasoconstriction in less active tissues, causes blood to be shunted

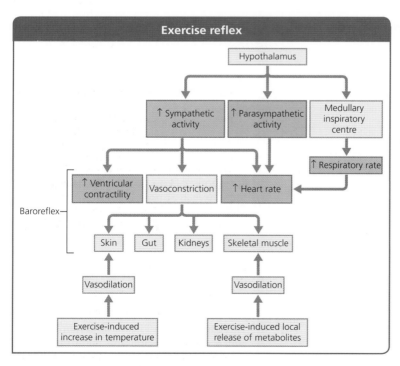

Figure 9.1 The hypothalamic–medullary output of the exercise reflex.

towards active muscles and away from areas of the body with lower energy demands and that can withstand temporary reductions in their blood supply. Vasoconstriction in the skin is overcome by thermoregulation(see page 275).

Effects of training

Physical training causes a number of changes which increase the ability of the body to perform exercise at a higher level or for longer. Repeated endurance training leads to changes in both the muscle itself and in the blood supply:

- Increased plasma volume and stroke volume, thus increased cardiac output
- Increased number of capillaries supplying the exercising muscles
- Muscles become hypertrophied and contain increased numbers of mitochondria
- Mitochondria use more fatty acids for energy, protecting glycogen stores
- Muscle glycogen stores are increased
- Increased maximal respiratory rate and tidal volume (V_T)

Together, these changes substantially increase the maximum amount of aerobic work that can be performed.

Blood gases in exercise

Each person has a set ability to deliver oxygen to, and remove carbon dioxide from, active muscle. The anaerobic threshold is the point at which demand for oxygen exceeds its delivery. Exercise affects arterial blood gases only when it continues past this threshold.

Exercise below the anaerobic threshold

Increased metabolic activity increases V_{O_2} and V_{CO_2}, which in theory would reduce arterial oxygen (P_aO_2) and increase arterial carbon dioxide (P_aCO_2). However, below the anaerobic threshold, arterial blood gases are unchanged. This is because the area of the hypothalamus that coordinates exercise drives the inspiratory centres to increase V_A to balance changes in V_{O_2} and V_{CO_2} (**Figure 9.2**).

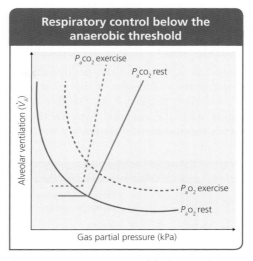

Respiratory control below the anaerobic threshold

P_aCO_2 exercise
P_aCO_2 rest
P_aO_2 exercise
P_aO_2 rest
Alveolar ventilation ($\dot{V}_A$)
Gas partial pressure (kPa)

Figure 9.2 Respiratory control during exercise below the anaerobic threshold. The vertical shift in both curves facilitates hyperpnoea without changes in blood gases.

This 'hyperpnoea' mediates an increase in VT while P_aO_2 and P_aCO_2 remain constant. Therefore, below the anaerobic threshold, there are no changes in these arterial blood gases for chemoreceptors to detect. Changes in oxygen and carbon dioxide occur in venous blood, but no venous chemoreceptors have been identified.

Exercise improves cardiac function, mood and life expectancy. For patients with ischaemic heart disease, gentle dynamic exercise is safest. The heart is under most strain when heart rate, contractility and total peripheral resistance are high. Static exercise causes the greatest increase in cardiac work. In contrast, the reduced total peripheral resistance in dynamic exercise is associated with less risk to the heart.

Exercise above the anaerobic threshold

Past the anaerobic threshold, the electron transport system in mitochondria fails, and intermediates in the citric acid cycle (also known as the tricarboxylic acid cycle or Krebs cycle) accumulate. One such intermediate is pyruvate. Lactate dehydrogenase converts the excess pyruvate into lactic acid (lactate).

The presence of lactate in the blood reduces its pH to cause metabolic (lactic) acidosis. The acidosis activates peripheral chemoreceptors to increase V_A by more than is required to balance P_aCO_2 (**Table 9.1** and **Figure 9.3**). The resultant hyperventilation causes hypocapnia and respiratory alkalosis, which partially counteracts the metabolic acidosis.

Hyperventilation slightly boosts P_aO_2 (remember that arterial oxygen is normally close to maximal anyway). However, this effect is insufficient to reverse the consequences of anaerobic respiration if the exercise continues. The accumulation of lactate and other metabolites produces muscle pain and fatigue, which encourages cessation of activity.

Blood gases and the anaerobic threshold	
Physiological variable	Change on exceeding the anaerobic threshold
Tidal volume	Increases
P_aCO_2	Decreases
P_aO_2	Increases (slightly)
Lactate	Increases
pH	Decreases (acidosis)

Table 9.1 Changes in blood gases in response to increasing exercise intensity past the anaerobic threshold

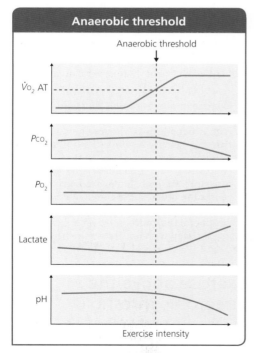

Figure 9.3 Effect of passing the anaerobic threshold on arterial blood gases. AT, anaerobic threshold.

Haemodynamic effects

The patterned response to exercise generated by the hypothalamus includes increased cardiac output and systemic vasoconstriction. These effects would be expected to increase both systolic and diastolic blood pressure, and consequently to produce a large increase in mean arterial blood pressure. However, changes in blood pressure are smaller than might be expected, because vasodilation in active muscle decreases peripheral resistance overall. Furthermore, changes in blood pressure are counteracted by the homeostatic baroreflex mechanism.

Static exercise

Muscle contraction occludes blood vessels, thus preventing the vasodilatory action of local metabolites and increasing total peripheral resistance. These effects increase mean arterial blood pressure in proportion to the percentage of maximum voluntary contraction.

On relaxation, there is sudden vasodilation in active muscle in response to metabolic hyperaemia. This causes a marked decrease in total peripheral resistance and a reduction in mean arterial blood pressure.

Dynamic exercise

Alternate contraction and relaxation in active muscle allows metabolic hyperaemia to cause vasodilation, as discussed above. Blood flow in active muscle decreases and increases accordingly, with an overall increase (**Figure 9.4**). Total peripheral resistance decreases, reducing diastolic blood pressure, and increased stroke volume

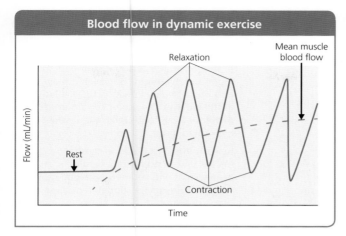

Figure 9.4 Blood flow through a muscle during dynamic exercise.

causes increased systolic blood pressure. Therefore mean arterial blood pressure remains about the same but pulse pressure increases.

Thermoregulation

The hypothalamus is the control centre for thermoregulation. It receives input from thermoreceptors both within the hypothalamus and peripherally, it determines the set point for core temperature, and its output maintains that temperature.

Disease can alter the thermoregulatory set point. In such cases, body temperature is increased in response to pyrogens (fever-producing substances) such as the interleukin-1 released during bacterial infection. An overview of thermoregulatory responses is shown in **Table 9.2**.

Response to heat

The skin is the key organ for heat loss. The dermis contains extensive superficial venous plexuses, which are not perfused when body temperature is normal. Their perfusion depends on arteriovenous anastomoses, which respond to temperature changes. When body temperature increases, the anastomoses open to increase blood supply to the peripheral venous plexuses, facilitating heat loss through conduction and radiation to the surrounding environment.

Heat is also lost from the skin by evaporation of sweat. The two types of sweat glands are apocrine and eccrine.

■ **Eccrine sweat glands** are exocrine glands controlled by muscarinic acetylcholine innervation from sympathetic neurones; increased sympathetic activity causes

Thermoregulatory responses	
Responses to heat	Responses to cold
Moving to a cooler area or removing some clothes	Seeking sources of warmth or donning more clothes
Opening of cutaneous arteriovenous anastomoses	Closure of arteriovenous anastomoses
Cutaneous vasodilation	Cutaneous vasoconstriction
Increased muscarinic acetylcholinergic stimulation of sweating	Reduced sweating
	Shivering
	Uncoupled ATP synthase spinning in brown adipose tissue

Table 9.2 The main processes in thermoregulation

more rapid sweat production and heat loss when the sweat evaporates

■ **Apocrine sweat glands** are predominantly in the axilla and groin and have no role in thermoregulation

> **Malignant hyperthermia (malignant hyperpyrexia) is a rare inherited autosomal dominant disorder that develops in response to certain anaesthetic drugs.** The administration of these drugs causes ryanodine receptors in skeletal muscle to remain open. Ryanodine receptors are a type of calcium channel in the sarcoplasmic reticulum; when open, they allow calcium ions to flow out into the cytosol. The high calcium concentration causes the muscle to contract, using up ATP and generating heat, which then stimulates further ATP synthesis and heat generation. Acidosis and rhabdomyolysis (breakdown of muscle tissue) develop and the condition is potentially life-threatening. The resulting high calcium concentration causes the muscle to contract, using up ATP and generating heat. This stimulates further ATP synthesis and heat generation. Acidosis and rhabdomyolysis (breakdown of muscle tissue) may develop as a consequence, and the condition is potentially life-threatening.

Response to cold

The body responds to cold by a reversal of its dermal responses to heat. When body temperature decreases, arteriovenous anastomoses close to reduce perfusion of peripheral venous plexuses and thus decrease heat loss to the surrounding environment. Also, sweat production decreases to reduce heat loss from its evaporation.

In addition to these heat-preserving processes in the skin, the body has two unique responses to generate heat:

■ shivering
■ non-shivering thermogenesis

> **Hypothermia is defined as a core temperature < 36°.** The condition commonly arises from exposure, for example when a person is stranded on moorland overnight. However, it may also be caused by infection (particularly in the elderly), the use of certain drugs and endocrine conditions (e.g. severe hypothyroidism).
>
> Rewarming must be done carefully, because it can precipitate cardiac arrhythmias and cutaneous vasodilation, which may trigger a sudden reduction in blood pressure.

Shivering

A sufficient, progressive decrease in body temperature triggers a reflex induction of rhythmic muscular contraction (shivering) of the trunk, head and upper limb muscles. The increased metabolism that shivering requires can increase total body heat production by up to fourfold for short periods, and double it for prolonged periods. Vigorous exercise can further increase heat production, generating the rough equivalent of the heat from a 1-kW electric fire.

Non-shivering thermogenesis

This is the process by which neonates use brown adipose tissue (brown fat) to maintain their temperature. Brown adipose tissue consists of adipocytes (fat cells) with a high density of specialised mitochondria. On the inner membrane of these mitochondria, ATP synthase uncouples the dissipation of the hydrogen ion gradient from the synthesis of ATP (see page 11). The consequence is spinning of the F0 domain, the rotary motor of the ATP synthase molecule, without synthesis of ATP; thus energy is generated as heat instead of being stored as ATP.

Non-shivering thermogenesis is particularly important in newborn babies, because their ability to shiver is limited.

Maintenance of effective circulating volume

The concept of an effective circulating volume (ECV) relates to the ability to perfuse the vital organs (heart, brain, lungs) adequately. ECV depends on the control of both blood volume and vascular volume, i.e. the fluid and the container. The heart must also be able to pump the blood and maintain adequate perfusion pressure.

Stimulus

Clinically, changes in effective circulating volume most often result from a decrease in blood volume (hypovolaemia). This occurs in cases of haemorrhage or dehydration.

In haemorrhage, less blood returns to the heart through the venous system; central venous pressure decreases in consequence. Through the Frank–Starlings law of the heart (see page 79), this translates into reduced stroke volume and arterial blood pressure. The latter is detected by high-pressure baroreceptors in the aortic arch, and this, together with detection by low-pressure baroreceptors in the atria, activates the main neurological component of the body's response to loss of circulating volume. In addition, reduced stretch of renal afferent arterioles, combined with sympathetic drive triggered by the baroreceptors, causes renin release, initiating the hormonal component of the response.

Immediate response

The immediate response to a reduction in volume is mediated by the nervous system (**Table 9.3**). Signals from the medulla increase sympathetic activity and reduce parasympathetic activity. These actions increase heart rate and stroke volume to increase both systolic and diastolic blood pressure.

Sympathetically mediated vasoconstriction in the skin, kidney, skeletal muscle and gut increases total peripheral resistance rapidly. This increases diastolic blood pressure and preserves perfusion pressure, so that the vital organs continue to receive blood. Venoconstriction helps maintain central filling pressure for stroke volume (according to the Frank–Starling law).

Early response

Over hours, hormonal factors play a role in the response to blood loss (**Table 9.3**). Renin release leads to generation of angiotensin II and aldosterone.

■ Angiotensin II causes arteriolar vasoconstriction and acts on the proximal tubules of the kidneys to promote reabsorption of sodium
■ Aldosterone causes sodium reabsorption from the distal tubules

Together, the effects of angiotensin II and aldosterone increase blood volume. The salt retained draws water from surrounding tissues, promotes thirst and increases antidiuretic hormone (ADH) secretion. Marked decreases in blood pressure or effective circulating volume also lead to ADH release through baroreceptor output, which is

Response to loss of effective circulating volume	
Timing	Response
Seconds	Sympathetic vasoconstriction and tachycardia (in response to signals from neurones and the adrenal medulla)
Minutes to hours	Release of angiotensin II, aldosterone and antidiuretic hormone, resulting in sodium and water reabsorption as well as vasoconstriction
	Reabsorption of fluid from the interstitial space
Days	Increase in red blood cell synthesis by erythropoietin

Table 9.3 Summary of the body's response to loss of effective circulating volume

enhanced by the presence of angiotensin II. Under the influence of antidiuretic hormone, water is then reabsorbed in the collecting ducts. As a result, only small amounts of highly concentrated urine are produced.

Thirst, which is normally stimulated by high plasma osmolality, can also be triggered by a large decrease in effective circulating volume. Therefore unexpected thirst in a patient is a clear warning sign of the loss of fluid, often blood.

Peripheral vasoconstriction and loss of venous pressure shift the balance of Starling's forces to promote reabsorption of fluid from the interstitial space.

Dangers of therapy

When blood is lost, plasma proteins are lost with it. If the lost blood is replaced with crystalloids (e.g. saline) to restore circulating volume, the plasma proteins remaining in the body are diluted and the reduction in oncotic pressure tends to lead to the movement of fluid out of the capillaries and into the interstitium. This effect can cause oedema, including pulmonary oedema.

Following significant blood loss, patients may need transfusions of packed red cells to maintain tissue oxygenation. Administration of blood products carries risks. All blood is screened for HIV and the hepatitis B and C viruses, but patients must be warned of the small risk of infection.

Transfusion reactions are more common; these occur when minor antigens on the surfaces of foreign cells trigger low-grade inflammatory reactions causing mild pyrexia and rash. Major transfusion reactions are rare; if they do occur, the reaction between foreign cells and preformed antibody can cause circulatory collapse, resulting in intravascular haemolysis and massive cytokine release.

A 71-year-old man is admitted to hospital with cough, fever and shortness of breath. He is drowsy, tachycardic (heart rate, 124 beats/min) and hypotensive (blood pressure, 84/34 mmHg). Despite the administration of 3 L of intravenous fluid and antibiotics, he requires a noradrenaline (norepinephrine) infusion to maintain a mean arterial blood pressure of 70 mmHg.

This patient has lost his effective circulating volume because of systemic vasodilation in response to bacteraemia (septic shock) from pneumonia. Without physical fluid loss, his body has increased its vascular space by opening capillary beds, and this action has reduced perfusion pressure to the vital organs. The physical response is the same regardless of the cause of the loss of effective circulating volume. Septic shock is defined as a requirement for vasopressors, such as noradrenaline (norepinephrine), to maintain blood pressure after adequate fluid resuscitation; the condition has a poor prognosis.

Late response

In the days to weeks after loss of circulating volume, and secondary to renal hypoxia, the production of erythropoietin by the tubular cells of the kidney is increased. Erythropoietin increases the rate of production of red blood cells from their myeloid precursors; these new cells replace the lost red cells and help improve oxygen delivery.

Stress

Stress has many definitions, depending on the aspect of stress in question, but has both physical and psychological components. The condition may be triggered by disturbances of:

- a person's psychological state, for example when they are undergoing examinations or experiencing difficulties with social relationships
- their physical state, for example at times of illness or poor nutrition

Short-term stress

In the short term, the body reacts to stress with the classic fight-or-flight response. This is predominantly mediated by the sympathetic nervous system and includes the release of adrenaline (epinephrine).

Activation of the sympathetic nervous system causes tachycardia (increased heart rate), increased blood pressure, cooling of the peripheral regions of the body and sweating; patients may also feel nauseous. These symptoms of stress are accompanied by the typical sensation of anxiety, which is mediated by the limbic system.

Long-term stress

As acute stress becomes chronic stress, the body's response shifts from being neurally mediated to being hormonally mediated. Chronic stress activates the hypothalamic–pituitary–adrenal axis, with a consequent increase in adrenocorticotrophic hormone and glucocorticoids such as cortisol. The glucocorticoids increase metabolic rate and cause the body to favour catabolism (breakdown of complex molecules and energy release) over anabolism (synthesis of complex molecules and energy storage).

Other results of activation of the hypothalamic–pituitary–adrenal axis are increases in the levels of adrenaline, glucagon and growth hormone.

These hormones help the body cope with stress by mobilising energy sources, but they also cause loss of muscle bulk and suppress the immune system.

Long-term stress also elicits a chronic emotional response mediated by the limbic system. The mechanism for this is not fully understood; however, the increased level of cortisol in people experiencing chronic stress has been implicated in the pathophysiology of depression.

> **One striking effect of cancer is the development of cachexia (physical wasting).** Patients often enter an extreme catabolic state, with little or no appetite; in this condition, their ability to tolerate treatment is reduced.
>
> It is unclear why cachexia develops, but it is thought to arise from a combination of the production of tumour-associated 'stress' factors and the immune response to the malignancy. If patients awaiting an operation are particularly cachectic, they may be fed by nasogastric tube in an attempt to maintain adequate nutrition.

High altitude

At high altitudes, atmospheric pressure is reduced. In accordance with Dalton's law (see page 107), this means that, although oxygen still represents 20% of the total system pressure, its partial pressure is lower.

This low partial pressure starts to affect humans at about 1500 m. Even people with a normal, healthy respiratory system become hypoxic at a high enough altitude.

Effect of high altitude on respiratory control

The partial pressure of inspired oxygen (P_iO_2) is a major determinant of both alveolar oxygen (P_AO_2) and arterial (P_aO_2) oxygen. Sufficient reduction of P_aO_2 activates peripheral chemoreceptors (see page 127) to cause hyperventilation. This mechanism helps maintain P_aO_2, but it is always limited by P_iO_2. Furthermore, hyperventilation causes hypocapnia (**Figure 9.5**).

Under normal circumstances, oxygen is a perfusion-limited gas, i.e. the rate of its transport from the lungs is limited by pulmonary blood flow (perfusion). However, when P_iO_2 is reduced, the gradient for oxygen exchange in the lungs is reduced to the point at which equilibrium is not achieved by time the blood reaches the ends of the pulmonary capillaries. In this situation, oxygen can be considered a diffusion-limited gas, i.e. the rate of its transport is limited by its diffusion from the alveoli to the blood, therefore pulmonary blood flow is less important for counteracting hypoxia.

Tissue oxygenation is likely to be maintained at high altitude, because of the properties of the haemoglobin–oxygen saturation curve (see page 120). Even with a PaO_2 of only 10 kPa, oxygen saturation is > 93%; at this level, a sufficient amount of oxygen is off-loaded when the blood reaches the tissues.

Hypoxia also stimulates production of erythropoietin, which increases production of red blood cells. This is why many endurance athletes use altitude training; with an increased haemocrit (the ratio of the volume of red blood cells to the total volume of blood), the oxygen-carrying capacity of their blood is enhanced. However, this is at the cost of greater blood viscosity, which increases the risk of stroke.

> **Hypoxia at high altitude causes headaches, fatigue and nausea; in severe cases, pulmonary oedema develops.** Acetazolamide, a carbonic anhydrase inhibitor, is used for symptomatic treatment. Carbonic anhydrase is needed for reabsorption and generation of HCO_3^- in the kidney, therefore acetazolamide produces a metabolic acidosis and corrects the pH disturbance caused by hyperventilation. This eases some of the symptoms associated with being at high altitudes.

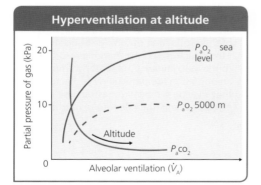

Figure 9.5 Effects on arterial blood gases of hyperventilation at altitude. Altitude reduces the maximum arterial oxygen (P_aO_2) that can be reached. Increased alveolar ventilation (V_A) brings PaO_2 closer to the partial pressure of inspired oxygen (P_iO_2) and reduces arterial carbon dioxide (P_aCO_2), because the partial pressure of inspired carbon dioxide is unaffected by altitude.

Acid–base disturbance

The hyperventilation caused by hypoxia produces hypocapnia. This condition reduces the P_aCO_2: bicarbonate (HCO_3^-) balance, resulting in respiratory alkalosis. Initially, this acidosis is buffered; however, blood pH increases once the body's buffering capacity is exceeded.

Consequently, the hydrogen ion concentration in renal tubular cells decreases, reducing the rate of reabsorption and generation of HCO_3^- (see page 158). This renal compensation helps correct the $P_aCO_2:HCO_3^-$ ratio and normalise serum pH.

Acutely, the decrease in hydrogen ions causes the haemoglobin–oxygen dissociation curve to shift to the left. This adjustment helps maximise oxygen uptake in the lungs despite severe hypoxia.

Answers to starter questions

1. After a haemorrhage the renin-angiotensin-aldosterone system is activated by several mechanisms: by reduced afferent arteriolar stretch, via the baroreflex, by the tubuloglomerular feedback mechanism and from sympathetic stimulation. This results in increased angiotensin-II and aldosterone, which act to reabsorb sodium (and water) and reduce the volume of urine. In addition, ADH is released as part of the baroreceptor response, which causes water reabsorption in the collecting duct and more concentrated urine.

2. During intense exercise, muscle requires energy at a rate greater than can be produced by aerobic respiration. Once the oxygen supply is depleted anaerobic respiration occurs, resulting in the formation of lactic acid. This, along with other metabolites, builds up in active muscle and causes pain by stimulation of metaboreceptors, which activate afferent pain fibres.

3. Infections, particularly gram-negative bacterial infections, are associated with the production of large amounts of inflammatory mediators. Some of these (e.g. IL-1) are pyrogens that increase the temperature 'set-point' of the hypothalamus. We then shiver and keep warm until our temperature is increased to that elevated set-point.

4. Altitude sickness is due partly to high blood pH (alkalosis) caused by hyperventilating in a low oxygen environment. The alkalosis is compensated for by reabsorption (from tubular fluid) and generation of HCO_3^- in the kidneys. A gradual ascent allows more time to correct the alkalosis, thus minimising pH changes and preventing sickness.

5. Chronic stress puts the body into a catabolic state mediated by cortisol, growth hormone, glucagon and adrenaline. The catabolic state promotes breakdown of macromolecules (e.g. fat stores) and suppresses their formation; as a result more energy stores are lost than generated, causing weight loss. Chronic stress also acts to suppress appetite, especially if associated with depression, causing weight loss from anorexia.

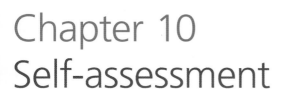

Chapter 10
Self-assessment

SBA questions

First principles

1. A 61-year-old man with Huntington's disease has an expanded cytosine, adenine, guanine (CAG) region.
   What single nucleotide triplet anticodon will be carried by the tRNA translating these bases?

   A Adenine, thymine, cytosine
   B Adenine, uracil, cytosine
   C Cytosine, adenine, guanine
   D Thymine, adenine, guanine
   E Uracil, thymine, cytosine

2. A 1-year-old boy has a severe skin condition where the epidermis and dermis separate with only minor trauma.
   What single cell junction type is most likely to be defective?

   A Adherens
   B Desmosomes
   C Gap junctions
   D Hemi-desmosomes
   E Occluding junctions

3. A 78-year-old man with advanced cancer is treated with vincristine, a microtubule inhibitor. During which single stage of mitosis are the tumour cells likely to arrest?

   A Anaphase
   B Cytokinesis
   C Metaphase
   D Prophase
   E Telophase

4. A 44-year-old woman has anxiety. She is treated with diazepam which hyperpolarises neurones.
   What single ion movement would cause neuronal hyperpolarisation?

   A Increased chloride influx
   B Increased sodium influx
   C Reduced calcium efflux
   D Reduced potassium efflux
   E Reduced sodium efflux

5. A 90-year-old woman with atrial fibrillation is treated with digoxin, which inhibits the Na$^+$/K$^+$-ATPase pump.
   What single effect will there be on intracellular ion concentrations?

   A Increased sodium
   B Increased potassium
   C Reduced calcium
   D Reduced chloride
   E Reduced sodium

6. A 51-year-old man with impotence is treated with sildenafil (Viagra), which causes a rise in intracellular cAMP.
   What is sildenafil's single mechanism of action?

   A 5'nucleotidase activator
   B Adenylate cyclase inhibitor
   C Guanylate cyclase activator
   D Phosphodiesterase activator
   E Phosphodiesterase inhibitor

7. A 72-year-old man has pancytopenia and requires a bone marrow biopsy for diagnosis.
   What single region of the bone must be sampled to obtain marrow?

   A Cancellous bone
   B Compact bone
   C Epiosteum
   D Haversian system
   E Periosteum

8. A 30-year-old man has anaphylaxis after a bee sting. He is treated with adrenaline to vasoconstrict his peripheral vasculature.
   Which single intracellular signalling pathway is activated to mediate this?

   A Arachidonic acid
   B cAMP-PKA
   C cGMP-PKG

D PIP$_2$-PKC
E Ras-MAPK

Neuromuscular systems

1. A 51-year-old man accidentally receives a signifi-
    cant dose of IV local anaesthetic. He develops
    tingling lips, becomes drowsy, and suffers a
    cardiac arrest.
    Which single ion channel has been affected?

    A Fast voltage-gated sodium
    B Slow voltage-gated sodium
    C Sodium leak
    D Voltage-gated calcium
    E Voltage-gated potassium

2. A 34-year-old woman has unilateral deafness and
    facial weakness. She is found to have a benign
    nerve sheath tumour of the VIII cranial nerve.
    What single cell is the origin of this tumour?

    A Astrocytes
    B Microglia
    C Oligodendrocytes
    D Pericytes
    E Schwann cells

3. A 31-year-old man has a peripheral neuropathy.
    Nerve conduction studies show that all impulses
    are transmitted but conduction is greatly slowed.
    What single nerve pathology is most likely to be
    present?

    A Congenital neuronal absence
    B Demyelination
    C Fibre-type grouping
    D Inhibition of sodium channels
    E Neuronal apoptosis

4. A 43-year-old woman has muscle weakness that
    is worse at the end of the day. She is positive for
    anti-nicotinic acetylcholine receptor antibodies.
    What is the single most appropriate treatment?

    A Acetylcholinesterase inhibitor
    B Choline acetyl-transferase activator
    C Neurosecretory vesicle fusion inhibitor
    D Uptake-1 inhibitor
    E Voltage-gated sodium channel blocker

5. A 71-year-old man has a left anterior cerebral
    artery infarction, causing ischaemia to the medial
    part of the frontal lobe.
    What single body part would be expected to have
    the greatest weakness?

    A Eyebrow
    B Hand
    C Leg
    D Tongue
    E Trunk

6. A 75-year-old man has an anterior spinal artery
    infarction at the T10 level.
    What single neurological deficit will he experi-
    ence?

    A Loss of motor activity on the left, pain on the
       right, below T10
    B Loss of motor activity, pain and temperature
       below T10 bilaterally
    C Loss of motor activity, proprioception and
       vibration below T10 bilaterally
    D Loss of proprioception and vibration below
       T10 bilaterally
    E Loss of proprioception on the right, pain on
       the left, below T10

7. A 21-year-old man has a severe traction and
    abduction injury to his right arm. He develops
    right-sided Horner's syndrome and Klumpke's
    palsy.
    What is the single most likely location of the
    sympathetic lesion?

    A Dorsal horn
    B Lateral horn
    C Superior cervical ganglion
    D Ventral horn
    E Ventral root

8. A 67-year-old patient is unwell with sepsis.
    What single autonomic transmitter is most crucial
    for maintenance of their systemic vasoconstric-
    tion?

    A Acetylcholine
    B Dopamine
    C Nitric oxide
    D Noradrenaline
    E Serotonin

Circulation and blood

1. A 61-year-old man with ischaemic heart disease
    has dull, central chest pain. His pain is improved
    by a sublingual spray. What is the mechanism of
    action of this drug?

    A Activation of adenylate cyclase
    B Activation of guanylate cyclase
    C Activation of phosphodiesterase
    D Activation of phospholipase
    E Activation of protein kinase C

2. An 82-year-old woman who has recently suffered
    a stroke is found to have an irregularly irregular
    pulse. ECG shows an absence of P-waves.
    What is single most likely pathological basis of
    her stroke?

    A Cholesterol embolus
    B Embolisation of cardiac thrombus
    C In situ thrombosis

D Paradoxical embolus
E Vasculitic

3. A 45-year-old man has stable congestive cardiac failure. His resting heart rate is 102 bpm.
What single factor mediates his tachycardia?

   A Decreased angiotensin-II
   B Decreased atrial naturietic peptide
   C Increased aldosterone
   D Increased anti-diuretic hormone
   E Increased sympathetic tone

4. A 67-year-old woman with end-stage congestive cardiac failure undergoes a follow-up echocardiogram.
What single ejection fraction is she most likely to have?

   A 5%
   B 20%
   C 45%
   D 55%
   E 70%

5. A 71-year-old man with cor pulmonale has troubling peripheral oedema.
What single change in the systemic capillaries mediates this symptom?

   A Increased tissue oncotic pressure
   B Increased venous hydrostatic pressure
   C Reduced capillary oncotic pressure
   D Reduced tissue hydrostatic pressure
   E Reduced tissue oncotic pressure

6. A 25-year-old man has sepsis due to cellulitis and a heart rate of 140bpm.
What single factor facilitates the increased myocardial blood supply required?

   A Adenosine
   B AMP
   C Carbon dioxide
   D Nitric oxide
   E Potassium

7. A 14-year-old girl has heavy menstrual bleeding. She has a prolonged bleeding time and normal APTT with normal levels of FVIII and FIX.
What is the single most likely diagnosis?

   A Factor V Leiden mutation
   B Factor XIII deficiency
   C Haemophilia A
   D Haemophilia B
   E von Willebrand factor deficiency

8. A 61-year-old man with hypertension has a calcium-channel blocker (amlodipine) added to his current medication.
By what single mechanism does it reduce blood pressure?

   A Decreases heart rate

B Decreases total peripheral resistance
C Decreases ventricular contractility
D Increases capillary permeability
E Increases ejection fraction

9. An 81-year-old woman has congestive cardiac failure and a raised JVP at 7 cm.
What single pathological change is her JVP a manifestation of?

   A Increased central venous pressure
   B Increased end-systolic volume
   C Reduced ejection fraction
   D Reduced end-diastolic volume
   E Reduced heart rate

10. A 51-year-old man has a myocardial infarction. He becomes bradycardic and hypotensive. His heart rate is 34 bpm. He is given two doses of atropine.
By what single mechanism does this drug act?

   A Increase AVN delay
   B Increase SAN depolarisation rate
   C Increase ventricular contractility
   D Reduce end-diastolic volume
   E Reduce stroke volume

Respiratory system

1. A 22-year-old man performs respiratory function tests. He is asked to breathe normally.
What is the single term for the volume of gas left in his lungs after a normal breath?

   A Functional residual capacity
   B Inspiratory reserve volume
   C Residual volume
   D Tidal volume
   E Vital capacity

2. A 52-year-old man has pyrexia, shortness of breath and right lobe consolidation on chest X-ray.
What single effect will this have on his dead space?

   A Increased alveolar dead space
   B Increased anatomical dead space
   C Reduced alveolar dead space
   D Reduced anatomical dead space
   E Reduced physiological dead space

3. A neonate born at 30 weeks has respiratory distress and requires oxygen. Pathologically, there is alveolar collapse and the air spaces are filled with a proteinaceous fluid.
What is the single most likely diagnosis?

   A Diaphragmatic hernia
   B Meconium pneumonitis
   C Pneumonia
   D Pneumothorax
   E Surfactant-deficient lung disease

4. A 71-year old man has COPD has peripheral oedema, a raised JVP and right upper quadrant pain. He is a lifelong smoker.
What single mechanism underlies the development his complications?

   A   Chronic pulmonary hypoxic vasoconstriction
   B   Chronic suppurative pulmonary infection
   C   Myocardial infarction
   D   Pulmonary embolism
   E   Spontaneous pneumothorax

5. A 75-year-old woman has an infective exacerbation of her severe COPD. She is given oxygen to achieve saturations of 99%. She becomes drowsy over the next 45 minutes.
What single change is most likely to be seen on a repeat arterial blood gas?

   A   Decreased CO_2
   B   Decreased O_2
   C   Increased CO_2
   D   Increased HCO_3^-
   E   Increased pH

6. A 27-year-old man with pancreatic cancer has sharp right-sided chest pain and haemoptysis. His chest X-ray is clear but a CT-scan confirms the diagnosis.
What single change in V/Q ratio will there be in the affected area of his right lung?

   A   Increased ventilation and increased perfusion
   B   No change in ventilation and reduced perfusion
   C   Reduced ventilation and increased perfusion
   D   Reduced ventilation and no change in perfusion
   E   Reduced ventilation and reduced perfusion

7. A 15-year-old boy with diabetic ketoacidosis has a respiratory rate of 34 breaths/min.
What single effect will this have on his acid–base balance?

   A   Fall in CO_2 causing decreased pH
   B   Fall in CO_2 causing increased pH
   C   Fall in HCO_3^- causing reduced pH
   D   Increase in CO_2 causing increased pH
   E   Increase in HCO_3^-- causing decreased pH

8. An 81-year-old man with stable pulmonary fibrosis is assessed for long-term oxygen therapy.
What single abnormality will be most prominent on his arterial blood gas?

   A   Decreased pH
   B   Raised base excess
   C   Raised HCO_3^-
   D   Raised PaO_2
   E   Reduced $PaCO_2$

9. A 14-year-old boy has exercise-induced asthma. He is started on montelukast which he is told will reduce the inflammation and narrowing of his airways.
What single mechanism is the action of this drug?

   A β_2-adrenoreceptor agonist
   B   Histamine receptor antagonist
   C   Leukotriene receptor antagonist
   D   Muscarinic acetylcholine receptor antagonist
   E   Prostaglandin receptor antagonist

Renal system

1. A 42-year-old man with dehydration has hyperkalaemia.
What single hormone is responsible for promoting excretion of the excess potassium?

   A   Aldosterone
   B   Angiotensin II
   C   Antidiuretic hormone
   D   Cortisol
   E   Renin

2. A 61-year-old man has type 2 diabetes. He is started on canagliflozin and is told he will lose glucose in his urine but not anywhere else. What single channel does this drug inhibit?

   A   GLUT-2
   B   GLUT-4
   C Na^+/K^+ ATPase
   D   SGLT-1
   E   SGLT-2

3. A 50-year-old woman has pulmonary oedema. She is treated with furosemide which blocks the $Na^+/K^+/2Cl^-$ co-transporter.
In what single area of the nephron does it exert most of its action?

   A   Collecting duct
   B   Distal tubule
   C   Glomerulus
   D   Loop of Henle
   E   Proximal tubule

4. A 33-year-old man has polyuria due to diabetes. What single serum electrolyte abnormality is a consequence of this?

   A   High Ca^{2+}
   B   High K^+
   C   High Na^+
   D   Low K^+
   E   Low Na^+

5. A 71-year-old man has an exacerbation of COPD. His blood pH is 7.15.
What single compensation do the kidneys make for this?

   A   Increased H^+ reabsorption
   B   Increased HCO_3^- generation
   C   Increased K^+ secretion

D Reduced HCO_3^- reabsorption
E Reduced Na^+ reabsorption

6. A 20-year-old man has a renal biopsy for suspected glomerulonephritis. It demonstrates expansion of the supporting cells within the glomeruli.
What single cell type has proliferated?

A Bowman's epithelial cells
B Granular cells
C Macula densa cells
D Mesangial cells
E Podocytes

Endocrine system and reproduction

1. A 52-year-old man with acromegaly secondary to a macroadenoma undergoes visual field assessment.
What single visual field defect is most characteristic of this condition?

A Binasal hemianopia
B Bitemporal hemianopia
C Loss of binocular vision
D Right-sided homonymous hemianopia
E Right-sided quadrantopia

2. A 32-year-old man has poor libido. Gynaecomastia is evident on examination. His partner has previously had a child with another partner.
What is the single most appropriate investigation to perform?

A Serum oestrogen
B Serum prolactin
C Serum testosterone
D Sperm analysis
E Ultrasound testes

3. A 41-year-old woman has anxiety, a tremor, goitre and exophthalmos. Against which single enzyme is drug treatment targeted?

A 1-α-hydroxylase
B 5-α-reductase
C 5'deiodinase
D Aromatase
E Thyroid peroxidase

4. A thin 73-year-old man has new-onset diabetes and a migratory necrolytic rash. He has no family history of diabetes.
From what single cell type does the underlying diagnosis arise?

A α-cells
B β-cells
C δ-cells
D Enterochromaffin-like cells
E L-cells

5. A 6-week-old boy has primary adrenal failure. He is hyponatraemic and volume depleted. Genetic testing demonstrates a deficiency of 21-α-hydroxylase.
What is the single most likely diagnosis?

A Addison's disease
B Congenital adrenal hyperplasia
C Conn's syndrome
D Cushing's syndrome
E Liddle's syndrome

6. A 63-year-old woman has excessive thirst and is generally feeling unwell. She has raised serum calcium and parathyroid hormone.
What is the single most likely diagnosis?

A Hypervitaminosis D
B Primary hyperparathyroidism
C Primary hypoparathyroidism
D Secondary hyperparathyroidism
E Tertiary hyperparathyroidism

7. A 50-year-old woman has intermittent hot flushes.
Which single set of results would suggest a diagnosis of menopause?

A High oestrogen, high LH, high FSH
B High oestrogen, low LH, low FSH
C Low oestrogen, high LH, high FSH
D Low oestrogen, high prolactin, high progesterone
E Low oestrogen, low LH, low FSH

8. A 30-year-old woman, at 41+3 weeks gestation, has been in the first stage of labour for over 36 hours. She undergoes a membrane sweep to stimulate cervical ripening and effacement.
What single hormone is the key mediator in this process?

A Cortisol
B Oestrogen
C Oxytocin
D Progesterone
E Prostaglandin E_2

9. An 89-year-old man with metastatic prostate cancer begins treatment with goserelin (a GnRH agonist).
What is the single aim of this treatment?

A Cytotoxic damage to adenocarcinoma cells
B Inhibit action of testosterone
C Inhibit bone resorption
D Stimulation of LH and FSH release
E Suppression of LH and FSH release

Gastrointestinal system

1. A 19-year-old man on a gap year in India eats at a local restaurant and subsequently suffers an

episode of vomiting.
What single form of gut motility is involved?

A Haustration
B Mass movement
C Peristalsis
D Retrograde peristalsis
E Segmentation

2. A 23-year-old woman is sitting her final exams. She notices that her mouth feels dry.
    Which single mechanism causes this sensation?

A Circulating adrenaline is increased, suppressing saliva secretion
B Parasympathetic activity is increased, increasing mucus secretion
C Parasympathetic activity is increased, suppressing saliva secretion
D Sympathetic activity is increased, suppressing saliva secretion
E Sympathetic activity is increased, increasing mucus secretion

3. An obese (BMI 32 kg/m²) 48-year-old man gets burning central chest pain after going to bed. His GP diagnoses gastro-oesophageal reflux disease (GORD).
    Along with weight loss, what is the single most appropriate treatment?

A 5-HT_3-receptor inhibitor
B H^+/K^+-ATPase inhibitor
C H^+/Na^+ exchanger inhibitor
D Na^+/K^+-ATPase inhibitor
E Nicotinic ACh-receptor agonist

4. A 28-year-old woman has epigastric pain, which has become more severe over the last couple of weeks. Endoscopy shows over 20 ulcers throughout the stomach.
    Which of these hormones is the cause of her multiple ulcers?

A Cholecystokinin
B Gastrin
C Glucagon-like peptide 1
D Secretin
E Vasoactive intestinal peptide

5. A 30-year-old man has become increasingly tired and lethargic. He had his distal ileum removed surgically 3 years ago. A blood test reveals a macrocytic anaemia.
    What is the single most likely diagnosis?

A Folate deficiency
B Iron deficiency
C Magnesium deficiency
D Vitamin B_{12} deficiency
E Vitamin K deficiency

6. A 22-year-old Chinese woman has 'windiness'. She has recently moved to the UK.

What single enzyme is she deficient in?

A Amylase
B Lactase
C Lipase
D Maltase
E Sucrase

7. A 3-year-old boy has cystic fibrosis. He is failing to thrive and is producing foul-smelling, pale stools which float.
    What is the single most appropriate treatment?

A Addition of pancreatic enzymes to the diet
B Addition of salivary amylase to the diet
C High-protein diet
D Low-fat diet
E IV antibiotic treatment

8. An obese (BMI 34 kg/m²) 40-year-old woman has recurrent epigastric pain and is diagnosed with gallstones. Her pain typically occurs after meals.
    What single hormone is responsible for the timing of her pain?

A Cholecystokinin
B Gastrin
C Secretin
D Somatostatin
E Vasoactive intestinal peptide

9. A 70-year-old man is treated with IV antibiotics for a chest infection. His infection is clearing but he has now developed profuse foul-smelling diarrhoea, pyrexia and severe abdominal pain.
    What is the single most likely causative organism?

A *Campylobacter jejuni*
B *Clostridium difficile*
C *Escherichia coli*
D *Salmonella enteritidis*
E *Shigella dysenteriae*

10 A 57-year-old man with alcohol-related cirrhosis has oedema and ascites.
    What is the single most likely cause of his symptoms?

A Reduced bile production
B Reduced fat metabolism
C Reduced glucose regulation
D Reduced hormone degradation
E Reduced protein synthesis

Higher neural functions

1. A 67-year-old man has progressive weakness affecting upper limbs, lower limbs and cranial nerves. Fasciculations are present. Sensation is normal.
    What is the single most likely cause of his symptoms?

A   Anterior spinal artery infarction
B   Motor neurone disease
C   Posterior spinal artery infarction
D   Tabes dorsalis
E   Vitamin B$_{12}$ deficiency

2. A cachectic 33-year-old refugee has poor night-time vision. She has loss of peripheral visual fields. Which cell type is most likely to be affected?

A   Amacrine cells
B   Bipolar cells
C   Cones
D   Ganglion cells
E   Rods

3. A 19-year-old woman is intubated on the ICU without sedation; she has suffered a major subarachnoid haemorrhage. When her head is turned to 90 degrees, the eyes turn with the head, remaining central in the orbit. Which part of her brain is affected?

A   Brainstem
B   Frontal lobe
C   Midbrain
D   Parietal lobe
E   Temporal lobe

4. A 28-year-old with Bell's palsy complains of hearing all noises at excessively loud volumes. What is the mechanism behind this feature?

A   Increased inner hair cell activity
B   Increased ossicle movement
C   Increased tympanic membrane movement
D   Reduced outer hair cell activity
E   Reduced round window movement

5. A 72-year-old diabetic man has suffered a right-sided stroke affecting his subthalamic nucleus. What clinical feature may he demonstrate?

A   Excessive left-side movement
B   Excessive right-side movement
C   Reduced movement bilaterally
D   Reduced left-side movement
E   Reduced right-side movement

6. A 23-year-old with epilepsy describes a sensation of strange tastes or smells just before she has a seizure. Where is her epileptogenic centre most likely to be found?

A   Brainstem
B   Frontal lobe
C   Occipital lobe
D   Parietal lobe
E   Temporal lobe

7. A 54-year-old treated for schizophrenia has uncontrollable, slow, writhing movements of the face and neck. Abnormal signalling by which neurotransmitter mediates these symptoms?

A   5-HT$_3$

B   Dopamine
C   GABA
D   Glutamate
E   Substance P

8. An 83-year-old man has a new ischaemic stroke. He is able to follow three-step commands but his speech is limited and does not make sense. Which area is most affected?

A   Arcuate fasciculus
B   Broca's area
C   Midbrain
D   Primary auditory cortex
E   Wernicke's area

9. A 32-year-old man suffers a traumatic injury to his frontal lobe. What clinical feature is he most likely to demonstrate?

A   Excess anger
B   Hypersomnolence
C   Increased hunger
D   Loss of inhibitions
E   Memory loss

Applied physiology

1. A 32-year-old man is running around the park. Which tissue is most sensitive to sympathetically-mediated vasoconstriction?

A   Brain
B   Genitalia
C   Gut
D   Heart
E   Liver

2. At the end of a series of sprints, a 28-year-old runner measures his lactate as 4.5 mmol/L (normal 0.2–2.5 mmol/L). Excessive levels of which precursor has lead to this raise lactate?

A   ADP
B   Citrate
C   Glucose
D   NADH
E   Pyruvate

3. A septic 4-day old boy is hypothermic on the neonatal intensive care unit. Why are neonates particularly susceptible to hypothermia?

A   Large amount of subcutaneous fat
B   Small surface area : weight ratio
C   Thick skin
D   Unable to shiver
E   Use of brown fat

4. A 41-year-old man suffers a 1 litre haemorrhage following a car crash. At a capillary level, what changes will occur?

A   Fall in capillary oncotic pressure
B   Fall in capillary hydrostatic pressure

C Fall in tissue hydrostatic pressure
D Rise in capillary oncotic pressure
E Rise in tissue hydrostatic pressure

5. A 30-year-old woman suffers a major post-partum haemorrhage. How do her stroke volume (SV) and heart rate (HR) change?

A Increased SV, increased HR
B Increased SV, reduced HR
C Reduced SV, increased HR
D Reduced SV, reduced HR
E Unchanged SV, increased HR

6. A 28-year-old woman has been very stressed with work over the last few months. Which hormone is most likely to be elevated?

A Adiponectin
B Cortisol
C Insulin
D Parathyroid hormone
E Somatostatin

7. A 31-year-old man has been living at 3000m altitude for several weeks. How would his blood gases be expected to differ from someone living at sea level?

A Increased HCO_3^-
B Increased $PaCO_2$
C Increased PaO_2
D Reduced HCO_3^-
E Reduced lactate

8. A 42-year-old man has ascended very rapidly to 4000m altitude, without any time for acclimatisation. How will this have affected his haemoglobin?

A Increased affinity for O_2
B Increased affinity for HCO_3^-
C Reduced affinity for CO_2
D Reduced affinity for O_2
E Reduced affinity for HCO_3^-

9. A 55-year-old man suffers a haemorrhage after a gardening accident. Assuming he is not given any intravenous fluid, what will be the effect upon his plasma osmolality (OSM) one day later?

A Increased OSM, due to ADH
B Increased OSM, due to aldosterone
C Reduced OSM, due to ADH
D Reduced OSM, due to aldosterone
E Reduced OSM, due to angiotensin-II

10. A 45-year-old man attends his GP for a blood test 1 week after an accident where he lost 1 litre of blood, but did not require a transfusion. What would his blood tests be expected to show?

A Increased haemoglobin
B Increased platelets
C Increased prothrombin time
D Increased reticulocytes
E Increased white blood cells

SBA answers

First principles

1. C

If the DNA sequence is cytosine-adenine-guanine, then the mRNA codon will be guanine-uracil-cytosine. The tRNA anti-codon that binds this will also be cytosine-adenine-guanine (coding for glutamine).

2. D

Hemi-desmosomes mediate the junction between basal epidermal cells and the basement membrane. Certain forms of epidermolysis bullosa have defective hemi-desmosomes, which causes skin loss on minimal trauma.

3. C

Microtubules are used to form the mitotic spindle, which is first used in metaphase for alignment of the chromosomes. It is also required for anaphase and cytokinesis but cells will arrest in metaphase before this.

4. A

Benzodiazepines increase the opening of chloride channels; the influx of chloride ions causes an accumulation of anions on the inside of the membrane and hyperpolarisation.

5. A

The Na$^+$/K$^+$-ATPase normally exports sodium from cells in exchange for potassium import. Inhibition of its action results in accumulation of intracellular sodium.

6. E

cAMP is broken down by phosphodiesterase; inhibition of its activity would increase cAMP levels. Increased activity of adenylate cyclase would also cause increased cAMP.

7. A

Bone marrow is contained in the centre of long bones, between the bony trabeculae of cancellous (spongy) bone.

8. D

Alpha-adrenoreceptors signal through G-protein q, which activates phospholipase C. This is the starting point for the PIP$_2$ pathway that results in PKC activation.

Neuromuscular systems

1. A

Local anaesthetics inhibit action potentials by preventing rapid depolarisation from blockade of fast voltage-gated sodium channels. It is normally given subcutaneously but when given intravenously it blocks the same channels in the heart and CNS.

2. E

This patient has a VII and VIII palsy due to an acoustic neuroma. The expanding tumour arises from VIII but also compresses VII. The supporting (glial) cells of peripheral nerves are Schwann cells, which myelinate fibres. Despite passing intracranially, the cranial nerves are part of the peripheral nervous system.

3. B

Demyelination causes a slowing of transmission but all action potentials should still be transmitted. The other options would cause an absence of transmission or larger potentials.

4. A

This patient has myasthenia gravis, in which autoantibodies block the acetylcholine (ACh) receptors which normally initiate muscle contraction. Acetylcholinesterase (AChEase) breaks down ACh and terminates its action at the neuromuscular junction. Inhibition of AChEase increases free ACh, increasing the signal from the remaining receptors, and helping with neuromuscular transmission.

5. C

Different areas of cerebral cortex are devoted to control of a particular body parts (somatotopic mapping). The medial aspect of the pre-central gyrus is supplied by the anterior cerebral artery and controls leg movement. The lateral part controls arm and face movements.

6. B

The anterior spinal artery supplies the anterior two-thirds of the spinal cord and will affect corticospinal and spinothalamic tracts. These carry the motor activity and pain/temperature, respectively. Proprioception/vibration are carried by the dorsal columns, which will be spared.

7. E

Severe traction to the arm can result in damage to the roots of the brachial plexus, causing a Klumpke's palsy. In addition, injury to the ventral roots will affect ascending sympathetic fibres, causing a Horner's syndrome.

8. D

Sympathetic vesicles release noradrenaline, which causes systemic vasoconstriction. This is the main mechanism for maintenance of vascular tone in systemic illness.

Circulation and blood

1. B

Glyceryl trinitrate (GTN) is a NO-releasing drug that is used to help relieve pain from myocardial ischaemia. NO activates guanylate cyclase, which increases formation of cGMP. This in turn activates PKG that causes smooth muscle hyperpolarization, and so relaxation.

2. B

This woman has atrial fibrillation: irregular, inefficient, chaotic contraction of the atria. It predisposes to formation of atrial thrombus, which may then embolise and cause stroke.

3. E

In order to maintain cardiac output in cardiac failure patients have a resting tachycardia, which is due to both a reduction in parasympathetic supply and an increase in sympathetic tone.

4. B

Ejection fraction (EF) is stroke volume expressed as a percentage of end-diastolic volume; it is a marker of ventricular function. As heart failure progresses the EF falls to below 50%, with under 30% being severe. An EF of 5% would not be compatible with life.

5. B

Right-sided heart failure causes increased pressure in the venous circulation as venous return is inefficiently cleared. This results in raised hydrostatic pressure in capillaries, favouring formation of tissue fluid.

6. A

Myocardial hypoxia, due to both sepsis and the tachycardia, increases 5'nucleotidase activity, which catalyses formation of adenosine. Adenosine dilates coronary arterioles.

7. E

von Willebrand factor (vWF) is needed for platelet adhesion and also carried FVIII in the blood. In the most common form of vWF deficiency, platelet aggregation is impaired but the clotting cascade functions normally.

8. B

Dihydropyridine-type calcium channel blockers (e.g. amlodipine) are selective for systemic arterioles, causing their vasodilatation and a reduction in total peripheral resistance with little effect on cardiac contractility.

9. A

In the early stages of heart failure the circulatory system compensates for the inadequate cardiac output by increasing central venous pressure (CVP). This, via the Frank-Starling law of the heart, increases stroke volume. The JVP is in direct communication with the right atrium and therefore indicates raised CVP.

10. B

Parasympathetic stimulation influences the potassium permeability of cardiac myocytes. Therefore, a muscarinic antagonist (e.g. atropine) reduces potassium permeability and increases the gradient of the pacemaker pre-potential, increasing SAN depolarisation and reducing AVN delay.

Respiratory system

1. A

Functional residual capacity (FRC) is the volume left in the lung at the end of passive expiration. There is no distending pressure over the lung at FRC.

2. A

In a healthy individual, there is no alveolar dead space. Alveolar dead space is an area normally involved in gaseous exchange that is not functional. This man has pneumonia, which will increase his alveolar dead space because gas exchange is impaired. Some anatomical dead space is normal; it represents the volume of the conducting airways.

3. E

Neonates born before 32 weeks are at risk of surfactant-deficiency lung disease. This makes their lungs poorly compliant, fill with fluid, and (according to Laplace's law) there is emptying of small alveoli into large.

4. A

Bronchioles and pulmonary arterioles can dilate or constrict to correct regional changes in V/Q ratio. Hypoxia causes pulmonary arteriolar vasoconstriction, which increases right-heart pressure. Chronically that can cause right-heart failure (cor pulmonale), as in this patient.

5. C

Under normal physiological conditions, CO_2 is the most important gas for controlling respiratory drive. However, in severe COPD patients with chronic hypercapnia the response to hypercapnia may be blunted: they rely instead on hypoxia as a respiratory driver. Therefore if they are given excess oxygen they may reduce their ventilation, retain CO_2, and become drowsy.

6. B

This man has had a pulmonary embolism, which causes a sudden reduction in perfusion to the area of affected lung, however ventilation will be relatively unaffected.

7. B

Hyperventilation secondary to metabolic acidosis causes a reduction in $PaCO_2$. This causes a reduction in H^+ and HCO_3^-, which increases the pH, helping to compensate partially for the metabolic acidosis.

8. E

Pulmonary fibrosis is characterised by impaired gas exchange: this affects oxygen more than CO_2. Consequently, patients hyperventilate to improve their oxygenation, but this results in hypocapnia. Chronically, they may have reduced HCO_3^-.

9. C

Asthma is driven by excessive, inappropriate inflammation. Leukotrienes are key mediators in the process and montelukast is known to be particularly effective in exercise-induced asthma.

Renal system

1. A

Aldosterone release is directly increased by hyperkalaemia; it acts on the distal tubule and collecting duct to promote potassium excretion.

2. E

SGLT-2 is a renal-specific sodium–glucose co-transporter that is used for uptake in the proximal tubule.

3. D

The $Na^+/K^+/2Cl^-$ co-transporter is the main route by which ions cross the apical plasma membrane in the thick ascending limb of the loop of Henle: the Na^+/K^+ ATPase on the basolateral side pumps sodium into the interstitium, while Cl^- follows through channels. This is used to establish the medullary interstitial gradient used to drive water reabsorption in the collecting duct.

4. D

Potassium excretion is regulated by flow rate: a greater flow of tubular fluid promotes increases potassium secretion. Therefore polyuria of any cause may result in hypokalaemia.

5. B

Acidosis increases the rate of renal bicarbonate reabsorption and generation, and H^+ secretion. This allows renal compensation for respiratory acidosis.

6. D

Proliferative glomerulonephritis (e.g. post-streptococcal) often affects the supporting, phagocytic cells of the glomeruli, the mesangial cells.

Endocrine system and reproduction

1. B

A macroadenoma (>1cm) may extend out of the pituitary and compress the optic chiasm. This contains fibres from the nasal retina, which perceive the temporal visual field, resulting in bilateral loss of temporal vision.

2. B

This man has features of hyperprolactinaemia (poor libido, infertility, gynaecomastia) due to raised prolactin, which also suppresses LH/FSH to cause infertility. Testosterone may be low but this will not give the diagnosis.

3. E

This lady has presented with features of Graves' hyperthyroidism (note involvement of the eyes). First-line treatment often involves thyroid peroxidase inhibitors (carbimazole or propylthiouracil).

4. A

Type 2 diabetes is uncommon in thin individuals without a family history. The rash described is typical of a glucagonoma, a tumour of alphacells from the pancreas.

5. B

A deficiency of 21-α-hydroxylase results in an inability to produce mineralocorticoids or glucocorticoids. Young infants present with adrenal failure in 'salt wasting crises'. Lack of negative feedback causes raised ACTH with secondary adrenal hyperplasia.

6. B

Raised (or even normal) PTH in the context of hypercalcaemia gives a diagnosis of hyperparathyroidism. Secondary hyperparathyroidism only occurs with hypocalcaemia, due to renal disease or vitamin D deficiency. Tertiary hyperparathyroidism requires a previous renal transplant.

7. C

The menopause is characterised by a fall in sex steroid concentrations, particularly oestrogen and progesterone. The loss of ovarian oestrogen production results in increased pituitary FSH and LH due to reduced negative feedback.

8. E

The first stage of labour involves dilatation of the cervix, which requires PGE_2-mediated degradation of extracellular matrix component by matrix metalloproteinases (MMPs).

9. E

Continuous stimulation of the pituitary by a GnRH agonist causes paradoxical suppression of LH and FSH release because GnRH is normally produced by the hypothalamus in a pulsatile manner. This subsequently leads to a fall in testosterone.

Gastrointestinal system

1. D

In vomiting retrograde peristalsis forces irritant material back along the gut and causes it to be expelled from the mouth.

2. E
Both parasympathetic and sympathetic stimulation increase salivary secretion, but while PS activity causes a watery secretion, SNS activity causes a thick, mucoid secretion.

3. B
Proton pump inhibitors (e.g. omeprazole) block the H^+-ATPase active transporter on parietal cells. This prevents HCl secretion into the gastric lumen, increasing stomach pH and reducing the symptoms of GORD.

4. B
Gastrin is the main hormonal driver for gastric acid secretion and this woman may have Zollinger–Ellison syndrome, a tumour of gastrin-secreting G-cells.

5. D
Vitamin B_{12} is absorbed mainly in the distal ileum, and deficiency causes a megaloblastic anaemia. Given the previous surgery, B_{12} deficiency is a more likely than folate deficiency, though both can cause a megaloblastic anaemia.

6. B
This lady describes classical symptoms of lactose intolerance. This is due to a relative deficiency of lactase and the condition is much more common in people with an oriental background.

7. A
CFTR is important in maintaining a good flow of pancreatic juice, and CF patients often have impaired enzyme secretion. Changing the diet will not help the nutritional defect, so supplementation with digestive enzymes is needed.

8. A
Epigastric pain occurring after meals is typical of gallstones. Presence of food, especially lipids, in the small bowel stimulates cholecystokinin release from L-cells. This causes gallbladder smooth muscle contraction over the contained stones, resulting in pain.

9. B
All are perfectly possible, but in this setting (hospital, and post-antibiotics that may have destroyed the normal gut flora) C. difficile is probably most likely.

10.E
Generalised oedema with ascites in liver failure is due to hypoalbuminaemia. This is a feature of loss of hepatic synthetic function, also responsible for the production of clotting factors, so such patients may bleed easily.

Higher neural functions

1. B
Motor neurone disease (MND) is characterised by damage to ventral horn cell bodies of lower

motor neurones. This results in a mixture of upper and motor neurone clinical signs. Sensation is spared, unlike in all the other options listed.

2. E
Patients with malnutrition may have vitamin A deficiency, which typically causes night blindness. Retinol (vitamin A) is a key component of rhodopsin, the photo-pigment in rods.

3. A
This woman has a negative doll's eye reflex, where the pupils stay fixed mid-orbit. It is due to severe brainstem dysfunction that results in bilateral loss of the vestibulo-ocular reflex.

4. B
A facial nerve palsy (as in Bell's palsy) can affect stapedius, which normally dampens ossicle vibration. In the absence of this effect, patients may complain of hyperacusis–excessively loud noises.

5. B
The subthalamic nucleus (STN) is one of the basal ganglia and part of the indirect pathway. A lesion results in predominance in the direct pathway, with ipsilateral hyperkinesia.

6. E
This patient has the classical features of temporal lobe epilepsy. They may be aware of strange tastes, smells, or sounds prior to their seizure. This is the 'aura' from epileptic activity in the gustatory, olfactory, or auditory cortices.

7. B
Tardive dyskinesia is an often-irreversible condition caused by chronic dopaminergic receptor blockage, classically in patients treated with typical neuroleptics for psychotic disorders. There is upregulation of striatal dopamine receptors, which causes the symptoms seen.

8. B
This man has features of an expressive aphasia; he is able to follow commands (therefore understand speech) but cannot talk fluently, this is due to a lesion of Broca's area.

9. D
The pre-frontal cortex is concerned with the 'executive functions', which include: social norms, personality, planning, organisation, and spatial orientation. Loss of inhibitions and change in personality are characteristic features of a frontal lobe syndrome.

Applied physiology

1. C
The coronary, cerebral, and reproductive circulations have very little autonomic innervation, whereas the gut, skin, and skeletal muscle

undergo sympathetic vasoconstriction during exercise. However this modulated by local
effects in the skin and muscle, which are the
dominant effects there.

2. E

During anaerobic respiration, metabolic intermediates back-up and excess pyruvate accumulates
because it cannot enter the TCA (Krebs) cycle.
Lactate dehydrogenase converts pyruvate into
lactic acid in muscle. This may cycle to the liver,
where it can be used for gluconeogenesis (the
Cori cycle).

3. D

Neonates are susceptible to hypothermia for a
number of reasons. They are unable to shiver,
have thin skin, have a large surface area to body
weight ratio, and are prone to infection. Brown
fat metabolism helps to counter this and raise
their temperature.

4. B

Haemorrhage is associated with reduced venous
pressure, reduced arterial pressure, and arteriolar
constriction will further reduce capillary hydrostatic pressure. Because whole blood has been
lost, there is no change in the oncotic pressure,
at least initially.

5. C

Blood loss causes a reduced stroke volume, predominantly due to loss of central venous filling
pressure. In order to maintain cardiac output, the
heart rate increases due to increased sympathetic activation.

6. B

Cortisol is the key 'stress' hormone and levels are
elevated in patients under chronic stress. Along
with adrenaline, growth hormone, glucagon, it
helps to maintain a high metabolic rate during
stress.

7. D

After living at altitude for weeks this man will
have had renal compensation for his respiratory
alkalosis; therefore he will have reduced HCO_3^-,
along with reduced PaO_2 and $PaCO_2$.

8. A

A rapid ascent will be associated with hyperventilation, a respiratory alkalosis and reduced
$PaCO_2$. Low CO_2 is associated with a leftwards
shift on the haemoglobin–oxygen dissociation
curve, and greater affinity for O_2.

9. C

There is release of ADH as part of the response
to a low ECV. ADH causes reabsorption of water
alone, which reduces the osmolality of blood.
However, aldosterone and angiotensin-II, also
increased in response to hypovolaemia, stimulate
reabsorption of sodium, so will tend to counterbalance the effects of ADH.

10. D

After a haemorrhage, there is release of
erythropoietin, which stimulates increased red
blood cell production. This is manifest as a raised
proportion of RBC precursors in the blood:
reticulocytes.

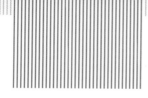

Index

Note: Page numbers in **bold** or *italic* refer to tables or figures, respectively.